Quick Reference to Adult and Older Adult Forensics

Kathleen M. Brown, PhD, APRN-BC, FAAN, is a practice assistant professor at the University of Pennsylvania School of Nursing as well as a practicing women's health nurse practitioner (NP) for 23 years and a sexual assault nurse examiner for the Philadelphia County, Pennsylvania, Sexual Assault Response Team. Additionally, she is a postgraduate student of Dr. Robert Sadoff at the University of Pennsylvania School of Medicine in the Applications of Forensic Psychiatry curriculum. She has been a coinvestigator in four funded research studies: two for the National Institute of Justice and two for the National Institute of Nursing Research. Her dissertation research on leaving abusive relationships was funded by American Women's Health, Obstetric and Neonatal Nursing (AWHONN).

Mary E. Muscari, PhD, CPNP, APRN-BC, CFNS, is an associate professor at the Decker School of Nursing, State University of New York (SUNY) at Binghamton (Binghamton University). Muscari has been a pediatric nurse practitioner (PNP) since 1980, when she earned her MSN/PNP from Columbia University. She earned a post-master's certificate in psychiatric nursing and a PhD, both from Adelphi University; a post-master's certificate in forensic nursing (2003) from Duquesne University; and has additional forensic education as a sexual assault nurse examiner, a legal nurse consultant, and a medicolegal death investigator. She attended the Sudden Unexpected Infant Death Investigation (SUIDI) Academy (2007) through the Centers for Disease Control and Prevention. Muscari has worked clinically as a PNP in a variety of environments, and has served on the Pennsylvania Sex Offender Assessment Board (2005–present) and as a private consultant on child health/mental health, parenting, and forensic issues.

Quick Reference to Adult and Older Adult Forensics

A Guide for Nurses and Other Health Care Professionals

KATHLEEN M. BROWN, PhD

MARY E. MUSCARI, PhD

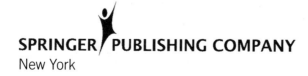

SPRINGER PUBLISHING COMPANY

New York

Springer Publishing Company, LLC
11 West 42nd Street
New York, NY 10036
www.springerpub.com

Acquisitions Editor: Margaret Zuccarini
Project Manager: Laura Stewart
Cover Design: Mimi Flow
Composition: Apex CoVantage, LLC
ISBN: 978-0-8261-2422-7
E-book ISBN: 978-0-8261-2423-4

10 11 12 13 / 5 4 3 2 1

The author and the publisher of this Work have made every effort to use sources be-lieved to be reliable to provide information that is accurate and compatible with the standards generally accepted at the time of publication. Because medical science is con-tinually advancing, our knowledge base continues to expand. Therefore, as new information becomes available, changes in procedures become necessary. We recommend that the reader always consult current research and specific institutional policies before performing any clinical procedure. The author and pub-lisher shall not be liable for any special, consequential, or exemplary damages resulting, in whole or in part, from the readers' use of, or reliance on, the information contained in this book. The publisher has no responsibility for the persistence or accuracy of URLs for external or third-party Internet Web sites referred to in this publication and does not guarantee that any content on such Web sites is, or will remain, accurate or appropriate.

Library of Congress Cataloging-in-Publication Data

Brown, Kathleen M., 1950–
    Quick reference to adult and older adult forensics : a guide for nurses and other health care professionals / Kathleen M. Brown, Mary E. Muscari.
        p. ; cm.
    Includes bibliographical references and index.
    ISBN 978-0-8261-2422-7 (alk. paper)
1. Medical jurisprudence.   2. Nurses.   I. Muscari, Mary E.   II. Title.
    [DNLM: 1. Forensic Medicine—methods.   2. Adult.   3. Aged.
4. Crime Victims.   5. Risk Assessment.   6. Violence—prevention & control. W 700 B8775q 2010]
    RA1053.B76   2010
    614'.1—dc22   2010002186

Printed in the United States of America by the Hamilton Printing Company

*This book is dedicated to
all health care professionals who work with victims and offenders;
to Ed for putting up with Kathy;
and to the Muscari Mob for putting up with Mary.*

This book is also dedicated to Margaret Zuccarini, the editor who has been with this project since it was just an idea and whose expert guidance and support have made it a reality. Margaret enabled this book to become a guide that can hopefully assist health care providers in working with victims and offenders.

Contents

Foreword by Ann Wolbert Burgess   *xiii*
Preface   *xv*
Acknowledgments   *xxi*

SECTION I: GENERAL PRINCIPLES

1   The Cycle and Continuum of Violence   3

2   Cultural Aspects of Forensics   9

3   Forensic Assessment and Documentation   21

4   Principles of Evidence   35

5   Navigating the Criminal Justice System   43

6   Expert Witness Testimony   49

7   Competency, Guardianship, and Civil Commitment   59

8   Violence in Health Care Settings   65

9   Professional Stress and Burnout   73

SECTION II: ADULTS AND OLDER ADULTS AS VICTIMS

10   Effects of Victimization on Adults and Older Adults   85

11   Victimization of Adults and Older Adults With Disabilities   103

12   Intimate Partner Violence in Adults   117

13 Intimate Partner Violence in Older Adults 131

14 Lesbian, Gay, Bisexual, and Transgender Intimate Partner Violence 139

15 Elders Abused by Family Members 147

16 Elders Abused by Health Care Workers 159

17 Female Victims of Sexual Assault 167

18 Male Victims of Sexual Assault 183

19 Elder Victims of Sexual Assault 191

20 Victims of Human Trafficking 199

21 Victims of Personal Injury 207

22 Stalking 217

23 Victim Services 227

SECTION III: ADULTS AND OLDER ADULTS AS OFFENDERS

24 Substance Abuse and Offending 235

25 Offenders With Mental Illness and Cognitive Impairment 245

26 Violence Risk Assessment 253

27 Long-Term Offenders 259

28 Offenders in Correctional Facilities 265

29 Offenders in the Community 275

30 Perpetrators of Intimate Partner Violence 285

31 Abusive Parents 297

32 Perpetrators of Elder Abuse 305

33 Adult Perpetrators of Sexual Violence 315

34 Older Adult Perpetrators of Sexual Violence 337

35   Female Offenders   341

36   Animal Cruelty   351

37   Parenting While Incarcerated   365

SECTION IV: UNNATURAL DEATHS

38   Medicolegal Death Investigation   373

39   Deaths of Elders in Long-Term Care Facilities   387

40   Suicide   391

41   Autoerotic Asphyxia   399

42   Homicide Survivors   405

Appendix A: Adult Body Diagrams   413

Appendix B: Crime Victim Compensation Programs   415

Forensic Glossary   419

Index   431

Contributor

Alison S. Cole, MS
Clinical Psychology PhD Candidate
Laboratory of Consciousness & Cognition
Binghamton University Psychology Department
Clearview Hall
Binghamton, NY

Foreword

Forensics is a cutting-edge topic, especially for today's health care providers who work with forensic clients regularly, sometimes without realizing it. Many health care clients have been victimized as children. Others are victimized by their intimate partner, their adult children, or strangers, and some are victimized by health care providers. Clients may also be the abusers: batterers, child abusers, elder abusers, or sexual predators, and many of these clients, such as female and older adult offenders, have special health care needs.

Health care professionals require information on forensics. Clients rarely present in health care settings with a chief complaint of victimization or offending. Instead they may manifest the signs of stress disorders or somatization, or present with no symptom at all, warranting advanced assessment skills on the part of health care providers. However, most providers lack these needed skills. While health care providers do learn the basics of intimate partner violence and elder abuse, they rarely learn how to conduct a forensic assessment, collect evidence, and testify as an expert witness. Concepts such as competency, human trafficking, stalking, sexual offending, and death investigation are rarely, if ever, mentioned in texts about adults and older adults.

This book provides health care providers with the tools they need to assess, manage, and prevent forensic problems within health care settings. The authors, Mary E. Muscari and Kathleen M. Brown, bring their years of experience to this book in a way that makes these challenging and often disturbing topics accessible to those providers on the front lines of violence recognition and management.

The authors have synthesized the key information on adult and older adult forensics and produced a "must read" text that needs to be on every person's bookshelf. I strongly recommend it!

Ann Wolbert Burgess, DNSc., APRN, BC
Professor of Psychiatric Nursing
Boston College
Chestnut Hill, MA

Preface

Forensic means "pertaining to the law" or "that which is legal." The word is derived from the Latin term *for ensis,* which means "open forum." Forensic health is the application of the heath care sciences to public or legal proceedings, and the application of the forensic aspects of health care combined with the biopsychosocial education of the health care professional in the scientific investigation and treatment of trauma and/or death of victims and perpetrators of abuse, violence, criminal activity, and traumatic accidents.

Health care practitioners frequently—and sometimes unknowingly— work with victims or offenders of intimate partner violence, elder abuse, sexual assault, workplace violence, and unnatural deaths. Emergency practitioners encounter the specialty of forensic science with increasing regularity, as many are now expected to know how to gather and preserve evidence from victims of gunshot or stab wounds and from those who have been victimized by sexual violence or other forms of abuse.

Clients who are victims require treatment using unique skills for competent medicolegal evaluation. Unfortunately, few practitioners have the education or resources to care for this population, a factor that impairs recognition of these problems when clients present with vague complaints or other agendas. Practitioners also receive little education on forensic assessment, principles of evidence, competency, guardianship, and navigating the justice system.

Violence is a health problem. Intimate partner violence, abuse between two people in an intimate relationship, can be very hazardous to health. The Centers for Disease Control and Prevention (CDC) note that physical abuse can cause anything from minor injuries to permanent disabilities to death. Emotional trauma could result in posttraumatic stress disorder (PTSD) and depression. Victims are also more likely to smoke, abuse alcohol, use drugs, and engage in risky sexual behaviors. Victims of sexual assault may be terrified of the offender and fear for their lives.

Victims may also feel humiliation, shame, and self-blame. If the assault is perpetrated by an acquaintance, friend, or lover, violation of trust can be an issue for the victim. Because of their shame and fear about how people will react, many victims keep their assault a secret. Male victims are more likely to suffer from depression and to develop antisocial personality disorder. Adult survivors of child sexual abuse may experience major depression, adjustment disorder, alcohol or other substance abuse, personality disorders, multiple personality disorder, psychosexual dysfunctions, and somatic symptoms.

Violence touches the lives of elders with alarming frequency. An estimated 2.1 million older Americans are victims of physical, psychological, or other forms of abuse and neglect each year. Most victims of elder abuse are mentally competent and reside in the community. But those with mental or physical disabilities are especially vulnerable. Some elders are the victims of battery by their husband or wife. Isolation and abuse go hand-in-hand. Most abused older people are isolated from their friends, neighbors, and other family members. Often the abuser will not let anyone visit or talk to the victim, in order to maintain a sense of isolation and helplessness. Elders with dementia are sexually abused more often by persons known to them (family member, caregiver, or another nursing home resident) than a stranger, and they present with behavioral signs of distress instead of verbal disclosures. These elders are easily confused, verbally manipulated, and pressured into sex by the mere presence of the offender. The ages of known sex offenders against elders ranges from 13 to 90.

Elders are also perpetrators, and the past decade has seen a drastic increase in the number of incarcerated elderly, due to mandatory minimum sentencing, longer sentences, and tighter parole policies. Offenders older than age 50 are the fastest growing subgroup within the inmate population. The health challenges experienced by older offenders are no different from those experienced by nonincarcerated elders. However, older offenders' situations are often complicated by their circumstances. As offenders age within the correctional system, changes that occur during their life spans create many challenges for prison authorities, health care personnel, and the offenders themselves.

This guide helps fill the forensic health information void by providing current, concise, and easy-to-use information that assists practitioners with the prevention, identification, and management of adult and older adult victims and offenders. The book is designed to be integrated into advanced adult, geriatric family, and forensic curriculums as a supplemental text, and to be utilized in primary, community, and acute care geriatric and family settings as an ongoing reference.

The book begins with a general principles section that describes the cycle, continuum, and cultural aspects of violence and discusses the mechanisms of forensic assessment and documentation, evidence collection, the criminal and family justice systems, expert witness testimony, and working with the multidisciplinary team. It also describes the issues of competence and guardianship, as well as violence in health care settings. Finally, it provides information on how professionals can manage their own mental health when working with these challenging issues.

The second section is devoted to adults and older adults as victims. The section begins with the effects on victims and how these impact on provider care. Other chapters provide information on intimate partner victimization, physical abuse, financial abuse, sexual assault, emotional abuse, human trafficking, personal injury, stalking, and resources for victims.

Section three focuses on adults and older adults as offenders. One chapter differentiates the lifelong offender from the new offender, with some emphasis on dementia and crime. Other chapters focus on perpetrators of intimate partner violence and sexual assault, offenders in institutions, offenders in communities, and the relationship of drugs and alcohol to offending in the older adult. There is also a chapter on parenting while incarcerated that addresses the issue of grandparents raising their grandchildren, often because the parents are incarcerated or unable to parent due to substance abuse problems.

The final section concentrates on medicolegal death investigations. The section explains the health care provider's role in elder death investigations and provides insight on topics that can better enable health care professionals to provide more detailed information to families undergoing these difficult times. There are chapters on suspicious deaths in long-term care facilities, autoerotic deaths, and homicide/suicide. This section ends with a chapter on working with grieving families who have lost a loved one to homicide.

Whenever possible, chapters are organized as follows:

■ Definition: This section provides definitions of pertinent terms, as well as more in-depth information on the subject matter of the chapter. Example: Stalking generally describes a pattern of overtly criminal and/or apparently innocent behaviors whereby an individual inflicts repeated, unwanted communications and intrusions upon another.

- Prevalence: This section provides statistics and relevant epidemiologic information. Example: Stalking is widespread, with nearly 1 in 12 women and 1 in 45 men stalked at least once in their lifetime. Most victims know their stalkers, and most stalkers (87%) are male.
- Etiology: This section addresses the cause or origin of the problem, as well as the factors that produce or predispose persons toward the problem, and/or issues found to correlate with the problem. Some chapters discuss typologies. Example: Stalking classifications or typologies vary. The National Center for Victims of Crime provides a typology that includes simple obsessional, love obsessional, and erotomanic stalkers.
- Assessment: This section guides health care providers to assessment issues relevant to the specific problem. Health care providers can then incorporate this information into their daily assessments as needed.

  - General Principles: This section provides information that helps guide assessments. Example: Most clients with psychotic disorders are not violent, but clients with acute psychosis who are paranoid and having command auditory hallucinations, or who have a history of being violent, being a victim of violence, or abusing alcohol or drugs are at high risk for violent behavior.
  - History and Physical Assessment: This section provides suggestions for problem-specific subjective and objective data collection that can be incorporated into comprehensive, episodic, or interval assessments. Example: Clients do not typically present with complaints of substance abuse problems; however, they can present with "red flags." Red flag symptoms include such issues as frequent absences from school or work, or history of frequent trauma or accidental injuries.
  - Diagnostic Testing/Screening Tools: When applicable, this section suggests testing that can help confirm specific diagnoses or, in most cases, provides a brief overview and access information for screening tools appropriate for settings such as primary care and emergency departments. Common tools, such as those used to screen for alcohol abuse and domestic violence, are included

in the chapter or appendix. This section also provides overview and access information on more advanced instruments, such as those used for assessing violence recidivism risk. These tools require specific educational backgrounds and training. However, it does benefit health care providers to have an understanding of these instruments since they relate to some of their clients.

- Intervention: This section provides information on therapeutic interventions and referrals.
- Prevention/Patient Teaching: This section is structured using the public health model of prevention. Patient teaching information is given when applicable.

  - Primary Prevention is concerned with health promotion activities that prevent the actual occurrence of a specific illness or disease. Primary prevention attempts to serve those individuals who are not yet part of the problem and strives to build skills and resiliency so that the problem will not develop.
  - Secondary Prevention promotes early detection or screening and treatment of disease and limitation of disability. By targeting individuals at high risk for the problem or who have displayed some form of antisocial or delinquent behavior, secondary prevention aims to keep these individuals from engaging in violent activity. Secondary prevention is also aimed at those who are at risk for becoming victims of violence to prevent the violence from occurring.
  - Tertiary Prevention is directed toward recovery or rehabilitation of a condition after the condition has been developed. Tertiary prevention is designed to serve those individuals who have already become violent or chronic offenders and emphasizes punishment and rehabilitation through the justice system. The objective is to help prevent future violent activity. Tertiary prevention for victims focuses on prevention of further damage from the victimization, as well as prevention of future victimization.

- Resources: This section provides readers with appropriate Web sites for further information.
- References: This section provides references used for that chapter.

The information in this guide comes from health care and criminal justice literature, as well as credible professional organizations. Many of the issues in this book have yet to be well researched, and some topics do not lend themselves to the rigor of random controlled trials. Readers will find rich information for their practices, as well as ideas for future research.

Acknowledgments

We would like to acknowledge all the forensic health students whose classroom contributions help to stimulate ideas for this book, as well as those students who assisted in the literature review:

Lauren Conaboy (University of Scranton)

Essie Lee (Binghamton University)

Carlotta Mendez (University of Scranton)

Jolynn Sannicandro (Binghamton University)

We would also like to extend thanks to Peter Rocheleau, Makeda Alexander, and Pam Amri of Springer Publishing, and Laura Stewart.

General Principles

1

The Cycle and Continuum of Violence

ADULT AND OLDER ADULT FORENSICS

Forensic means "pertaining to the law" or "that which is legal." The word is derived from the Latin term *for ensis,* which means "open forum." Adult and older adult forensics are the application of heath care sciences to public or legal proceedings; the application of the forensic aspects of health care combined with the biopsychosocial education of the health care professional in the scientific investigation and treatment of trauma and/or death of victims and perpetrators of abuse, violence, and criminal activity.

According the Centers for Disease Control and Prevention (CDC, 2009) violence is a serious public health problem that affects people in all stages of life: in 2006, more than 18,000 people were victims of homicide and more than 33,000 took their own lives. However, violent death numbers are only a fraction of the problem. Many more people survive violence with permanent physical and emotional damage, and communities erode due to reduced productivity, decreased property values, and disrupted social services.

Victims of violence are also more likely to smoke, abuse alcohol, use drugs, and engage in risky sexual behaviors. Victims of sexual assault may be terrified of the offender and fear for their lives. Victims may also feel humiliation, shame, and self-blame. If the assault is perpetrated by an acquaintance, friend, or lover, violation of trust can be an issue for the victim. Because of their shame and fear about how people will react, many victims keep their assault a secret. Male victims are more likely to suffer from depression and to develop antisocial personality disorder. Adult survivors of child sexual abuse may experience major depression, adjustment disorder, alcohol or other substance abuse, personality disorders, multiple personality disorder, psychosexual dysfunctions, and somatic symptoms.

Violent offenders are usually from high-risk groups and have poor health histories, increasing their susceptibility to disease. But offender health problems are not contained within correctional facilities. Prisoner health problems are public health problems. Infectious diseases common in the incarcerated population include human immunodeficiency virus (HIV), tuberculosis, hepatitis, and sexually transmitted diseases. Mental health problems also abound in offenders. Persons with mental illness are more likely to be victims of a crime than to commit one; however, approximately half of all prisoners have mental health problems (James & Glaze, 2006).

Health care practitioners frequently—and sometimes unknowingly—work with victims of intrafamilial abuse, sexual assault, and unnatural deaths, as well as criminal offenders. Emergency practitioners encounter the specialty of forensic science with increasing regularity, as many are now expected to know how to gather and preserve evidence from victims of gunshot or stab wounds and from those who have been victimized by sexual violence or other forms of abuse. Primary care and other providers often see clients who present with vague symptoms that may indicate the hidden agenda of abuse. Therefore it is critical that forensic issues become a component in the education of health care providers.

VIOLENCE AS A HEALTH PROBLEM

Violence is a public health problem that affects all people, regardless of socioeconomic class, racial or ethnic background, educational level, or sexual preference. Some violent crime rates, including murder and sexual assault, have declined over the past decade; however, violence crime rates in the home, workplace, community, and schools have increased. Approximately 899,000 children were victimized by child abuse or neglect in 2005, and one to two million individuals age 65 and older were mistreated by those on whom they depended for their care and safety.

Intimate partner violence is responsible for 5.3 million victimizations among women, 2 million injuries, and 1,300 deaths per year, with an annual cost of $4.1 billion.

The cycle of violence refers to a sociological theory about violence that explains violence as a learned behavior passed down from one generation to the next. According to this theory, this learned behavior can explain all forms of violence. The person committing the violent act chooses violence as a response to a stimulus because violence is the behavior that has been modeled to the person. In other words, the person reacts to a situation with violence because this is the reaction the person has "learned" via family, peers, and community.

Children in the United States are more likely to be exposed to violence than are adults, and millions of children and adolescents in the United States are exposed to violence in their homes, schools, and communities, as both victims and witnesses. The recent Comprehensive National Survey on children's exposure to violence confirms that most of the children in the United States are exposed to violence on a daily basis. More than 60% of the children surveyed were exposed to violence within the past year, either directly or indirectly; and 46.3% were assaulted at least once in the past year. A little more than 25% witnessed a violent act, and 9.8% saw one family member assault another (Finkelhor, Turner, Ormrod, Hamby, & Kracke, 2009).

Violence exposure can have significant effects on children as they develop and as they form their own intimate relationships throughout childhood and adulthood. Some children experience chronic community violence and are exposed to guns, knives, drugs, and random violence in their neighborhoods; some are exposed to witnessing violence against their mother perpetrated by their father or her paramour on a regular basis; some children are exposed to a plethora of violent acts on the screens of televisions, computers, video games, and other media. Many children are exposed to all of these. Risk factors are cumulative, and thus the risk of negative outcomes multiplies, putting children in "double jeopardy," such as those exposed to both domestic and community violence. Children who are direct victims of assault and who witness repeated violence are more likely to have significant negative outcomes than children who are exposed to a single instance.

Dauvergne (2002) states that intimate partner violence and sexual assault are leading causes of injury-related death in women. Of solved crimes in 2001, 52% of all female homicide victims were killed by someone with whom they had an intimate relationship at one point in time, either through marriage or dating, compared to 8% of male victims. The World Health Organization (WHO, 2009) notes that there are many forms of violence against women, including sexual, physical, or emotional abuse by an intimate partner; physical or sexual abuse by family members or others; sexual harassment and abuse by authority figures (such as teachers, police officers, or employers); and trafficking for forced labor or sex. Violence can result in long-term health consequences for women. Physical and sexual abuse is associated with injuries, as well as sexually transmitted infections such as HIV/AIDS, unintended pregnancies, gynecological problems, induced abortions, and adverse pregnancy outcomes, including miscarriage, low birth weight, and fetal death. Abuse can result in many physical health problems, including headaches, back pain, abdominal pain, fibromyalgia, gastrointestinal disorders, limited mobility, and poor overall health, and violence increases the risk of depression, posttraumatic stress disorder, sleep difficulties, eating disorders, and emotional distress (WHO, 2009).

Men's health can be significantly affected by violence. The World Health Organization (2002) states that males account for three-quarters of all victims of homicide, and that males also have higher rates of suicide. Male survivors of violence may also face non–life threatening injury, mental health problems, reproductive health problems, and sexually transmitted diseases. The Mayo Clinic (2009) notes that intimate partner violence against males may lead to depression and anxiety, as well as suicide. Male victims are also more likely to engage in substance abuse and unprotected sex that males who have not been abused. Men are also less likely than women to report intimate partner violence in a heterosexual relationship because of embarrassment or fear of ridicule, and similarly, a man being abused by another man may be reluctant to talk about the problem because of how it reflects on his masculinity.

As the number of older adults increases, the number of elder abuse cases will increase as well, and the impact of elder abuse as a public health issue will grow. Elders who are victims of physical abuse or neglect have triple the mortality of those who were not abused. Mortality rates in physically abused elders are also significantly higher than for younger adults. Even with correction for severity of injury, elders are five to six times more likely to die of similar injuries than younger people. The Coalition to Eliminate the Abuse of Seniors (2005) points out that older adults have less physical strength and are less able to defend themselves from physical abuse. Additionally, older bones break more easily and take longer to heal. Abused elders may suffer from psychological distress or depression, worry, and anxiety that may be mistaken for dementia. They may also feel shame, guilt, or embarrassment, especially when the abuser is a family member. Some older adult victims turn to alcohol or drugs, including the abuse of prescription medication, sometimes to the point of dependency.

THE HEALTH CARE ROLE

Health care providers can use the theory of violence as learned behavior to develop risk assessments based upon exposure to violence. If a client is determined to be a victim of violence, health care interventions would include counseling for psychological processing of the violent event with the goal of preventing the victim from reexperiencing violence or perpetrating violence. It is well known in the forensic community that the strongest correlate to victimization is past victimization, and that the best predictor of future violence is past violence. Victims and offenders require referrals to provide sufficient interventions to break the cycle of violence. The overall intervention for proponents of the cycle of violence theory is a strong public health initiative for reduction of violence in American culture. Cycle of violence theorists recommend interventions for young people who witness violence, are exposed to violence, and live in violent neighborhoods. Cycle of violence theorists recommend early detection and interventions to alter violent homes and neighborhoods.

Primary prevention methods include school and workplace programs designed to teach children or adults nonviolent strategies for managing conflict, as well as programs that provide support to young first-time mothers to prevent child abuse. Secondary prevention that requires early recognition of child abuse, intimate partner, and gang-related behaviors would facilitate referral into a system of support that will prevent further victimization and offending.

Tertiary prevention impacts on violence that has already occurred. Interventions are planned to decrease the probability that these clients will be revictimized or offend again. The juvenile justice system in the United States is based upon the theory that intensive rehabilitation will prevent juveniles from reoffending. Juveniles are treated by the justice system very differently from adults, based upon the theory that violence is learned and can therefore be unlearned through rehabilitation. Public health initiatives to stop drug dealing in neighborhoods are an overall effort to reduce violence in communities and stop the lessons drug dealing delivers about violence as a means to control territory.

RESOURCES

American Academy of Psychiatry and the Law: http://www.aapl.org
Bureau of Justice Statistics: http://www.ojp.usdoj.gov/bjs
FBI Uniform Crime Report: http://www.fbi.gov/ucr/ucr.htm
Office for Victims of Crime: http://www.ojp.usdoj.gov/ovc
U.S. Department of Defense Sexual Assault Prevention and Response: http://www.sapr.mil

REFERENCES

Bureau of Justice Statistics. (2003). *Crime characteristics: Summary findings.* Retrieved from http://www.ojp.usdoj.gov/bjs/cvict_c.htm
Centers for Disease Control and Prevention (CDC). (2009). *Violence prevention.* Retrieved from http://www.cdc.gov/ViolencePrevention/index.html
Child Welfare Information. (2007). *Child maltreatment 2005.* Washington, DC: Children's Bureau, U.S. Department of Heath and Human Services. Retrieved from http://www.acf.dhhs.gov/programs/cb/pubs/cm05/index.htm
Coalition to Eliminate the Abuse of Seniors. (2005). *Health effects of abuse and neglect of older adults elder abuse prevention series: Number 93d.* Retrieved from http://www.healthlinkbc.ca/healthfiles/pdf/hfile93d.pdf
Dauvergne, M. (2002). Homicide in Canada—2001. Canadian Center for Justice Statistics: Juristat 22 (7). Retrieved from: http://www.statcan.gc.ca./pub/85-002-x/85-002-x2002007-eng.pdf
Finkelhor, D., Turner, H., Ormrod, R., Hamby, S., & Kracke, K. (2009). Children's Exposure to Violence: A Comprehensive National Survey. Office of Juvenile Justice and Delinquency Prevention Juvenile Bulletin. NCJ 227744. Retrieved from: http://www.ncjrs.gov/pdffiles1/ojjdp/227744.pdf
Freedberg, P. (2008). Integrating forensic nursing into the undergraduate nursing curriculum: A solution for a disconnect. *Journal of Nursing Education, 47*(5), 201–208.
James, D., & Glaze, R. (2006). *Mental health problems of prison and jail inmates.* Bureau of Justice Statistics Special Report, NCJ 213600. Retrieved from http://www.ojp.usdoj.gov/bjs/pub/pdf/mhppji.pdf
Mayo Clinic. (2009). *Domestic violence against men: Know the signs, seek help.* Retrieved from http://www.mayoclinic.com/health/domestic-violence-against-men/MY00557
National Center on Elder Abuse. (2005). *Fact sheet: Elder abuse prevalence and incidence.* Washington, DC: Author. Retrieved from http://www.ncea.aoa.gov/NCEA root/main_site/pdf/publication/FinalStatistics050331.pdf
National Institute of Justice. (2001). *An update on the cycle of violence. U.S. Department of Justice Research in Brief.* Retrieved from http://www.ncjrs.gov/pdffiles1/nij/184894.pdf
Sellas, M., & Krouse, L. (2009). Elder abuse. *Emedicine.* Retrieved from http://emedicine.medscape.com/article/805727-overview
WHO. (2002). *World report on violence and health: Summary.* Geneva: Author. Retrieved from http://www.who.int/violence_injury_prevention/violence/world_report/en/summary_en.pdf
WHO. (2009). *Violence against women.* Retrieved from http://www.who.int/mediacentre/factsheets/fs239/en/

2   Cultural Aspects of Forensics

DEFINITIONS

Twenty-five percent of the U.S. population identifies themselves as belonging to one of the federally defined minority groups, and almost 20% of the American population speaks a language other than English as their primary language. And the American population is becoming even more diverse. It is predicted that shortly after 2050, no single racial-ethnic group will hold a majority population position.

The increasing diversity of Western society adds an important dimension to forensic practice. The understanding of cultural differences can aid health care providers in managing the cycle of violence, and the utilization of culturally competent health care can facilitate recovery from trauma. An example would be interpreting the meaning of a man disallowing his wife to answer questions. Western cultural may lead the health care provider to interpret this as controlling behavior. However, this behavior may be acceptable in some cultures to the point where the woman is comfortable with it and not comfortable with answering the questions.

The Merriam-Webster Dictionary (http://www.merriam-webster.com) defines *culture* as the integrated pattern of human knowledge, beliefs, and behaviors that depend on transmission to succeeding generations, and the traditional beliefs, social manner, and material traits of a racial, religious, or social group. Culture extends beyond ethnicity and religion to include elements such as gender identity (e.g., lesbian, gay, bisexual, transgender) and location (e.g., rural or urban), and it encompasses an array of values, beliefs, and customs.

- Values act as the foundation for culture. Values are acquired through socialization in early childhood and guide people's goals, aspirations, and behaviors. For example, people value time differently. Some are present-oriented, accepting each day as it comes with little regard for the past and future; others are past-oriented, maintaining traditions and worshiping ancestors. Still others are future-oriented, with a high value for change.
- Beliefs include knowledge, opinions, and faith about the world. Witchcraft and the "evil eye" are two personalistic folk beliefs.
- Customs are learned behaviors that are easily assessed through questioning and observation. Problems can develop if professionals do not validate the meaning of observed behaviors. For example, most health care providers consider lack of eye contact abnormal behavior; however, some cultures consider eye contact a sign of disrespect or even hostility.

Race is a social and political construct rather than a biological one. Ethnicity is a term used to describe a common heritage, history, and worldview. The U.S. Census Bureau combines race and ethnicity into the following categories: American Indian, Alaskan Native, Asian, Black or African American, Hispanic or Latino, Native Hawaiian or Pacific Islander, and White. The purpose of this categorization is to help the government understand the needs of its citizens, including mental health care. However, this classification can be confusing and inadequate. There are more than 40 Asian and Pacific Island Countries, and over 560 Native American and Alaskan Native tribes. African Americans whose ancestors lived in the United States centuries ago have different cultural norms than those from Africa or the Caribbean today. Latinos may be from different racial groups, and the White group includes a very diverse population of Americans of European descent, as well as people from the Middle East. Biracial persons have no unique category.

Culture also includes immigration status, an issue critical in forensics since foreign-born women are over-represented among intimate partner female homicide victims when compared to the general population.

- Permanent residents or immigrants are persons who come to the United States to remain permanently or for an indefinite period of time. The United States is their primary place of residence, and their permanent resident status is shown by possession of an identification card (green card).
- Refugees are those persons living outside of their country of nationality and who are unable or unwilling to return because of persecution or fear of persecution on account of race, religion, nationality, membership in a particular social group, or political opinion.
- Refugees make an application to U.S. authorities outside the United States and are approved for such status before coming to the United States. They are eligible to apply for permanent resident status after one year of continuous stay in the United States.
- Asylees must meet the definition for a refugee but differ because they make an application for asylum (protection) after arriving in the United States.
- Naturalization is the process of becoming a U.S. citizen. Lawful permanent residents may apply for U.S. citizenship by filing an application with the U.S. Citizenship and Immigration Services. It usually takes six months to two years to become naturalized.
- Undocumented immigrants are those who entered the country without valid documents, as well as those who entered with valid visas but overstayed their visas' expiration or otherwise violated the terms of their admission.

CULTURE AND FORENSICS

Certain cultural beliefs and customs have implications in the legal system, and health care professionals can assist law enforcement by performing detailed assessments to ascertain whether beliefs and behaviors are related to culture, mental health issues, or other factors. This may be important in cases where family violence is suspected or other violence has taken place.

Culture-Bound Syndromes

Culture-bound syndromes (culture-related syndromes) are folk illnesses with prominent alterations of behavior and experience. They usually do not conform to conventional diagnostic syndromes; however, they have cultural validity in the societies in which they occur. Some culture-bound syndromes involve somatic symptoms (pain or disturbed function of a body part), while others are purely behavioral. The ones noted here are those that may have legal implications:

- *Amok* or *mata elap* (Malaysia) is probably the most known in this category and is a dissociative episode characterized by an outburst of violent, aggressive, or homicidal behavior directed at people and objects. The episode is usually triggered by a perceived insult or slight and seems to be prevalent among males. Persons who "run amok" usually experience persecutory ideas, automatism, and amnesia during the episode, and a return to premorbid state following the episode. A similar behavior pattern is found in Laos, the Philippines, Polynesia (*cafard* or *cathard*); New Guinea and Puerto Rico (*mal de pelea*); and among the Navajos (*iich'aa*).
- *Ataquque de nervios* (Latinos from the Caribbean, and other Latino groups) manifests in symptoms of uncontrollable shouting, crying, trembling, and verbal or physical aggression. The individual may also experience dissociative experiences, seizure-like or fainting episodes, and suicidal gestures. These symptoms frequently occur after a stressful event relating to the family, such as separation, divorce, or an accident.
- *Boufée deliriante* (West Africa and Haiti) is a sudden outburst of agitated and aggressive behavior, marked confusion, and psychomotor excitement. *Boufée deliriante* may sometimes be accompanied by visual and auditory hallucinations or paranoid ideation.
- *Hi-Wa itck* (Mohave American Indians) is associated with the unwanted separation from a loved one, resulting in insomnia, depression, loss of appetite, and sometimes suicide.
- *Latah* (Malaysia and Indonesia) is characterized by hypersensitivity to sudden fright, often with echopraxia, echolalia, command obedience, and dissociative or trancelike behavior. The Malaysian syndrome is more common in middle-aged women. Similar syndromes are found in Siberian groups (*amurakh, irkunii, ikota, olan, myriachit,* and *menkeiti*); Thailand (*bah-tschi, bah-tsi,* and *baah-ji*); Japan (*imu*); and Philippines (*mali-mali* and *silok*).
- *Locura* (Latin America) is a severe form of chronic psychosis that is attributed to an inherited vulnerability, the effect of multiple life difficulties, or a combination of the two. Manifestations include incoherence, agitation, auditory and visual hallucinations, inability to follow social interaction rules, unpredictability, and possible violence.

- *Pibloktoq* or Arctic hysteria (Greenland Eskimos) is an abrupt dissociative episode accompanied by extreme excitement lasting up to 30 minutes and frequently followed by seizures and coma lasting up to 12 hours. The affected individual may be withdrawn or slightly irritable for a period of hours or days before the attack and typically reports complete amnesia for the attack. During the attack, the individual may shout obscenities, eat feces, flee from protective shelters, tear off his or her clothing, break furniture, or perform other irrational or dangerous acts.
- Qi-gong psychotic reaction (China) is an acute, time-limited episode characterized by dissociative, paranoid, or other symptoms that occur after participating in the Chinese folk health-enhancing practice of qi-gong. Individuals who become overly involved in the practice are especially vulnerable.
- *Shenkui* (China) is characterized by marked anxiety or panic symptoms with accompanying somatic complaints without obvious physical cause. Symptoms include dizziness, backache, fatigability, general weakness, insomnia, frequent dreams, and complaints of sexual dysfunction (such as premature ejaculation and impotence). Symptoms are attributed to excessive semen loss from frequent intercourse, masturbation, nocturnal emission, or passing of "white turbid urine" believed to contain semen. Similar symptoms are found in India (*dhat* and *jiryan*); and Sri Lanka (*sukra prameha*).
- *Tabanka* (Trinidad) is characterized by depression associated with a high rate of suicide and is usually seen in men who have been abandoned by their wives.
- *Zar* (North Africa and the Middle East) is an experience of spirit possession with symptoms that include dissociative episodes with laughing, shouting, hitting the head against a wall, singing, or weeping. Individuals may show apathy and withdrawal, refusing to eat or carry out daily tasks, or may develop a long-term relationship with the possessing spirit.

Cultural Customs Related to Female Reproduction

Female Genital Mutilation (May Mimic Intimate Partner Violence)

Female genital mutilation (FGM) refers to procedures that intentionally alter or injure female genital organs for nonmedical reasons. FGM is usually performed when a girl is between 4 and 8 years old. It is practiced in about 28 African countries, Asia, the Middle East, and increasingly in Europe, Australia, Canada, and the United States. The World Health Organization (WHO), which promotes the elimination of FGM, has estimated that between 100 and 140 million women have undergone FGM, and that two million more undergo some form of FGM every year.

The WHO has identified four types of FGM.

- Type I is a clitoridectomy, which is the only type that can accurately be referred to as female circumcision and involves the removal of the prepuce and all or parts of the clitoris. This procedure typically does not result in long-term complications.
- Type II involves removal of the clitoris and inner labia, possibly resulting in pain during intercourse and other long-term problems.
- Type III is an extreme form of circumcision that involves removal of the clitoris, at least two-thirds of the labia majora, and the entire labia minora. Incisions are made in the labia majora to create raw surfaces, which are then stitched or held together (sometimes by tying the woman's legs together), until a hood of skin grows to cover the urethra and vagina. Afterward, a tiny hole is made to allow for menstrual flow and urination.
- Type IV involves piercing or incising the clitoris and/or labia, and cauterization by burning of the clitoris and surrounding tissue.

Health care providers are likely to encounter women who have had FGM in their clinical practice, possibly for one of the adverse effects, which include: cysts, abscesses, and scar tissue; sexual dysfunction; dysmenorrhea; chronic pelvic infections; damage to the urethra; incontinence; chronic pelvic and back pain; chronic urinary tract infections; and difficulties with childbirth. It is important that health care providers not assume that all these women want this condition reversed. Women who have undergone FGM have been taught to believe that this rite of passage is normal. Their culture may believe that reversal of circumcision makes a woman unsuitable for marriage, liable for divorce, and virtually an outcast in their communities. Instead, providers should ask how this alteration has affected the woman's life, urination, and menstruation. Health care professionals can also refer these women to a counselor from the same cultural background to discuss deinfibulation or other possible treatments, if needed.

Practices Around Menstruation

Beliefs about the cause and purpose of menstruation vary among cultures. For example, Navajo culture views menarche as a symbol for passage into adulthood, whereas both Iranian and Orthodox Jewish cultures view menstruation as a period of uncleanness. Extremely Orthodox Jewish women separate themselves from all men during menses, and no man is allowed to touch or even sit where a menstruating woman has sat. Women are considered to be in a state of impurity for at least 12 days (5 days from the onset of the menstrual cycle and 7 clean days following it). They then must attend a *mikvah* (ritual bath) before engaging in sexual intercourse with their husbands.

Practices Related to Illness Treatment (May Mimic Child or Elder Abuse)

Coining, or *CaoGio* (Southeast Asia) is one of the most commonly practiced cultural folk remedies. Coining is rubbing or scratching with a coin on the skin of the back, neck, upper chest, and arms. Before or during rubbing, Tiger Balm (a mentholated ointment), Ben-Gay, an herbal liquid medicine or water is applied on the skin. The skin is then rubbed in a downward, linear fashion with the edge of the copper coin or a silver spoon until dark lines appear. These marks can persist for several days and have the appearance of being struck with a stick or whip.

Cupping (Hmong, Vietnamese, ethnic Chinese) or *bahnkes* (Russians, Koreans, and others) is performed on the chest, back, abdomen, and/or back of legs for pain, and the forehead and temples for headaches. A glass is held upside down, and a lit match, candle, or lighter is held under it in order to burn off the oxygen, creating a vacuum. The cup is quickly placed on the skin and the vacuum effect pulls the skin up, creating a mark that looks like a bruise and that may last for several days.

Stick burns and moxibustion, also called *poua*, are remedies used in certain cultures to relieve a variety of illness symptoms. These remedies are related to acupuncture; however, they cause a circular, cigarette-tip-size burn. The procedure calls for an incense-like stick to be lit and placed on the palms of the hands, soles of the feet, and genital area. Moxa herbs, usually mugwort (*Artemisia vulgaris*), or yarn are rolled into a pea-sized ball, placed on the skin, lit, and allowed to burn to the point of pain.

Pinching, or *bat gio* (Southeast Asia) is used to treat pain and a variety of conditions. For example, the area between the eyebrows, upper nose, and temples is pinched to relieve headaches. Tiger balm may be massaged into the area before pinching. The pressure from the pinching leaves a reddened area that may give the appearance of having been struck.

Air suctioning (Southeast Asia) is used to relieve headaches. The cut end of a bull or goat horn is placed on the patient's forehead and/or temples, and the practitioner sucks the air out of the other end. The horn sticks to the application site and is then plugged with wax and left on the forehead for 10 to 15 minutes. Blood drawn to the surface of the skin leaves a round, bruiselike mark after the horn is removed. The marks may persist for several days.

Fallen fontanel or *caida de la mollera* (Latino populations), a challenging and potentially fatal pediatric folk illness, may develop from any severe illness (such as gastroenteritis) resulting in a 10% body weight loss in an infant. Children with *caida* are believed to be neglected, creating a high degree of maternal guilt. The cause is believed to be mechanical, such as the soft palate pulling down the fontanel when the feeding nipple is suddenly pulled out of the infant's mouth. Folk remedies include: pressing upward on the soft palate with thumbs or fingers, sucking the anterior fontanel, holding the baby upside down over water with or without shaking or hitting the feet. Poultices may be applied to the fontanel with raw egg, oil, or liniment and the hair is pulled up (so that the roots will raise the skin back up).

Culture and Intimate Partner Violence

Intimate partner violence (IPV) seems to be more prevalent and more lethal among immigrant women than among U.S. citizens. The Office for Victims of Crime notes that there are several factors that may make this type of victimization more likely, as well increase the difficulty immigrant victims face in seeking safety and using the justice system effectively:

- Cultural barriers: Cultural beliefs and practices may make it difficult for a victim to leave an abusive relationship and may even reinforce the idea that violence against a spouse is acceptable.
- Fear of deportation: Immigrants may fear being deported and losing custody of their children. Perpetrators of domestic violence and other crimes may use the fear of deportation to thwart the victim from reporting the crime. Lack of proper legal documentation (social security number, green card, or employment authorization)

to work or live in the United States can contribute to immigrants staying with abusive partners and not seeking outside help.

- Language barriers: Lack of or limited English proficiency keeps victimized immigrants from seeking protection with the police, the court system, social service agencies, and shelters.
- Misinformation about the legal system: Many immigrants come from countries where women cannot receive justice. Immigrant victims may be wary of seeking assistance from official institutions based on real or imagined experiences.
- Fear of the police: Immigrants may come from countries where police repress citizens, respond only to bribes, or believe women should be subordinate to men.
- Economic barriers: An abusive spouse may be a woman's only means of support, and her immigrant status may make it impossible for her to legally obtain work or find child care.

The Violence Against Women Act (VAWA) of 1994 addresses the needs of immigrant women who are victimized by their spouses. This law created two ways for women who are married to U.S. citizens or lawful permanent residents to get their residency without having to rely on their abusive spouse: (a) Self-petitions allow a victim of IPV to file for and obtain permanent resident status without the knowledge, cooperation, or participation of the perpetrator. These petitions are applicable to victims of IPV who would have lawful immigration status through their spouses. These women should first consult a shelter worker, immigration attorney, or domestic violence or immigration agency for assistance. (b) Undocumented immigrant victims of IPV may be able to obtain U.S. residency through VAWA cancellation of deportation, if they are currently in or can be placed into deportation proceedings. Victims who qualify for cancellation may have their deportation waived by the court and may be granted residency. These women should consult an immigration attorney before proceeding.

Culture and Human Trafficking

The United Nations defines human trafficking as

The recruitment, transportation, transfer, harbouring or receipt of persons, by means of the threat or use of force or other forms of coercion, of abduction, of fraud, of deception, of the abuse of power or of a position of vulnerability or of the giving or receiving of payments or benefits to achieve the consent of a person having control over another person, for the purpose of exploitation. (United Nations, n.d.)

Many victims have language barriers and are isolated and unable to communicate with service providers, law enforcement, and others who might help them. They are often subjected to debt-bondage, usually in the context of paying off transportation fees into the destination countries, and are often threatened with injury or death or threats to the safety of their family back home. Please see chapter 20 for more on human trafficking.

Immigration Consultant Fraud

Scam artists prey upon immigrants seeking assistance in obtaining legal residence, work authorization, or citizenship. Many claim that they are attorneys or that they have close connections to the Immigration and Naturalization Service (INS). Others use titles such as notary public to deceive people into believing that they are lawyers. Typical scams include: charging excessive fees for immigration services and then failing to file any documents; filing false asylum claims; and charging fees to prepare applications for nonexistent immigration programs or for legitimate programs for which the client does not qualify.

CULTURAL COMPETENCY

Cultural competence goes beyond cultural sensitivity. It implies moving beyond awareness about different cultures to in-depth knowledge, and from sensitivity to issues to commitment to change situations of oppression. Culturally competent providers move beyond awareness about different cultures to an in-depth knowledge of them.

To provide culturally competent care, health care providers should:

- Develop knowledge about the norms of the ethnic and cultural groups they are likely to encounter in everyday practice
- Have the ability to perform a cultural assessment
- Make a commitment to spend time with diverse groups outside the health care setting

- Understand the political and social issues that affect these groups
- Understand how various groups react to stress

To provide culturally competent care:

- Become aware of your own professional and personal values about cultural practices. Ethnocentrism is common in all cultural and social groups, but health care professionals must transcend this bias. Health care professionals do not need to abandon personal values, beliefs, and cultural practices; however, they do need to understand how their personal perspectives may impact on their responses and assessments of diverse patients.
- Identify cultural nuances when assessing behaviors considered abnormal by Western society, such as lack of eye contact or an unresponsive or flat affect. These signs are often associated with mental illness or deceptiveness, yet in some cultures these are normal behaviors. Be sure to compare the patient's behavior with normative standards of his or her cultural group, not only with the Westernized diagnostic system.
- Try to understand patients and their situations within the context of their cultural group. Ask questions about beliefs, perceptions about the cause of a problem, and how this type of problem is usually addressed in their culture. Ask about religious and spiritual beliefs and experiences.
- Realize that not all members of a particular cultural group are the same. Information about cultural trends should not overshadow the understanding of the individual person. Avoid stereotyping.
- Empathy can bridge cultural differences. Convey a caring attitude toward patients, and show interest in cultural differences and acknowledge these with the patient.

The U.S. Department of Justice's Office of Victims of Crime presents five core tenets to providing high-quality multicultural victim assistance services:

- Develop the cultural awareness and competency
- Acknowledge the different and valid cultural customs of recovery from traumatic events
- Support cultural pathways to mental health and incorporate these into victim services and referrals

- Rely on multiethnic and multilingual teamwork to implement and monitor effective victim services
- Develop a cross-cultural perspective

RESOURCES

National Center for Cultural Competence: http://www.11.georgetown.edu/research/guc chd/nccc

Office for Minority Health Cultural Competency Section: http://www.omhrc.gov/tem plates/browse.aspx?lvl=&lvlID=3

Program for Multicultural Health: http://www.med.umich.edu/Multicultural/ccp/in dex.htm

Think Cultural Health (U.S. Department of Health & Human Services): http://www. thinkculturalhealth.org/

REFERENCES

Administration for Children's Services, U.S. Department of Health and Human Services. Human trafficking fact sheet. Retrieved from http://www.acf.hhs.gov/traffick ing/about/factsheets.html

American Psychiatric Association. (2000). *Diagnostic and statistical manual of mental disorders* (4th ed.). Washington, DC: Author.

Child Abuse Prevention Council of Sacramento, Inc. (n.d.). *Cultural customs.* Retrieved from http://www.capcsac.org/cultural-customs

Femicide in New York City: 1995–2002. New York City Department of Health and Mental Hygiene, October 2004. Retrieved from http://www.nyc.gov/html/doh/downloads/pdf/ip/femicide1995–2002_report.pdf

Gerace, L., & Salimene, S. (2009). *Cultural competence for today's nurses, part two: Culture and mental health.* Retrieved from http://www.nurse.com/ce/CE399-60/Course Page/2009

Salimene, S., & Gerace, L. (2009). *Cultural competence for today's nurses, part one: Culture and women's health.* Retrieved from http://www.nurse.com/ce/CE398-60/Course Page

Simons, R. (2001). Introduction to culture-bound syndromes. *Psychiatric Times, 18*(11). Retrieved from http://www.psychiatrictimes.com/display/article/10168/54246

United Nations. (n.d.). *Gender and human trafficking.* Retrieved from http://www.unes cap.org/esid/Gad/Issues/Trafficking/index.asp

U.S. Census Bureau. (2004). *U.S. interim projections by age, sex, race, and Hispanic origin.* Retrieved from http://www.census.gov/ipc/www/usinterimproj

U.S. Citizenship and Immigration Services. (n.d.). Glossary and acronyms. Retrieved from http://www.uscis.gov/graphics/glossary4.cfm#U

3

Forensic Assessment and Documentation

DEFINITION

Forensic assessments are those assessments performed for legal purposes. Health care providers who perform these assessments may be evaluating victims (as in sexual assault evaluations) or offenders (as in criminal competency evaluations). Forensic assessment differs from clinical assessment. Clinical assessments are confidential. Forensic assessments have limited confidentiality, because the assessment information may be used in court or for other purposes (such as parole evaluation). Thus, the forensic assessment requires that the client and collateral sources be informed of the limitations on confidentiality.

When performing clinical assessments, the health care provider listens empathetically to the subject in a nonjudgmental attitude, focuses on the subject's needs, facilitates the subject's ability to verbalize distressing feelings, and assists the subject with problem solving. When performing a forensic assessment, the health care provider must remain unbiased, objective, and void of emotional attachment to the subject. The focus is on gathering information in a methodical and purposeful manner. When conducting the forensic assessment, the subject is not the health care professional's client; the client is usually the state (if assessing for the prosecution), the plaintiff attorney (in civil cases), or the defense attorney (in civil and criminal cases).

ETIOLOGY

Health care providers frequently encounter clients whose clinical situation includes a legal component. Victims of crime, accident victims, and perpetrators of crime are frequently seen in health care settings. The role in forensic assessment is to help ensure that the legal aspects of their cases are appropriately addressed.

ASSESSMENT

General Principles

The purpose of a forensic assessment depends on the legal situation. If the subject warrants assessment for issues such as competency or risk, the purpose is usually to collect pertinent information from the subject and collateral sources (persons and documents relevant to the case) and perform specific psychological testing. For example, forensic assessment of a sex offender may warrant an interview with the subject, interviews with the victims and family, assessment of all past and present juvenile and adult criminal records, and performance of risk assessments such as the Static 2002.

These assessments are usually carried out by professionals with advanced psychological/psychiatric education and experience. The purpose of forensic assessment of crime victims is to gain facts for the legal investigation. This is achieved though obtaining the victim's account of the incident and identifying and collecting evidence that has transferred from the perpetrator and/or crime scene to the victim. For example, the forensic assessment of an elder-abuse victim would include an interview of the elder (if possible), a review of the elder's medical records, a physical examination to determine the extent and type of injuries, and pertinent diagnostic tests that would be used in this case to further diagnose elder abuse. This chapter focuses on forensic assessment of the crime victim.

The Forensic Interview

Whenever possible, health care providers interview the victim with a law enforcement professional present to avoid subjecting the victim to an additional interview process. The victim account of what occurred during the commission of the crime, in as much detail as possible, is most helpful for evidence collection and preservation. For example, in a sexual assault case, knowing where the suspect placed his mouth on the victim is likely to enhance the accuracy of the search for saliva. In cases of dating violence, knowing exactly what areas of the body may be injured makes the search for early bruising and patterns of bruising more likely to be successful. Knowing that the victim was restrained in any way during an assault, allows the examiner to carefully search for signs of restraint, such as bruising and tape marks.

Health care providers should record what the client/victim recalls in his or her own words as often as possible. An ideal victim interview is recorded in a series of quotes, in quotation marks, about what the victim recalls. Statements made by the victim to the health care provider can be used in court. The forensic role in interviewing is not to analyze or place judgment on the words of the victim, but simply to record them, in writing, exactly as stated, such as "He shoved his penis in my mouth," "He burned me with the curling iron," or "I was beat up by John." The victim's description should not be sanitized or interpreted, just recorded with as many exact quotes as possible.

An interview conducted with law enforcement present prevents the client/victim from the need to retell the account multiple times. Law enforcement must determine what crime or crimes were committed, gather information related to the crime scene, and obtain as much information as possible about the suspect(s) from the victim. Health care providers are seeking information about possible injury and possible evidence transfer from the suspect to the victim. Information desired by law enforcement and by health care personnel can be derived from the victim's description of the events preceding his or her entry into the health care system.

Because health care concerns are always a priority, the interview may be delayed until the victim is medically stable; but examination, evaluation, and treatment may proceed without the interview. The interview may also be delayed if the victim is unconscious or semiconscious, and/or under the influence of alcohol or drugs. Evaluation, treatment, and testing should proceed in these situations without an interview. The interview can be conducted at a later time. When the victim cannot speak for himself or herself, as in the case of confused elders, careful documentation of any and all observations of the victim by health care personnel becomes crucial.

Consent to collect forensic evidence and submit the evidence to law enforcement should be obtained. This consent is different from consent for medical treatment. Consent for photography should also be obtained.

The Forensic Physical Examination

The forensic examination is performed to gain facts for the investigation, specifically evidentiary information. A general assessment should be conducted, noting the physical and emotional state of the victim, as well as hygiene and appropriateness of the clothing. For nonfamilial abuse cases (e.g., sexual assault cases), the examiner should focus on the areas appropriate to the interviewing information about the incident. For elder abuse cases, a complete physical examination should be conducted, including nutritional assessment measurements. (More specific information on different aspects of elder abuse can be found in their appropriate chapters.) One of the critical aspects of the forensic physical examination is the differentiation of wounds.

Types of Body Injury

Injury or tissue damage occurs when some quantity or quality of force is applied to the body. Force can be applied to tissue either by a moving object impacting the body or by the body contacting an object. Blunt force trauma is the term associated with injury created by force applied with a blunt object. Blunt force trauma is divided into four types: contusions, lacerations, abrasions, and fractures.

The amount of force applied influences the trauma. Also, identical applications of force do not result in the identical injury in every person. The quality of the tissue subjected to blunt force trauma influences the injury. Several factors may contribute to increase bruising in older adults, including: fragility of capillary walls, thinning skin with loss of the protective fatty layer, and consumption of certain medications, including anticoagulants. Any disease of the skin and or any systemic disease may alter the body's response to blunt force trauma.

Patterned Injury. A patterned injury is a representation of the shape of the object that caused the injury. It is important to recognize and document patterns. The pattern can resemble the exact shape of the object that impacted the skin. The pattern can be represented by abrasions, contusions, or lacerations, or all of these.

The different types of injuries are defined by the layer of tissue they affect. The anatomy of the skin includes three layers of tissue: the epidermis, which includes the stratum corneum (keratinized cells) and the basal cell layer; the dermis, which forms the greater part of the skin and contains blood vessels, hair follicles, cutaneous glands, and nerve fibers; and the subcutaneous or fatty layer. Deep fascia or connective tissue and muscle lie beneath the three layers of the skin. The mouth and vaginal vault are lined with mucosal tissue. These areas do not have the same protective layers as the epidermis (keratinized cells) or fatty tissue; therefore, mucosa is more vulnerable to injury. (See the figures at the end of this chapter for examples of injuries.)

Abrasions. Abrasions are superficial injuries to the skin, limited to the epidermis and superficial dermis. An abrasion is scraping and removal of the superficial layers of the skin. Small flaps of the uppermost layer of skin may remain attached to the area. These small flaps may indicate the direction in which the scraping occurred. Abrasions may also be called scratches when the injury is caused by a fingernail. Abrasions may also be called brush burns if the injury is caused by frictional force against a rough surface or by dragging along coarse carpet. Rope burns are abrasions caused by friction of rope against the skin. Abrasions can be caused by handcuffs and by tying and binding. Such abrasions are usually found on wrists and ankles. Abrasions can have patterns that reflect abrasive clothing or a textured object.

Some materials used to restrain the victim are more likely to create abrasions than others. For example, abrasive clothing is more likely to cause an abrasion than a towel or smooth articles of clothing. Bleeding does not usually occur with an abrasion. The superficial nature of the abrasion precludes bleeding. Abrasions begin to heal within several hours of injury. A fresh abrasion usually oozes fluid from the tissues for a day or two. Gradually the abrasion is covered with a crust or scab under which the healing proceeds until it is complete. The duration of healing is dependent upon factors such as the extent of the injury and repeated trauma in the same area. Infection can also alter the healing of an abrasion.

Contusions and Bruises. Bruises lie below the intact epidermis and consist of an extravascular collection of blood that has leaked from ruptured capillaries or blood vessels. A contusion or bruise is hemorrhage into the skin and the tissues under the skin or both. The bruise usually comes from a blow or a squeeze that crushes the tissue and ruptures the blood vessels. The quantity and quality of the force applied dictates the extent of the contusion. A contusion can occur in any tissue—skin, brain, or lungs. The following discussion will concern contusions of the skin. In contusions of the skin, the blood is trapped under the skin because the skin does not break.

Bruises can resemble the object that created the bruise, such as whips, shoes, boots, fists, hands, pipes, and gun handles. The forensic examiner should note any patterns within a bruise that may be indicative of the object used to create the bruise. Parallel tracklike lines of hemorrhage result from a blow with a rod or a stick or an object with a similar shape. The skin between the lines looks pale, because the force of the blow displaces the blood sideways.

Bruises do not occur immediately but may take hours or longer to develop. Several factors can influence the size, color, and appearance of a bruise: available space for blood to collect, weight of the force, vascularity of the area, fragility of the blood vessels, and the location of the bruise. Areas that do not have a hard structure such as a bone beneath may result in less trauma.

The color of a bruise changes over time. Fresh injury ranges in color from light bluish red to purple. In time the bruise changes to green and yellow and brown. This change proceeds from the periphery of the bruise toward the center. Light red usually becomes noticeable within a few hours. The change to purple occurs over time. The color of a bruise is affected by time, size and extent of the bruise, its depth, and the victim's circulatory efficiency and local circulation. No solid studies to date provide an accurate analysis related to age and color of bruising. Research has identified other factors influencing the color of bruising, such as impaired blood clotting, immunosuppression, certain diseases, diabetes, alcoholism, malnutrition, and age. Even the temperature of the environment has been noted to influence the appearance of a bruise.

Bruising occurs when blunt force trauma is applied to an area of the body. However, a contusion or bruise does not necessarily indicate the exact point of force. Blood can shift under the skin due to gravity. For example, if the victim is in a recumbent position, the blood can gravitate to the posterior. Petechiae are tiny red or purple spots on skin or other tissue. Petechiae less than 3 millimeters in diameter are pinpoint-sized hemorrhages of small capillaries in the skin or mucous membranes. In all situations, petechiae, ecchymosis, and bruises do not blanch when pressed.

Superficial face and scalp wounds generally bleed more profusely than similar injuries elsewhere. Also, people often get superficial hemorrhages in the skin following minor injury, due to age-linked fragility of the small blood vessels. Kicking can create minimal bruising on the skin, but deep organ damage may be under the bruises. Nurses must carefully appraise bruising in the abdomen, back, and chest related to kicking.

Erythema. Erythema, or redness of the skin, should not be mistaken for bleeding under the skin. Erythema blanches with gentle pressure. Erythema is usually diffuse and does not have a pattern. The cause of redness can be a forceful slap or pressure to the skin. With sudden pressure, the blood is momentarily forced out of the capillaries in the area of contact. When the pressure is withdrawn, the blood returns to the capillaries, which may then dilate. The result is redness or flushing of the skin.

Lacerations. A laceration occurs when the continuity of the skin is broken or disrupted by blunt force. It is a tear created by blunt trauma. Tissue opens due to force applied. The amount of force and its direction create the appearance of the laceration. The impact creates crushing and tearing of tissue. Lacerations can occur in any tissue, but the following discussion is confined to the skin. Between the sides of a laceration run multiple threads of tissue called tissues bridges. Theses bridges are tissue that remains connected after the blow. The bridges are made up of fiber and blood vessels. The wound edges of a laceration are usually abraded. The abraded area may resemble what made contact with the impacting surface. Lacerations are not cut injuries; rather, they are breaks in tissue from blunt force trauma applied to tissue with enough force to overcome the strength of the tissue. Lacerations sustained by falling are generally located on protuberant parts such as knees and cheekbones and jaws. Thus, in a fall, the eyes are typically spared and the rims of the eye socket are commonly abraded or torn.

A blow with a blunt object can produce a tear with finely abraded edges. Lacerations can indicate the point of force on the skin. Therefore, it is important to carefully examine and document all lacerations. Trace evidence from the crime scene such as dirt and fibers may be found in lacerations.

Cut Wounds. A cut wound occurs whenever a sharp object is drawn over the skin with sufficient pressure to produce an injury. The wound edges can be straight or jagged depending upon the shape of the cutting instrument. The edges of a cut wound are not abraded, and tissue bridging is not present in the wound. Cut wounds of the upper extremities, especially on the forearm and hands, are referred to as defensive wounds. These occur when the victim raises his or her arms in an effort to protect the face and chest. Defensive wounds can also be found on the legs of a victim if she or he was on the ground during the assault and was using the legs for defense.

If the examiner notes interruptions in cutting patterns, movement of the victim usually causes these. Fingernails can create breaks or cuts in the skin. Fingernails marks are usually superficial, semicircular, and irregularly shaped. These breaks in tissue are superficial. However, gouges corresponding to fingernails can be noted. Bruising may accompany fingernail cuts.

Stabbing. A stab wound results from penetration by an instrument into the body. A stab wound is deeper than it is long. The thrust of a weapon such as a knife produces the injury; however, any object that can be thrust into the body can create a stabbing injury. The edges of a stab wound are sharp, and the wound is deeper than the length on the skin. The edges of the wound may be abraded from the hilt of a knife. The amount of blood at the crime scene may be minimal because most of the bleeding is internal.

Bite Marks. Human bites seldom cause tears in the skin. Most often biting injuries result in semicircular or crescentic patterned abrasions. Bite marks create underlying hemorrhages. In cases of sexual assault, biting is generally located on breasts and on or near genitalia. Health care providers should note that the skin could become twisted or distorted during the act of biting, thus distorting the pattern. Expert dental consultation is advised in cases in which the victim experiences biting.

Strangulation. The hallmarks of manual strangulation are fingertip bruising and fingernail marks on the neck. In some cases there is extensive external injury and in other cases the external injury is minimal. Fingertip bruising is circular and oval, produced by pressure from the fingertips on the skin of the neck. Underlying muscles are usually bruised. Fingernail marks are thin linear or crescentic marks.

Strangulation by ligature creates a ligature mark resembling the ligature itself. Pinpoint and larger areas of hemorrhage are often noted on the face of the strangled victim. These areas of hemorrhage are often noted in the conjunctiva and on the eyelids. The offender may employ the use of a chokehold. In this form of restraint a forearm is placed across the front of the neck while the other hand pulls the forearm back. The chokehold causes airway compression. Chokeholds can cause serious damage and death. Petechial hemorrhage can be found in the eyes and face after application of the chokehold. Injury to the skin is usually absent.

Blockage of the nose and mouth can create asphyxia. This can occur by gagging the victim, holding a pillow over the victim's mouth and nose, or placing a hand over the mouth and nose.

Gunshot Wounds. Firearms are classified as either small arms or artillery, depending on the size of the projectile that they fire. Handguns, the most common firearm in gunshot injuries, are usually low-energy weapons with muzzle velocities less than 1,400 feet per second. There are three basic types of handgun: single-shot pistols, revolvers, or semiautomatics. Rifles are named for their rifle barrel and are grouped as single-barrel sporting, double-barrel sporting, or high-powered military assault-type rifles. Common types include the single-shot automatic and the lever, bolt, and pump action. Shotguns look like rifles; however, they lack rifling inside the barrel. Shotguns fire a missile that consists of a fuse of hundreds of pellets with muzzle velocities of 1,000 to 1,500 feet per second. Even though they are technically considered low-velocity weapons, they are definitely the most destructive of all small arms at close range. Common types include the single-shot, double-barrel, and also the automatic and pump action.

Range of fire is essentially the distance from the barrel or muzzle of the firearm to the target. In contact or near-contact range, the firearm is very close to or touching the victim's skin or clothing. Wound features would be the bullet hole, tearing of soft tissue from gases that escape behind the bullet under pressure, and powder or soot. They may also exhibit the barrel of the weapon in skin-contact injuries. Short or close-range shots are a few inches away from the victim. The wound would exhibit the bullet hole, powder grains or powder markings (fouling), and powder soot. Medium-range shots come from within a few feet of the victim. The wound contains the bullet hole and stippling or tattooing made by gunpowder residue. In distant or long-range shots, which are fired from more than a few feet away from the victim, only the bullet reaches the target. The type of weapon and ammunition also play a role in the wound appearance. When documenting the appearance of gunshot wounds, do not attempt to differentiate entrance and exit wounds.

DOCUMENTATION

Documentation consists of the narrative report, diagrams, and photographs.

The Narrative Report

The narrative report begins with a carefully documented history. Remember to use the subject's own words as often as possible and to document these with quotation marks. Accurately describe each injury and be sure to use the proper medical terminology. Measure all wounds in centimeters and describe wound size, shape, appearance, and location using readily recognized anatomic landmarks.

Diagrams

Each injury should be placed on a trauma diagram. Each injury should be drawn on the diagram and described in writing next to the drawing. Multiple front and back blank drawings are required for documentation. Utilize age-appropriate diagrams whenever possible. (See Appendix A for adult body diagrams.)

Photographs

It is difficult to document injury related to assault in words alone. Photography is required. Injuries to the body, including the genitalia, are photographed with a digital camera. Photo documentation is an important function; however, health care providers need not be professional photographers.

The purposes of forensic photography are to record injury, and to provide photographic evidence. Trauma to the body is of importance to legal proceedings, making it critical that evidence of injury be documented via photography. Injury to the body should be documented in color photographs.

If the victim is suffering from injury that will heal in time, injuries must be accurately preserved photographically. It takes months or years until any evidence is presented in a court of law, and injuries may be minimal or completely healed by that time. Photographs are all that will remain of the victim's injuries.

Digital photography is advantageous in forensic work. Images are recorded on a removable disk or memory card or memory stick. There is no film to be processed. Chain of custody can be simplified. Images can be transmitted instantly. The camera and computers process the pictures. Federal Rules of Evidence allow the admission of digital photography.

Authenticity of color in digital photographs can be assured with the use of a gray scale. Digital photographs should include a gray scale to ensure color accuracy. Scales that include reassurance of 90-degree angle are also recommended.

Consent for Photography

Consent for photography must be obtained by the client or guardian. In urgent cases where a signature is unobtainable, consent is implied. "Client consents to treatment and documentation of injury with photographs" is a typical statement found on a consent form given to sexual assault victims.

Taking Photographs

There are two kinds of light important to photography: ambient and artificial. Indoor artificial light must be added to the natural or ambient light in the room in order to get clear photographs of injury. Fluorescent light commonly found in hospitals tends to give photos a washed out or yellow or green hue. This can be eliminated by adding more artificial nonfluorescent light and by using a flash.

A full-body photograph should be taken first, ensuring that the face is included. This full-body photo will identify the victim and demonstrate the presence or absence of any overall injury. The overall photo often may also serve as photo documentation of "demeanor of the victim." Modesty must be considered in taking this first photo. Providing the victim with something to cover may be necessary.

After the overall photo, a far-away, midrange, and close-up photo of each injury should be taken. For example, injury on the back should be documented with first an overall photo of the entire back of the victim. Then a midrange picture is taken of the injury in a context of other body parts such as buttock or shoulder or waist. A close-up photograph is then taken of each injury. One close-up photo of each injury is taken with a scale and one is taken without the scale.

Recommended background for forensic photos of a person is non-cluttered and of a soothing color. The color white tends to be stark and does not demonstrate injury well. The colors back and red are also not good background colors for photographing injury. The colors light blue and light green make excellent backgrounds for photographing injury.

Flat surfaces as opposed to shiny surfaces make better backgrounds for photographing injury. Shiny surfaces reflect back light. A blue pad with the shiny side down and the dull side under the victim makes a good background for photographing injury.

Health care providers should be aware of the clutter in the workspace when taking photographs of injury. Covering or removing clutter will enhance photographs by placing emphasis on the injury and not on the clutter.

A 90-degree angle is recommended for photographing injury. Using a 90-degree angle eliminates distortion of size of the injury. Angling a photograph off 90 degrees can distort size. The scale placed in the photographs of injury should include a gray scale to ensure accurate color and symbols to ensure 90-degree angle.

Photo Log

The set of photographs represents a record of the event experienced by the victim. The full-body photo is the introduction to the photo log. This photo is listed as the number one photograph. Each photo of every injury is then listed, including all midrange and close-up photos.

Chain of Custody

Chain of custody or chain of evidence must be followed for photographs, as it is followed for all evidence. Photographs should be turned over to law enforcement, along with all other evidence collected. If photographs are saved to a computer, they must be encrypted so that only the medical team has access to the photographs. Law enforcement must sign the chain of custody forms, including the photo log.

Photography Review

Take photographs before and after cleaning up the victim. This is most important in cases with bleeding, blood spatter, gunshot residue, and excessive dirt. Take a full-length photo of the person that captures the person's face and overall injuries. Respect the client's privacy and allow her or him to cover up for this photograph. Take a far-away, midrange, and close-up photograph of each injury. Close-up photos should be taken with and without a scale. Label each photograph with date and time, medical record number or case number, name of the hospital, and the photographer's name.

Follow-Up Photographs

Follow-up photographs of injury may be required to document the progress of an injury. Photographs of healing may be desired. Injury that may heal without scarring may be photographed over time. Sexual assault examinations may be performed within hours of the event. At times, injury is not identified at early intervals because it is not yet evident. For example, fingertip bruising of the neck may not be evident in the first few hours after an assault. Dependent upon the amount of pressure applied to the neck, the bleeding from the ruptured vessels may be slow and take time to be obvious.

RESOURCES

American College of Forensic Examiners: http://www.acfei.com/programs.php
American Forensic Nursing (AFN): http://www.amrn.com
The Differences Between Forensic Interviews & Clinical Interviews: http://www.icctc. org/Resources/forensic.pdf
Duma, S., & Ogunbanjo, G. A. (2004). Forensic documentation of intimate partner violence in primary health care. *South African Family Practice, 46*(4), 37–39. http:// www.safpj.co.za/index.php/safpj/article/viewFile/64/64
Patterns of Tissue Injury: http://library.med.utah.edu/WebPath/TUTORIAL/GUNS/GUNINJ.html

REFERENCES

Evans, M. (2004). *Gunshot wound ballistics.* Baylor College of Medicine. Retrieved from http://www.bcm.edu/oto/grand/02_12_04.htm
Hazelwood, R., & Burgess, A. (2001). *Practical aspects of rape investigation.* New York: Elsevier.
McCans, J. (2009). Forensic evidence: Preserving the clinical picture. *RN, 69,* 28–44.
Olshaker J., Jackson, M., & Smock W. (2001). *Forensic emergency medicine.* Philadelphia: Lippincott Williams & Wilkins.

Porteous, J. (2005). Don't tip the scales! Care for clients involved in police investigation. *Canadian Operating Room Nursing Journal, 23*(3), 12–144.

Ribaux, O., Walsh, S., & Margot P. (2006). The contribution of forensic science for crime scene analysis and investigation. *Forensic Science International, 156*(2–3), 171–181.

Saferstein, R. (2008). *Criminalistics: An introduction to forensic science* (9th ed.). Englewood Cliffs, NJ: Prentice Hall.

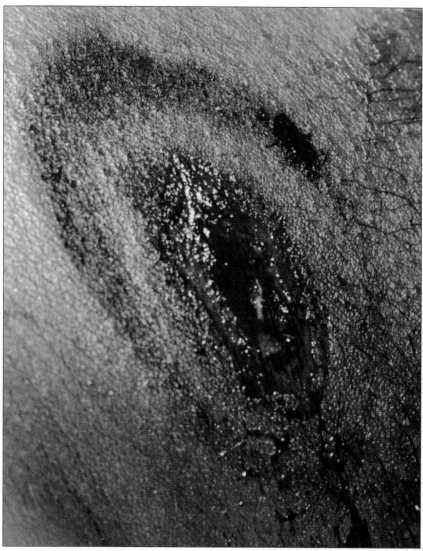

Figure 3.1 Gunshot wound. Notice the pattern of discoloration around the wound, probably from the gun muzzle.

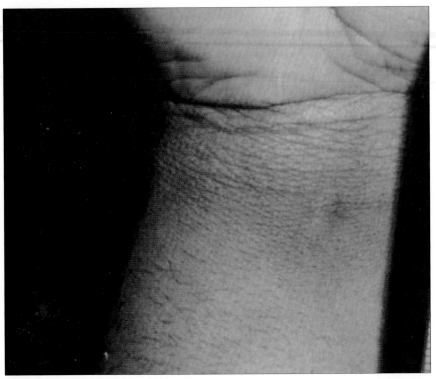

Figure 3.2 Bruising of the wrist. This bruising pattern is commonly seen as a result of forceful restraint.

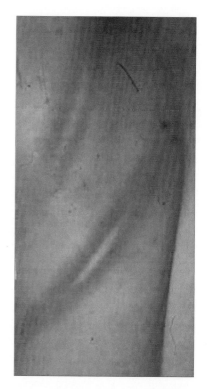

Figure 3.3 Patterned injury. Note the area of central clearing on the inside of the pattern.

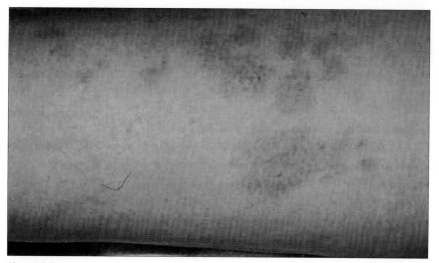

Figure 3.4 Bruising. Multiple bruises related to blunt force trauma that created bleeding under the skin.

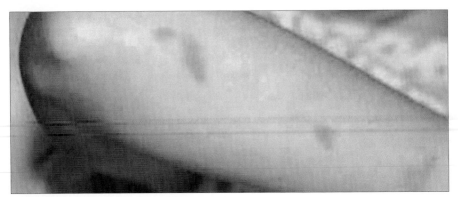

Figure 3.5 Bruising. A common area for bruising is the forearm. This type of injury is called a defensive injury.

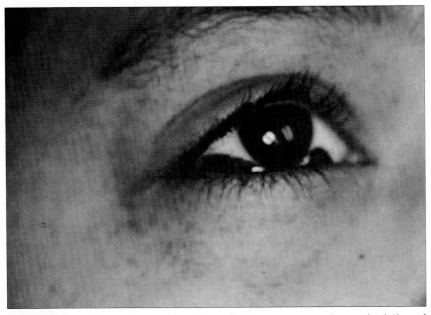

Figure 3.6 Petechiae and hemorrhage. These findings are commonly seen in victims of strangulation.

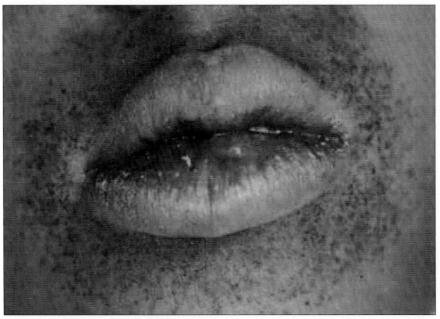

Figure 3.7 Abrasion. Note the removal of the most superficial tissue on the lips. Note the lack of bleeding.

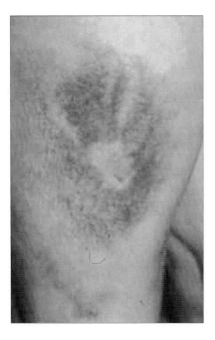

Figure 3.8 Patterned injury. Note that the area of central clearing in this photo resembles an open hand.

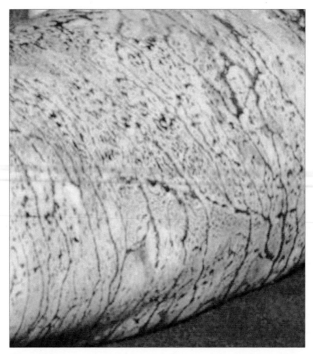

Figure 3.9 Blood spatter. Spatter, as seen in this photo, can and does occur on the body of the victim or the offender.

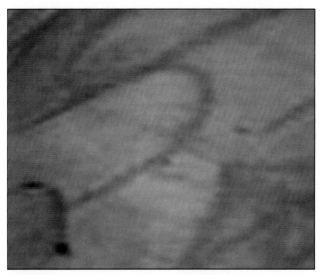

Figure 3.10 Pattern of injury. Note that the pattern of injury in this photo resembles the weapon used.

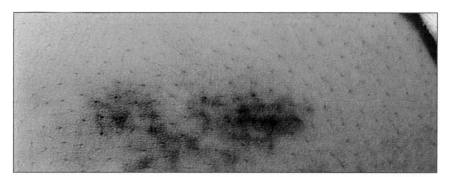

Figure 3.11 Bruising. This pattern of bruising is commonly seen as a result of a bite.

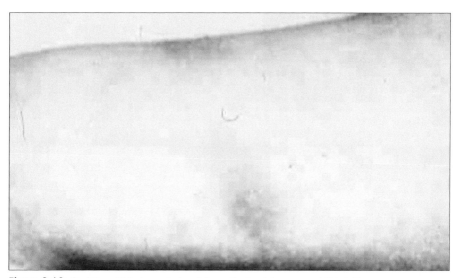

Figure 3.12 Bruising. This is a photo of fingertip bruising on a child victim.

4 Principles of Evidence

DEFINITION

Forensic evidence is physical or trace evidence that is scientifically matched with a known individual or item. Crime laboratories analyze specimens retrieved from a suspect or a crime scene and compare the specimens with control specimens retrieved from the suspect in order to determine whether or not they have a common origin.

Individual evidence is defined as evidence that can be associated with a common source with an extremely high degree of probability. This evidence is analyzed at a crime laboratory and used by law enforcement to identify a suspect. Individual scientific evidence includes: fingerprints, DNA, tool marks, tire marks, and footprints.

Class evidence is evidence that is associated only with a group and never with a single course. This evidence is analyzed at a crime laboratory and used by law enforcement to associate a suspect with a crime or crimes. Class scientific evidence includes: paint, blood, hairs, and fibers.

Crime laboratories also determine the identity of a physical or chemical substance with as near absolutely certainty as analytic techniques permit.

Types of Evidence

Circumstantial: Facts of circumstances that tend to implicate a person in a crime. Forensic science results do not enter into circumstantial evidence. Examples of circumstantial evidence are: a person owns a vehicle similar to one used in crime; the suspect has made threats to the victim; the suspect has been known to engage in similar behavior. Circumstantial evidence has been described as: the person has motive, means, and opportunity to commit crime.

Eyewitness testimony: Interviewing a witness to a crime is eyewitness testimony. In recent history, the credibility of eyewitness evidence is questioned. Criticism is particularly focused on the ability to identify a suspect via an eyewitness encounter. Witnesses have been known to make false identifications. False identification may be related to an eyewitness telling an untruth in a purposeful manner, but in most cases misidentification occurs via an eyewitness without specific intent. The psychological trauma of witnessing appears to be related to misidentification. In other words, the eyewitness, due to the trauma of witnessing, is not able to accurately identify the suspect.

Direct evidence: Evidence found in the suspect's possession that was taken from the victim or taken from the crime scene is called direct evidence. This type of evidence is commonly called "fruits of the crime." This evidence may be items stolen from the victim(s) that have monetary value. This evidence may also be a token or trophy taken from the victim by the suspect that has little monetary value. This trophy or token has value only to the suspect and serves as a reminder of the criminal activity. Direct evidence indicates a direct connection between the suspect and the victim or the suspect and the crime scene.

Collateral evidence: Evidence obtained about the suspect via investigation is collateral evidence. Forensic science is not a component of collateral evidence. Collateral evidence is commonly called "intelligence." A portion of any investigation is interviews of people who know the suspect. Any information obtained about the suspect is collateral. Interviews are collateral information, but information found on computers and in books and journals is also collateral information. Finding information about the planning of crimes is considered collateral evidence.

PRINCIPLES OF EVIDENCE

Health care providers collect what the crime lab calls trace evidence. Trace evidence means a small amount. Health care providers collect trace evidence from a person's body. Law enforcement collects from the crime scene and from the suspect's residence. Law enforcement collects trace evidence and also collects large pieces of evidence such as computers, furniture, and automobiles. All forensic evidence is submitted to the crime laboratory via law enforcement.

The most important health care forensic skill associated with collection of evidence is observation—health care professionals need to be able to recognize potential evidence. Evidence can be anything on a client, but the most common types of evidence are clothing, bullets, bloodstains, hairs, fibers, and small pieces of material such as fragments of metal, glass, paint, and wood.

When evidence is identified it should be collected and preserved. All evidence should be submitted to the crime laboratory reasonably dry. Trace evidence collected on swabs dries quickly. Specimens that are wet by nature, such as urine for a toxicological screening, must be handed to law enforcement identifying verbally and in writing that the specimen is wet. Any trace evidence collected by health care professionals must be clearly identified. On each specimen a label must be attached that gives the name of the patient, the date and time, and who collected the specimen. The specimen should be labeled indirectly, meaning not written on the evidence itself. Rather, the evidence should be put in an envelope or a container and a label added to the envelope. Noting on the label the body part from which the evidence was retrieved is necessary.

Chain of Custody

Each item that may be evidentiary in nature must be held in the presence of the person who collected the evidence until that evidence is given to law enforcement. If law enforcement is not present when evidence is collected, evidence must be held in a locked location until law enforcement arrives to retrieve the evidence.

The chain begins with the person who collects the evidence, who may be the health care provider. The links in the chain are individuals having control or custody over evidentiary or potentially evidentiary material or personal property. This chain of custody should be defined in forensic protocol and generally requires a form of written documentation. Generally, the rules of establishing the chain of custody include the following:

- Rules of evidence require a chain of custody for each item recovered from the patient, including trace and physical evidence, laboratory specimens of blood/body fluids, clothing, and personal articles.

- The integrity of every piece of evidence seized must be ensured to protect the admissibility in a court of law.
- Failure to maintain the chain of custody renders potentially important evidence worthless if lost, damaged, or unaccountable from the hands of the nurse to the police officer.
- The examiner should remain in control of the collected evidence at all times. Nothing can be left unattended. All evidence must be remain in plain view of the collector.
- Evidence that is to be used in court must be appropriately packaged and given to law enforcement to maintain a continuity or chain of custody. In an ideal situation, the examiner maintains custody of all evidence until it is collected by law enforcement. All personnel who handle or examine evidence must be acknowledged via signature on the chain of custody form to establish its integrity for presentation in a court of law.
- If evidence cannot be maintained in the sight of the examiner, it must be locked in a secure area at room temperature away from anyone not in the chain of custody.

Locard's Exchange Principle

Locard's principle essentially states that whenever two objects come into contact, a mutual exchange of matter takes place. This principle is used to link the suspect to the victim, the suspect to the crime scene, and the victim to the crime scene through forensic evidence. Most forensic scientists accept Locard's Exchange Principle, which was enunciated early in the twentieth century by Edmund Locard, the director of the first crime laboratory, in Lyon, France. Every contact leaves a trace.

EVIDENCE COLLECTION

Forensic evidence collection is a methodical process that follows state and federal requirements. Evidence collection kits usually contain instructions for use, but evidence collection procedures should be written and readily available in health care settings for reference when needed. Health care providers must wear gloves during handling of all physical evidence, and they should change gloves often during evidence collection. All packages used to collect evidence must be sealed and labeled with the client's name, the date and time of collection, the description and source of the material (including anatomic location), the name of the health care provider, and the names and initials of everyone who handled the material.

Clothing

Health care professionals should be taught to recognize and preserve vital fragments of trace evidence by careful handling of the patient's clothing and personal property. Clothing worn at the time of the incident may contain trace evidence useful in linking the victim with the assailant or crime scene. Locard's general procedure for examining clothing includes the following:

- Check clothing for defects. Defects in clothes can be compared to wounds of the victim, and often clothes provide insight as to the type of weapon or wounding instrument used.
- Check clothing for blood, semen, gunshot residue, or trace materials such as hair or fibers: document, diagram, photograph, collect, and preserve. The clothing may contain fragments from the assailant. If the assailant was injured, his or her blood may be on the victim's clothing.
- Treat clothing from accidents the same as you would from possible crime. Garments from automobile/pedestrian accidents may display tire impressions or conceal trace evidence such as paint chips or broken glass that could identify the vehicle that struck the victim.
- Check for laundry marks (which are not very common these days). Laundry markings may offer a clue to identification or origin of an unknown, unconscious, near-death, or deceased individual.
- Give special attention to the examination and security of clothing from a gunshot victim. Gunshot residues surrounding bullet holes in the clothes may determine the distance of the firearm from the victim at the time of firing (range of fire).
- Carefully remove clothing to protect any foreign fragments adhering to them. Do not shake clothes.
- Clothing is frequently cut away for emergency treatment, sometimes loosing the article itself and/or evidentiary materials. When this happens, try to avoid cutting through tears, rips, and holes that may have resulted from the weapon or the assault.

- Do not discard clothing or throw it on the floor, which can result in cross-contamination of trace evidence with debris from the treatment environment.
- A clean, white sheet can be placed on an empty trauma table, mayo stand, or on the floor in the corner of the room for clothing to be placed until time permits for effective packaging.
- If possible, allow the victim to remove his or her clothes, while standing on a clean sheet or a large sheet of paper. This will collect any microscopic evidence that may become dislodged during removal. The sheet must be placed in a separate paper bag for transfer to the crime laboratory.
- If possible, hang up moist clothing to dry in a secure area. Tell police if clothing they are to retrieve is in a damp condition.
- Clean white paper should be placed over stains to avoid cross-contamination.
- Each item of clothing should be stored in separate paper, not plastic, bags.

  - Plastic bags are inappropriate because there is a tendency for condensation to accumulate, resulting in a degradation of the integrity of the evidence.
  - Each bag should be sealed and clearly marked with the date, time, and signature or initials of the individual doing the sealing. Fortunately, a hospital is an excellent place to find all manner of containers (bags, bottles, boxes, and tubes) for properly storing evidence.

- Document, document, document!

Hair, Fiber, Debris, and Solid Objects

Carefully comb the victim's hair to remove evidence that may not be visible. Use forceps with plastic-coated tips to carefully remove hairs, fibers, or other debris from the client's body and place each collected item into a paper envelope. Dry surface debris can be gently scraped onto a glass slide. Place sharp objects (needles, blades, knives, glass fragments) in double peel-packs (heavy-gauge polyethylene pouches with tamper-evident adhesive closures) or in plastic, glass, or cardboard containers.

Preserve evidence on the victim's hands until collected by securing paper bags over each hand (this should also be performed on deceased victims). Scrape or swab beneath fingernails, or clip off fingernails, and

Exhibit 4.1

PROCEDURE FOR CREATING A "DRUGGIST-STYLE" ENVELOPE

1. Place evidence in the center of clean, white paper.
2. Fold paper in thirds.
3. Turn folded paper 90 degrees and fold in thirds again.
4. Tuck one edge into the other to form a closed package.

package and label as right or left hand. If envelopes are unavailable, place fingernails, scrapings, and the orange stick or swab used to collect them in the center of a clean piece of paper, which is then folded "druggist style" and sealed (see Exhibit 4.1).

Wrap bullets in gauze to preserve trace evidence and place in a peel-pack, cup, or envelope. Do not touch bullets with metal instruments, and do not write on them. Gunpowder residue can be removed with tape that is then applied to a glass slide.

Body Fluids

Use a high-intensity lamp to visualize stains or biological secretions including saliva, semen, urine, and blood that have been determined of significance through the history. Collect dried secretions or fluids with a slightly moistened sterile swab, and air dry the specimen before packaging. Swab bite marks (after photographing) for biological specimens. In sexual assault cases, swab body orifices for biological specimens, and collect as much as possible. Biological samples should be collected before contamination by drinking, eating, smoking, or voiding. Collect laboratory specimens for toxicology screens and control, or reference, samples to be used in DNA analysis.

RESOURCES

DNA: What Every Law Enforcement Officer Should Know: http://www.ncjrs.gov/pdf files1/jr000249c.pdf

Evidence Collection and Care of the Sexual Assault Survivor: The SANE-SART Response: http://www.mincava.umn.edu/documents/commissioned/2forensicevidence/ 2forensicevidence.pdf

Hairs, Fibers, Crime, and Evidence: http://www.fbi.gov/hq/lab/fsc/backissu/july2000/ deedric4.htm

REFERENCES

McCans, J. (2006). Forensic evidence: Preserving the clinical picture. *RN, 69*(9), 28–44.

Olshaker, J., Jackson, M., & Smock. W. (2001). *Forensic emergency medicine.* Philadelphia: Lippincott Williams & Wilkins.

Porteous, J. (2005). Don't tip the scales! Care for patients involved in police investigation. *Canadian Operating Room Nursing Journal, 23*(3), 12–14.

Ribaux, O., Walsh, S., & Margot, P. (2006). The contribution of forensic science for crime scene analysis and investigation. *Forensic Science International, 156*(2–3), 171–181.

Saferstein, R. (2008). *Criminalistics: An introduction to forensic science* (9th ed.). Englewood Cliffs, NJ: Prentice Hall.

Stokowski, L. (2008, March 6). Forensic nursing. Part 1. Evidence collection for nurses. *Medscape Nurses: Nursing Perspectives.* Retrieved from http://cme.medscape.com/viewarticle/571057

Navigating the Criminal Justice System

Navigating the criminal justice (CJ) system is a very different process for offenders than it is for victims. For offenders, the process begins when the person, still called a suspect or person of interest (a term that can apply to anyone related to the case that the police wish to interview) is arrested. For the victim, the process begins when that person reports the crime to law enforcement. This chapter discusses both pathways, beginning with the offender.

THE OFFENDER PATH IN THE CRIMINAL JUSTICE SYSTEM

The CJ system contains safeguards to protect the civil rights of people caught up in an inquiry. Law enforcement officers should ensure that their preparation of a case is fair and unbiased. They need to comply with certain rules to avoid giving a prime suspect legal grounds to escape conviction, and they also should assure that any evidence in favor of the accused is presented to the lawyers so the defense can use it. To make an arrest, law enforcement officers need probable cause, a sufficient reason based on facts and observations that the suspect committed the crime.

Probable Cause

The Fourth Amendment to the Constitution of the United States reads:

> The right of the people to be secure in their persons, houses, papers, and effects, against unreasonable searches and seizures, shall not be violated, and no warrants shall issue, but upon probable cause, supported by oath or affirmation, and particularly describing the place to be searched, and the persons or things to be seized.

Probable cause is the largest foundation and requirement for arrest. Probable cause for arrest exists where facts and circumstances within law enforcement officers' knowledge and of which law enforcement has reasonably trustworthy information are sufficient in themselves to warrant a person of reasonable caution in the belief that an offense has been or is being committed. Probable cause does not require that law enforcement possess knowledge of facts sufficient enough to establish guilt; however, it does require more than mere suspicion. Probable cause must be demonstrated before a search or arrest warrant can be issued.

Arrest and the Miranda Warning

The Fifth Amendment to the Constitution of the United States reads:

> No person shall be held to answer for a capital, or otherwise infamous crime, unless on a presentment or indictment of a grand jury, except in cases arising in the land or naval forces, or in the militia, when in actual service in time of War or public danger; nor shall any person be subject for the same offence to be twice put in jeopardy of life or limb; nor shall be compelled in any criminal case to be a witness against himself, nor be deprived of life, liberty, or property, without due process of law; nor shall private property be taken for public use, without just compensation.

The Sixth Amendment to the Constitution of the United States reads:

> In all criminal prosecutions, the accused shall enjoy the right to a speedy and public trial, by an impartial jury of the State and district wherein the crime shall have been committed, which district shall have been previously ascertained by law, and to be informed of the nature and cause of the accusation; to be confronted with the witnesses against him; to have compulsory process for obtaining witnesses in his favor, and to have the assistance of counsel for his defense.

The rights outlined in the Fifth and Sixth Amendments to the U.S. Constitution form the basis for the Miranda warning. Before a suspect can be questioned in custody, law enforcement must inform him of his rights via the Miranda Warning. There are various versions of the Miranda, but at minimum it must include the following statements:

1. You have the right to remain silent.
2. Anything you say can and will be used against you in a court of law.
3. You have the right to speak to an attorney, and to have an attorney present during any questioning.
4. If you cannot afford an attorney, one will be provided for you.

The Miranda Warning came out of the *Miranda v. Arizona* case. In 1963, Ernesto Miranda was accused of kidnapping and raping an 18-year-old, mildly retarded woman. He confessed to the crime but was not told that he did not have to speak or that he could have an attorney present. His lawyer tried to get the confession thrown out, but the motion was denied. In 1966, the case came in front of the Supreme Court, which ruled that the statements made to the police could not be used as evidence, since Miranda had not been advised of his rights as outlined in the Fifth and Sixth Amendments.

Ever since this landmark decision, and before any pertinent questioning of a suspect commences, law enforcement has been required to recite the Miranda warning, also referred to as Miranda rights. It should be noted that a person does not have to be Mirandized to be arrested, since there is a difference between being arrested and being questioned. Basic questions, such as name, address, and Social Security number do not need to be covered by a Miranda warning, and law enforcement need not Mirandize someone who is not a suspect in a crime.

Postarrest

Once a suspect is in custody, he will be booked. Booking may involve searching, fingerprinting, and photographing of the suspect. In homicide cases, suspects may be required to await the filing of the initial charge document, which must take place in a reasonable period of time, before appearing before a judge or magistrate. The magistrate usually assesses the evidence to ensure that probable cause has been established. At this point bail may be granted. Bail is generally unavailable for people charged with capital crimes.

Most states require that person be indicted (formally charged by a grand jury) before the trial. Procedures in other states include a preliminary hearing. The question for the grand jury or presiding judge is whether there is sufficient probable cause to justify continuing the proceedings. The grand jury usually only hears the prosecutor's evidence. The accused does not have the right to be present, to submit evidence, or to cross-examine witnesses for the prosecution. An arraignment will then take place in the court in which the accused is to be tried. Here the accused has to answer the charge and is required to plead "guilty" or "not guilty."

A plea bargain may be negotiated between the prosecution and the defense. This is an agreement whereby the defendant pleads guilty to a lesser offense or to one of multiple charges in exchange for some concession by the prosecutor, usually a more lenient sentence or dismissal of the other charges. However, every suspect has the right to a trial if he or she wishes to have a trial.

Trial

A bench trial is held before a judge without a jury; the judge decides questions of fact as well as questions of law. A jury trial is one where the factual issues are decided by a jury, not a judge.

Persons involved in the trial are:

- Prosecutors: In most states, local district attorneys are elected officials who have a team of prosecuting attorneys (depending on the size of the jurisdiction). The prosecution is responsible for representing the state in presenting the case against an individual suspected of breaking the law.

- Defense attorneys: The defense represents the accused. The Supreme Court ruled that felony defendants have the right to competent counsel in 1970 in *McMann v. Richardson.* Judges can overturn convictions because of public defender incompetence.

- Judges: Judges are either elected or appointed. The judge, who is impartial, hears both sides of the case and makes a ruling—sometimes with a jury.

- Court clerks: Clerks handle a variety of duties, including preparing daily calendars, calling cases before the judge, and controlling the evidence.

- Bailiffs: Bailiffs perform a variety of duties, including maintaining order in the court.

- Court reporters: Also called court stenographers, these professionals record everything said in court. Some courts have replaced them with voice-activated video and computers.

- Witnesses: Fact witnesses testify to something relevant they saw or experienced (in the case of the victim) and are unpaid. Expert witnesses provide information on a special topic of interest. They are usually paid professionals with degrees, experience, and publication background. Both sides can bring in either type of witness.

- Jurors: Jurors are citizens selected to render a verdict on the case.

- Victim: Victims can present potent evidence; however, the defense may cross-examine and test the victim's truthfulness.

The standard of proof in a criminal trial is *beyond a reasonable doubt*. Most states require that a criminal verdict be unanimous. A hung jury results when the jury is unable to agree on its verdict. If this happens, the defendant may be retried by another jury.

After the suspect is found guilty, the judge must decide on a sentence using established sentencing guidelines. If the defendant is found guilty, he or she may seek a new trial on the basis that the conduct of the trial was prejudicial.

THE VICTIM PATH IN THE CRIMINAL JUSTICE SYSTEM

Victims are not the focus of this criminal justice system—it is a criminal justice system, not a victim justice system. Victims have very little input into the suspect's navigation through the criminal justice system. The case at hand is not the victim versus the offender. Rather it is the commonwealth, the state, or the federal judicial system versus the individual being charged with the crime, for example, *The Commonwealth of Pennsylvania v. John Smith*. Victims of crime move through the criminal justice system as witnesses. Law enforcement requires reporting of crime before an investigation can begin. The person who reports can be someone in the neighborhood who witnessed a crime, a person in a work environment who notices a discrepancy in the books, or a mandated health care reporter; however, it is usually the victim who reports a crime.

Victims may or may not be asked to testify at the preliminary hearing or grand jury hearing. Victims are usually asked to testify at the trial. The Sixth Amendment to the Constitution of the United States guarantees offenders the right to "be confronted with the witnesses against him," meaning, the right of the victim to "face the accuser" and other witnesses. Victims make impact statements at the sentencing portion of any trial. Here victims may testify as to how the crime has impacted their lives. Families of the victim can also testify at sentencing hearings. Victim impact statements are developed by victims and families via court advocacy workers and are read in court. These statements are usually designed to influence the judge to consider a longer rather than a shorter sentence. Prosecutors' offices do inform victims when incarcerated offenders are placed on work release and when offenders are released on parole or released after the sentence is served.

RESOURCES

Constitution of the United States: http://www.archives.gov/exhibits/charters/constitution_transcript.html

Criminal Justice System Handbook: http://www.courts.state.ny.us/litigants/crimjusticesyshandbk.shtml.

Victim Impact Statements: http://www.ncvc.org/ncvc/main.aspx?dbName=DocumentViewer&DocumentID=32515

REFERENCES

Albanese, J. (2007). *Criminal justice* (4th ed.). Boston: Pearson.

Bureau of Justice Statistics. (2004). *The criminal justice system.* Retrieved from http://www.ojp.usdoj.gov/bjs/justsys.htm

6 Expert Witness Testimony

Expert witness testimony is a method of enabling attorneys, judges, and juries to better understand the evidence presented in a case. An expert can also help get things into evidence that would otherwise be inadmissible. Expert witnesses differ from fact witnesses. Fact witnesses, also called eyewitnesses or percipient witnesses, can give a firsthand account of something seen, heard, or experienced. Expert witnesses are allowed to do the one thing that all other types of witnesses cannot: offer opinions. These opinions must be reliable and not based on subjective belief or unsupported speculations.

Health care providers may be subpoenaed (a subpoena is a court order) as fact witnesses to testify in court about an event that occurred in their presence. For example, a health care provider could be called to testify about the quality of a person's parenting skills in a failure-to-thrive case. Another health care provider may be subpoenaed as an expert in that same case. This health care provider would be called to provide his or her expert opinion about the person's parenting skills based on the expert's assessment of the case and the expert's knowledge of parenting.

EXPERT WITNESS QUALIFICATIONS

An expert is someone who knows something beyond common experience. Most expert witnesses are professionals, but there are also non-degreed experts whose background and experience qualifies them. Qualifications include technical and academic training, degrees, licenses, certificates, postgraduate training, membership in professional or industry organizations, titles, belonging to specific staff, writing and speaking professionally, positions held throughout one's career, and dealing with the same or similar issues as the one at hand.

Voir dire, French for "to speak the truth," is the term used in court proceedings for the questions to determine the competence of the expert witness. As an expert, a health care provider may be asked for the following information to determine you're his or her qualifications as an expert. In the following example, a pediatric nurse is being questioned:

1. Describe your current position and background as a pediatric nurse.
2. How long have you been a nurse and in what areas have you practiced?
3. How long have you been working as a pediatric nurse? What education prepared you for this specialty? Describe your work as a pediatric nurse.
4. What continuing education have you had in this specialty?
5. What professional organizations do you belong to?
6. Are you certified in your field?
7. Have you published any material in your field?
8. How does a forensic nurse conduct an examination (step-by-step)?
9. Pediatric sexual assault nurse examiners (PSANEs) may be asked to describe sexual assault response team (SART) team members or examination equipment.
10. How many cases have you done?
11. Have you qualified as an expert witness in court before? Which courts?

Health care providers should make sure their curriculum vitaes (CVs) or résumés that are accurate, up-to-date, and error-free, as they need to present them to the court before testifying. The term CV is often used interchangeably with the term *résumé*. Sometimes these are differentiated by length (a CV is comprehensive and long; a résumé is pertinent and brief), and sometimes differentiated by style, with the CV written in outline format and the résumé written as a narrative. In any case, the CV should include the following information:

Name and contact information

Licenses and national/state certifications: (include state, license/certification number, expiration date)

Employment history: (current employer/dates of employment; previous relevant employment/dates of employment)

Education: (name of school/location of school/name of degree/date of degree)

Training and certificates: (includes conferences, workshops, training, in-services, seminars, and so on, with the name of training, dates of training, and type of certifications)

Professional organization affiliations

Research: (include current and past project titles)

Grants: (include name of grant, granting organization, and whether or not funded)

Publications: (include articles for newspapers, newsletters, professional journals, brochures, academic publications, etc.; listed should be name of article, name of publication, date of publication)

Presentations: (include in-service, community presentations, conferences, etc.; listed should be name of presentation, name of conference, date of presentation)

Awards: (service-related and community-related; include name of award, presenting agency, date of award)

Community Service: (volunteer activities)

Prior testimony as an expert witness: (name of the court, year of testimony, party for which you testified, type of case)

Do not underestimate opposing counsel, who may check into the background and representations of the CV.

RULES OF EVIDENCE

Health care providers should familiarize themselves with the Federal Rules of Evidence. The Federal Rules of Evidence govern the introduction of evidence in proceedings, both civil and criminal, in federal courts. The rules of many states have been closely modeled on these provisions. The following are the rules as they apply to expert witness testimony as of December 2008.

Rule 702. Testimony by Experts

If scientific, technical, or other specialized knowledge will assist the trier of fact to understand the evidence or to determine a fact in issue, a witness qualified as an expert by knowledge, skill, experience, training, or education, may testify thereto in the form of an opinion or otherwise, if (1) the testimony is based upon sufficient facts or data, (2) the testimony is the product of reliable principles and methods, and (3) the witness has applied the principles and methods reliably to the facts of the case.

Rule 703. Bases of Opinion Testimony by Experts

The facts or data in the particular case upon which an expert bases an opinion or inference may be those perceived by or made known to the expert at or before the hearing. If of a type reasonably relied upon by experts in the particular field in forming opinions or inferences upon the subject, the facts or data need not be admissible in evidence in order for the opinion or inference to be admitted. Facts or data that are otherwise inadmissible shall not be disclosed to the jury by the proponent of the opinion or inference unless the court determines that their probative value in assisting the jury to evaluate the expert's opinion substantially outweighs their prejudicial effect.

Rule 704. Opinion on Ultimate Issue

(a) Except as provided in subdivision (b), testimony in the form of an opinion or inference otherwise admissible is not objectionable because it embraces an ultimate issue to be decided by the trier of fact.

(b) No expert witness testifying with respect to the mental state or condition of a defendant in a criminal case may state an opinion or inference as to whether the defendant did or did not have the mental state or condition constituting an element of the crime charged or of a defense thereto. Such ultimate issues are matters for the trier of fact alone.

Rule 705. Disclosure of Facts or Data Underlying Expert Opinion

The expert may testify in terms of opinion or inference and give reasons therefore without first testifying to the underlying facts or data, unless the court requires otherwise. The expert may in any event be required to disclose the underlying facts or data on cross-examination.

Rule 706. Court Appointed Experts

(a) Appointment

The court may on its own motion or on the motion of any party enter an order to show cause why expert witnesses should not be appointed, and may request the parties to submit nominations. The court may appoint any expert witnesses agreed upon by the parties, and may appoint expert witnesses of its own selection. An expert witness shall not be appointed by the court unless the witness consents to act. A witness so appointed shall be informed of the witness' duties by the court in writing, a copy of which shall be filed with the clerk, or at a conference in which the parties shall have opportunity to participate. A witness so appointed shall advise the parties of the witness' findings, if any; the witness' deposition may be taken by any party; and the witness may be called to testify by the court or any party. The witness shall be subject to cross-examination by each party, including a party calling the witness.

(b) Compensation

Expert witnesses so appointed are entitled to reasonable compensation in whatever sum the court may allow. The compensation thus fixed is payable from funds which may be provided by law in criminal cases and civil actions and proceedings involving just compensation under the fifth amendment. In other civil actions and proceedings the compensation shall be paid by the parties in such proportion and at such time as the court directs, and thereafter charged in like manner as other costs.

(c) Disclosure of appointment

In the exercise of its discretion, the court may authorize disclosure to the jury of the fact that the court appointed the expert witness.

(d) Parties' experts of own selection

Nothing in this rule limits the parties in calling expert witnesses of their own selection.

ADMISSIBILITY OF SCIENTIFIC EVIDENCE

Admissibility is the legal concept that determines what evidence, both testimonial and physical, will be admitted by the court and what the jury will be permitted to hear. Admissibility is determined by statute, rules of evidence, and case law. This aspect of admissibility relates solely to the admissibility of the science/subject at issue and not to the qualifications of the individual. Three distinct "tests" or "standards" have evolved with respect to scientific evidence: Frye, Daubert or hybrid. States opt for Daubert, Frye, or a method of their own, and the number of states that uses either the Frye or the Daubert standard fluctuates over time.

1. Frye rule (Kelly-Frye from *United States v. Frye,* 1923): This case established, in the rules of evidence, that the results of scientific tests or procedures are admissible only when the tests or procedures have gained general acceptance in the particular field to which they belong. The Frye is also referred to as the "general acceptance" standard.
2. Daubert test (*Daubert v. Merrell Dow Pharmaceuticals,* 1993): Daubert shifted the determining factor of admissibility away from the general acceptance of the relevant scientific community to the "gatekeeper" concept. Under Daubert the presiding judge would act as the gatekeeper and determine whether or not the proposed evidence was relevant and applicable to the case, and would be helpful to the jury. Expert opinion must be based on reliable methodology or analysis and not subjective belief or unsupported speculation. The reliability of the expert testimony is as important as the relevance of the expert testimony. All evidence can be challenged, but Daubert made criteria more rigorous.
3. Hybrid states have either adopted legislation or rules of evidence that modify or alter in some way either the Frye or Daubert standards.

EXPERT WITNESS PROCESS

While there is no specific expert witness process, there are suggestions for the pretrail, trial, and posttrial periods.

Pretrial

Trial preparation should be done relatively close to the trial. If done too early, you may forget important details. Remember, as an expert witness, you are unbiased. Your role is to present scientific information and your opinion on a specific matter of the case. You are not there to "win" the case.

1. Obtain important documentations (reports, diagrams, photographs, etc.) relating to the case. What you get depends on the case.

2. Study all documents thoroughly to the point of memorization. Records may be accessed in the courtroom, but you will look more like an expert if you know all your details prior to testifying. Focus on significant information and be able to retrieve it from your memory promptly if questioned on it during testimony.

3. Take notes about the case. But remember that everything recorded, including your notes, may be discoverable (may be submitted as evidence in court). Write notes as if they may be used in court. You most likely will also be asked to prepare a report for the court. This will be admitted into evidence. You may refer to your report during the trial.

4. Never make notes on original documents. Make them on copies.

5. Prepare a series of questions for the attorney of record for your side of the case to ask you. Attorneys do not have medical knowledge, and it is very helpful for you to prepare this list. You may also need to educate the attorney—and the judge and jury—as to your health care specialty.

6. As an expert witness, you assist the attorney in making testimony demonstrable and illustrative. Therefore, prepare "show and tell"—computerized slides, charts, or whatever is needed to illustrate your important testimony.

7. Meet with the attorney before the court date. This is not a rehearsal, but it gives you time to give the attorney your questions and to review your résumé/qualifications.

8. Ascertain the identity of the opposing expert witness and what that witness will be testifying about. Whenever possible, obtain a copy of the opposing expert's report and review it before the trial. The attorney may ask you to review the report for assistance with cross-examination questions. (The opposing attorney and expert will most likely do the same with your report.)

9. If possible, observe the courtroom before the trial. This is especially helpful for your first few cases as it will help decrease your anxiety.
10. Check out all your equipment ahead of time and make sure it works. Bring back-up equipment if you have it.

Depositions

You may be asked for a deposition. A deposition is the testimony of a witness taken outside the court, where the witness is subject to both direct and cross examination. It is usually reduced to writing and taken under oath and is a prediscovery method, whereby a witness statement concerning the case is taken under oath with all parties and their attorneys present.

Trial

Voir Dire

After you are called to the witness stand and are sworn in, you begin the voir dire process. You must qualify as an expert prior to giving testimony. The attorney you are working with will present your CV or résumé and ask questions that will demonstrate your expertise. The opposing counsel may ask questions to try to disqualify you. After questioning, the judge determines if you qualify as an expert. Once qualified, testimony begins as the attorney you are working with asks you questions.

Testimony

Direct examination is what occurs as the attorney you are working with asks you questions. This is when you will present any material you have developed, including your report. The attorney may also ask you to describe evidence.

Cross-examination is when the opposing attorney questions you. This can be very stressful. Be aware of leading questions that suggest an answer, especially answers you would not otherwise give.

In redirect, the direct examiner asks questions after the cross-examiner. (This process can continue back and forth.)

Posttrial

Contact the attorney you worked with once the trial has concluded to find out the outcome. Juries are often interviewed to see how they reached

Exhibit 6.1

HELPFUL HINTS FOR COURT APPEARANCES

Dress professionally.
Relax.
Walk into the courtroom with authority.
Sit up straight and look attentive.
Do not fidget.
Speak clearly.
Make eye contact with those you are speaking to, as well as the judge and jury.
Exude confidence.

their conclusions. Find out what the strongest and weakest evidence was; what helped the case most and least; whether there were any shortcomings that failed to support the evidence; if the defendant was found guilty, what was the most compelling evidence. If the defendant was found not guilty, what motivated the jury to acquit? (See Exhibit 6.1.)

REFERENCES

American Academy of Pediatrics Committee on Medical Liability. (2002). Guidelines for expert witness testimony in malpractice litigation. *Pediatrics, 109*(5), 974–979.

DiLuigi, K. (2004). What it takes to be an expert witness. *RN, 67*(2), 65–66.

Federal Rules of Evidence. (2008, December). Retrieved from http://www.uscourts.gov/rules/EV2008.pdf

National Institutes of Justice Firearm Examiner Training Court Room Testimony. (n.d.). Retrieved from http://www.ojp.usdoj.gov/nij/training/firearms-training/module14/fir_m14_t08.htm

7 Competency, Guardianship, and Civil Commitment

DEFINITION

Competency is a legal, not clinical, concept that becomes relevant when important legal decisions need to be made regarding an individual's ability to make critical decisions. Adults are generally presumed competent; however, others, typically family members, and the state may raise an issue about a person's competence when evidence points to their inability to make decisions.

Most people are able to act or make decisions in a particular context, and most possess the cognitive resources to understand the likely consequences of those decisions. The reference to "particular context" is an important one, because an individual's competence pertains to specific acts or situations, not general ability. Therefore, one may be competent for one level of employment but not another, or be competent to live independently but not to refuse medical treatment.

Formally defined areas of competency include fiduciary competency (the ability to make financial decisions, such as the allocation of financial resources), testamentary competency (the ability to sign legal documents such as a will, and understand the implications and potential ramifications of providing the signature), and criminal competency (competency at the time of the offense, appreciation of the illegality of the offense, ability to waive Miranda Rights, competency to stand trial, ability to consult with or refuse legal counsel, and presence of mind to understand the proceedings and sentencing). Other areas in which issues of competency are raised include the acceptance or rejection of medical treatment (competence to consent to treatment), competence to live independently, and competence to maintain employment and perform the tasks satisfactorily.

Just as an individual's competence is situation-specific, it is also temporally specific. Depending on the nature of the condition responsible for the compromised functioning, the individual's competence may be reevaluated and reinstated. Situations in which the stability of the impairment can change include, but are not limited to, medical decisions, independent living, employment, and child custody.

GUARDIANSHIP

If the court determines an individual to be incompetent, a legal guardian is appointed as a surrogate decision maker. The appointed guardian is responsible for the best interests of the individual (the ward) and has the legal authority to make decisions concerning the ward. The purview of the guardian's responsibilities and decision-making authority is dependent upon the extent of the ward's impairment. A guardian who is responsible for the personal, legal, and financial well-being of the individual is a general guardian (such as the parent of an underage child). An individual with circumscribed impairment may be assigned a special guardian, who would have only limited decision-making authority.

An example of this may be a guardian responsible for the financial interests of the ward, but who has no authority over the living arrangement of the individual. A guardian who has power over only a single interest of an individual (e.g., a will) or a single action in litigation is a guardian ad litem. Ad litem guardians are often called upon in legal proceedings in which children are involved and are appointed to represent the best interests of the child. Examples include divorces, child custody hearings, abuse or neglect allegations, and juvenile delinquency.

The interests of the ward for which a guardian may be responsible are generally dichotomized as those involving the person (e.g., medical treatment, living arrangements) and those involving the property assets of the person (e.g., inheritances, settlements). A guardian responsible for the physical well-being of the ward is referred as a "guardian of the person," whereas a guardian responsible for the financial and property resources of the ward is referred to as a "conservator" or "guardian of the property."

For cases in which legal guardians were not appointed by the self or the responsible family members, the court will appoint a guardian. These individuals are often volunteers, social workers, or attorneys, depending on the area of interest. Instances in which family members may request guardianship include the parents of an adult child with a developmental disability, or the adult child of a parent with declining cognitive functioning who failed to complete a power of attorney. Power of attorney is a legal instrument executed (signed) by a person called the principal and used to delegate legal authority to another (the agent or attorney-in-fact) to make legal decisions for the principal. Three types of power of attorney exist:

- *Nondurable power of attorney* takes effect immediately and remains in effect until it is revoked by the principal, or until the principal becomes incompetent or dies. A nondurable power of attorney is usually used for a specific transaction, like the sale of a house.
- *Durable power of attorney* allows the agent to act for the principal even after the principal is not mentally competent or physically able to make decisions. It may be used immediately and is effective until it is revoked by the principal, or until the principal's death.
- *Springing power of attorney* becomes effective at a future time upon the happenings of a specific event (illness or disability of the principal) chosen by the power of attorney. The springing power of attorney frequently allows the principal's physician to determine whether the principal is competent to handle his or her financial affairs, and it remains in effect until the principal's death, or until revoked by a court.

A problem in many jurisdictions is that guardianships are plenary, that is, they do not distinguish between different types of competencies (medical, marital, financial), and they do not include time limits. A person that has recovered from a brain injury, for example, may now have the burden of proof of demonstrating restoration of competency and setting aside the guardianship. Guardians may not always be willing to relinquish their control.

CONDITIONS OF IMPAIRMENT

The nature of the clinical syndrome that produces the incompetency falls into three major classes.

1. The first category includes stable conditions such as severe mental retardation and autism. In these conditions the impairment is stable and significant, and improvement is not likely; thus the appointment of a permanent guardian is likely.
2. The second category includes slow and progressive illnesses such as schizophrenia and degenerative diseases such as Huntington's chorea, Alzheimer's disease, or HIV/AIDS. In these cases, impairment worsens, but determining incompetency may not be clear-cut.
3. The third class of conditions for which competency hearings are performed involve sudden-onset diseases or abrupt impairments. Examples of this class of conditions may include neurological disease or dysfunction (e.g., cerebral vascular accident), motor vehicle accidents involving brain injury or coma, certain forms of mental illness (e.g., bipolar disorder), and treatable infections or diseases for which cognitive impairment is sustained. This class of impairment differs from the others in that prognosis may include substantial recovery to the point where the determination of incompetence would be overturned.

COMPETENCY EVALUATION

In order to determine the competency of the individual, the court hears medical testimony and considers all pertinent information that may influence the court's decision. These factors include the debilitation condition, the nature of the impairment, and the cognitive resources and adaptive functioning of the individual. Given the restriction of rights that may result from the evaluation, the clinician should make every effort to ensure that the information obtained is accurate and thorough, so that recommendations and predictions made on the basis of that information are appropriate and serve the best interests of the individual.

Of particular importance is the nature of the debilitative condition. A psychological expert assists in the determination of incompetency by conducting an evaluation of the individual's mental function via a thorough clinical examination, review of records, interview of family members or other collaterals, and the administration of a number of psychological and neuropsychological tests.

Among the factors considered during the competency evaluation is the nature of the impairment, with particular emphasis on the likely course of the condition responsible for the impairment. Information that is typically obtained includes current cognitive functioning of the individual. If the impairment is progressive in nature, such as in the case of an AIDS or Alzheimer's patient, then the recent cognitive functioning is also relevant. Cognitive functioning is often determined through neuropsychological assessment batteries administered and interpreted by a neuropsychologist or other professional trained in the administration of such assessments.

In addition to assessments of cognitive functioning, the adaptive functioning, or ability to perform day-to-day tasks is also assessed. This level of functioning is determined through behavioral observations, corroborative materials obtained from individuals who have regular contact with the subject, and interviews with the subject. Again, the evaluation of competency must take into account the skills being questioned, such that deficits in other, irrelevant areas are not influential in the decision-making process.

Other Factors to Consider

Other factors that might be taken into account during the evaluation include the etiology of the impairment (e.g., stable vs. progressive vs. treatable condition), and subsequently, the likely prognosis of the subject. Impairments that are severe, stable, and degenerative should be interpreted differently than those that are acute, unstable, and treatable. The history of functioning of the individual should be incorporated, as well as the resources available to the subject (e.g., social supports, financial situation, treatment options). However, although historical information is often reviewed, the competency determination is based on current functioning (Abrams, 2002).

An additional factor to consider in such an evaluation is the validity of the information obtained from the subject, as well as the corroborating sources. The subject may be motivated to perform poorly or otherwise inaccurately, depending on the possible outcomes of the evaluation. If, for instance, the subject's ability to stand trial is in question, he or she may be motivated to appear more impaired so as to avoid being tried as a competent defendant. On the other hand, an individual attempting to maintain an independent living situation would be motivated to perform to the best of his or her ability. Several assessment instruments exist to measure the validity of the subject's performance, but an awareness of the various motivational factors at work is also necessary.

Restoration of Competency

For individuals with treatable conditions for which improvements in functioning are conceivable, the restoration of competency as determined by the court may be possible. In such cases the court would order a hearing, and the reasons for the request to restore competency would be heard. Should the court find the evidence of improvement to be compelling, then the need for guardianship may be dismissed or modified. The decision to restore competency is based on the degree of improvement. If the ward has fully regained his or her capacity to make decisions, then the full rights of the individual would be restored. If the improvements were circumscribed to a few areas but some deficiencies remained, then the order of incompetency would be modified, and the rights would be restored to the ward to the extent possible. Given that the ward's decision-making abilities may improve, the assessment of his or her functioning is ongoing, with regular reviews being held before the court (e.g., annually).

REFERENCES

Abrams, A. A. (2002). Assessing competency in criminal proceedings. In B. V. Dorsten (Ed.), *Forensic psychology: From classroom to courtroom* (pp 105–142). New York: Kluwer Academic/Plenum Publishers.

Franzen, M. D. (2003). Neuropsychological evaluations in the context of competency decisions. In A. M. Horton Jr. & L. C. Hartlage (Eds.), *Handbook of forensic neuropsychology* (pp 505–518). New York: Springer Publishing.

Nicholson, R. A., & Kugler, K. E. (1991). Competent and incompetent criminal defendants: A quantitative review of comparative research. *Psychological Bulletin, 109,* 355–370.

Perlin, M. (1995). *1995 cumulative supplement to* Mental disability law: Civil and criminal (Vol. 1). Charlottesville, VA: Michie.

Slovenko, R. (2006). Civil competency. In I. B. Weiner & A. K. Hess (Eds.), *The handbook of forensic psychology* (3rd ed.) (pp 151–170). Hoboken, NJ: John Wiley & Sons.

8 Violence in Health Care Settings

DEFINITION

The National Institute for Occupational Safety and Health (NIOSH) defines workplace violence as "violent acts (including physical assaults and threats of assaults) directed toward persons at work or on duty." The University of Iowa developed a workplace violence typology for researchers and policy makers. However, this categorization also allows clinicians to better understand the different types of potential victim/perpetrator relationships:

> Type I (Criminal Intent): Violence is the result of a criminal activity such as a robbery. The perpetrator commits the crime and has no relationship to the workplace. (Example: A health care worker is injured when a perpetrator breaks into the hospital pharmacy to steal medications.)

> Type II (Customer/Client): The perpetrator is a customer or client at the workplace who becomes violent while being served by the worker. (Example: A psychotic client attacks and injures a health care worker in the emergency department.)

Type III (Worker-on-Worker): The perpetrator is an employee or past employee of the workplace. (Example: A disgruntled health care worker shoots his boss after being fired.)

Type IV (Personal Relationship): The perpetrator and health care victim have a personal relationship. (Example: A health care worker is attacked by her estranged husband in the pediatric department where she works.)

Scope of Employer Responsibility

The Occupational Safety and Health Administration (OSHA) does not have specific current standards regarding workplace violence. However, federal regulations have been interpreted to include workplace violence. Section 5(a)(1), often referred to as the General Duty Clause, of the Occupational Safety and Health Act of 1970 (OSH Act), requires employers to provide employees employment and a place of employment that are free from recognized hazards that are causing or are likely to cause death or serious physical harm to the employees. Section 5(a)(2) mandates that employers comply with occupational safety and health standards promulgated under this act. OSHA relies on the General Duty Clause for enforcement authority. Failure to implement these guidelines is not in itself a violation of the General Duty Clause. However, employers can be cited for violating the General Duty Clause if there is a recognized hazard of workplace violence in their establishments, and they do nothing to prevent or abate it.

PREVALENCE

The Bureau of Labor Statistics (BLS) reports that there were 69 homicides in the health services from 1996 to 2000. Homicides in the workplace attract more attention; however, the vast majority of workplace violence consists of nonfatal assaults. BLS data show that in 2000, 48% of all nonfatal injuries from occupational assaults and violent acts occurred in health care and social services. Most of these occurred in hospitals, nursing and personal care facilities, and residential care services. Nurses, aides, orderlies, and attendants suffered the most nonfatal assaults resulting in injury.

Injury rates also reveal that health care and social service workers are at high risk of violent assault at work. In 2000, health service workers overall had an incidence rate of 9.3 for injuries resulting from assaults and violent acts. The rate for social service workers was 15, and for nursing and personal care facility workers 25.

The Department of Justice's (DOJ) National Crime Victimization Survey for 1993 to 1999 lists average annual rates of nonfatal violent crime by occupation. The average annual rate for nonfatal violent crime for all occupations is 12.6 per 1,000 workers. The average annual rate for physicians is 16.2; for nurses, 21.9; for mental health professionals, 68.2; and for mental health custodial workers, 69. BLS and DOJ data do not directly compare, because DOJ presents violent incidents per 1,000 workers and BLS displays injuries involving days away from work per 10,000 workers.

However, both sources reveal the same high risk for health care and social service workers. As significant as these numbers are, the actual number of incidents is probably much higher. Incidents of violence are likely to be underreported, perhaps due in part to the persistent perception within the health care industry that assaults are part of the job. Underreporting may reflect a lack of institutional reporting policies, employee beliefs that reporting will not benefit them, or employee fears that employers may deem assaults the result of employee negligence or poor job performance.

According to Lussier (2004), 25% of workplace violence occurs in health care settings—75% of physical assaults that occur in health care are committed by males and 25% are perpetrated by women. Hewlett and Levin (1997) noted that incidents of physical assault in health care residential facilities is ten times more likely than assaults in any other industry.

RISK FACTORS

OSHA and the Department of Justice note that health care workers face an increased risk of work-related assaults due to several factors:

- Prevalence of handguns and other weapons among patients, families, or friends
- Increasing use of hospitals by police and the criminal justice system for criminal holds and the care of acutely disturbed, violent individuals
- Increasing numbers of mentally ill clients being released from hospitals without follow-up care
- Availability of drugs or money at hospitals, clinics, and pharmacies
- Unrestricted movement of the public in clinics and hospitals and long waits in emergency or clinic areas that lead to frustration over an inability to obtain needed services promptly

- Increasing presence of gang members, substance abusers, trauma patients, and distraught family members
- Low staffing levels during times of increased activity such as mealtimes, visiting times, and client transport
- Isolated work with clients during examinations or treatment
- Solo work, often in remote locations with no backup or way to get assistance, such as communication devices or alarm systems (this is particularly true in high-crime settings)
- Lack of staff training in recognizing and managing escalating hostile and assaultive behavior
- Poorly lit parking areas

ASSESSMENT

A general assessment of the health care environment is needed to evaluate the risk for violence in the setting. Analysis of past violent episodes that have occurred in the setting should begin the evaluation. Following a review of the history of violence in the setting, the health care environment should be evaluated, including

- Workplace security system
- Presence of metal detectors
- Video camera placement
- Safe rooms available for health care staff
- A flag system (chart tags) for patients who have been violent in the past
- A system that does not require health care workers to be alone with potentially violent people
- A fair and just system that restricts visitors
- A close alignment with law enforcement

INTERVENTION

Physical violence in any health care setting should not be tolerated or viewed as "part of the job." There is a duty to protect on the part of health care institutions. These duties including the following:

- Every health care system should have a zero tolerance policy toward physical violence.

- Every health care system should have a workplace violence policy.
- Every incident of physical violence in a health care setting should be reported to law enforcement. A law enforcement investigation will follow the report and the offender, in some fashion, will be held accountable for his or her behavior.
- Adequate security teams should be in placed in every health care setting. The security system should include guards, security cameras, and metal detectors.
- Training of health care workers on methods to reduce incidents of physical violence should be in place in all health care settings. Training should focus on identification and intervention of conflict and anger in the health care setting.
- An alarm system and a safe area for retreat should be in place for employees who feel threatened.
- Staffing in all health care systems, 24 hours a day every day of the week, should be sufficient. Adequate staffing reduces the incidence of physical assault occurring to a health care worker interacting with a patient alone. Many physical assaults of health care workers occur during the night shift when staffing is low.
- Adequate lighting is essential near entrances, walkways, and parking lots.

PREVENTION/PATIENT TEACHING

Primary Prevention

Several strategies that health care employers can use to reduce workplace violence include the following measures:

- A criminal background check and references should be required of each employee. These very simple procedures can reduce the incidence of worker-on-worker assault.
- Screening procedures of all patients and visitors who enter a health care facility should be implemented. This procedure would serve to reduce the incidence of physical assault on health care workers by patients and their visitors.
- Screening for weapons is necessary in both rural and urban settings.
- Training related to prevention of violence from patients and visitors should be implemented in every health care setting, including:

emergency departments, psychiatric settings, medical settings, surgical settings, obstetric departments, and pediatric departments.

- Every clinical setting should have a policy and procedure for health care workers who are assaulted or believe that they are in danger of being assaulted.
- Every clinical setting should have a security system in place that includes security guards.
- Every clinical system should have adequate staffing during operating hours.

Secondary Prevention

Every health care setting should have in place a policy about intimate partner violence (IPV) offenders. IPV offenders should be restricted from entering health care settings where their victims are being treated. IPV offending partners of health care workers should also be restricted from entering health care settings.

Tertiary Prevention

Health care institutional policies are for both the victims of assault and the offenders of this form of violence and should be in place in all health care settings. Law enforcement should be included in policies and procedures after the assault of a health care worker.

RESOURCES

OSHA Workplace Violence: http://www.osha.gov/SLTC/workplaceviolence/
USDA Handbook on Workplace Violence: httpa://www.usda.gov/news/pubs/violence/wpv.htm
Workplace Violence: Issues in response (FBI): http://www.fbi.gov/publications/violence.pdf

REFERENCES

Bureau of Labor Statistics. (2001). *National crime victimization survey 1993–1999*. Retrieved from Bureau of Labor Statistics.

Duhart, D. (2001).*Violence in the workplace* (1993099 NCJ 190076). Washington, DC: U.S. Department of Justice.

Fitzgerald, S., Dienenam, J., & Cadorette, M. (1998). Domestic violence in the workplace. *AOHN Journal*, 46(7), 345–353.

Gaci, S., Juarez, A., Bayett, L., Homoyer, D., Robinson, L., & McLean, S. L. (2009). Violence against nurses working in U.S. emergency departments. *Journal of Nursing Administration, 39*(7/8), 340–349.

Green, K. (2000). Workplace violence in health care. *Wyoming Nurse, 12*(3), 14–15.

Hewlett, J. B., & Levin, P. F. (1997). Violence in the workplace. *Annual Review of Nursing Research, 15*, 81–99.

Lussier, R. (2004). Dealing with anger and preventing workplace violence. *Clinical Leadership and Management Review, 8*(21), 117–119.

McPhaul, K., & Lipscomb, J. (2004, September 30). Workplace violence in health care: Recognized but not regulated. *Online Journal of Issues in Nursing, 9*(3), Manuscript 6. Retrieved from http://www.nursingworld.org/MainMenuCategories/ANAMarketplace/ANAPeriodicals/OJIN/TableofContents/Volume92004/No3Sept04/ViolenceinHealthCare.aspx

Occupational Safety and Health Administration. (2004). *Guidelines for preventing workplace violence for health care and social service workers.* Retrieved from http://www.osha.gov/Publications/OSHA3148/osha3148.html

Pazzi, C. (1998). Exposure of prehospital providers to violence and abuse. *Journal of Emergency Nursing, 24*(4), 320–323.

U.S. Department of Labor. (n.d.). Occupational Safety and Health Act (OSHA 314-01R2004). Retrieved from http://www.osha.gov/pls/oshaweb/owasrch.search_form?p_doc_type=oshact

U.S. Department of Labor, Occupational Safety and Health Administration. (2007). *Workplace violence.* Retrieved from http://www.osha.gov/SLTC/workplaceviolence/index.html

9 Professional Stress and Burnout

The work environment can significantly affect one's physical, psychological, and/or spiritual health, and professional job stress can be quite apparent among those working in health care professions. Health Care Professionals deal with life-threatening injuries and illnesses, complicated by overwork, understaffing, tight schedules, paperwork, intricate or malfunctioning equipment, complex authority hierarchies, dependent and demanding clients, and client deaths, all of which contribute to stress. Those who work with victims of violent crimes and/or offenders face the additional stressors that come from working with these challenging populations. The consequences of stress can be devastating to health care professionals and can result in decreased professional effectiveness, delivery of inadequate client care, the destruction of home life, and overall burnout.

TYPES OF PROFESSIONAL STRESSORS

Working with forensic clients exposes forensic health care professionals to specific types of stressors. All face the same stressors faced by other health care workers. However, they face the additional issues of compassion fatigue and vicarious trauma. While all of these issues affect overall job satisfaction and functioning, they are inherently different. Research on work life and the work environment has demonstrated that the professional/client relationship may not play a central role in the onset of burnout. On the other hand, trauma research suggests that interpersonal relationships, particularly the concept of empathy and emotional energy, may play a key role in the development of compassion fatigue or vicarious traumatization. When working with clients who are experiencing pain, suffering, or trauma, the health care professional may experience adverse effects similar to that of their clients, frequently resulting in professionals reassessing their reality and creating a new reality based upon what they have been exposed to.

Traditional Stress

According to the National Institute of Occupational Safety and Health, job stress results from a poor match between job demands and the capabilities, resources, or needs of workers. Job stress can also result from fear of job loss and unsafe working conditions. And even the best jobs have stress from performance evaluations, deadlines, and other responsibilities.

In addition, a poor economy can mean both downsizing and increased crime, adding to workload demands. Technological advances including smart phones and netbooks have made it possible to take work everywhere, and far too many jobs are expecting just that. Many health care professionals find that the only way to stay on top of things is to arrive at work early, stay late, work through lunch and on weekends, and bring work home. This leaves little time for self, family, and pleasurable pursuits, leaving professional lives seriously out of balance.

Images of acts of terrorism and mass shootings lurk in the back of most people's minds. Such images can contribute to the fear experienced by many health care professionals who work in places where the possibility of violence is a more common event, such as emergency departments and community centers. Violence in the health care workplace is a serious safety and health issue. The media tends to over-sensationalize some rare types of violent assaults, such as mass shootings by disgruntled employees, but less dramatic risk factors can be just as dangerous. One example is domestic violence that surfaces when angry spouses act out at the workplace. Other examples include:

■ Threats: Communications of intent to cause harm, including verbal threats, threatening body language, and written threats.

- Physical assaults: These may range from slapping to rape and homicide.
- Muggings: Aggravated assaults that are usually conducted by surprise and with intent to rob.

For more information, please see chapter 8 on workplace violence.

Compassion Fatigue

One can care too much. Compassion fatigue can result from helping or wanting to help a traumatized or suffering person. It tends to happen more suddenly than burnout. This phenomenon seems to be connected to the therapeutic relationship between the health care professional and the client, whereby the experience of the client triggers multiple responses in the health care provider. Factors such as poor collaborative work environments, lack of support, and the blur between work and home caring roles, as well as societal and organizational factors, may be associated with an increased risk. This concept is not new, and most of what is known comes from the hospice literature. However, providing effective victim intervention requires tremendous emotional energy and resilience, which can be a near-constant source of stress. Compassion fatigue is connected to posttraumatic stress disorder (PTSD), because it is a very intensive psychological assault on an individual that is almost immediately overwhelming.

Compassion fatigue creates a deep physical, emotional, and spiritual exhaustion accompanied by acute emotional pain. Health care providers with burnout tend to adapt to their exhaustion by becoming less empathetic and more withdrawn, while those with compassion fatigue continue to give themselves fully to their clients, finding it difficult to maintain a healthy balance of empathy and objectivity. They often describe this state as being sucked into a vortex that pulls them slowly downward, leaving them with no idea of how to stop the downward spiral, so they work harder and continue to give to others until they are completely drained.

Vicarious Traumatization

Vicarious traumatization refers to the negative transformation in the health care provider's inner experience, resulting from empathic engagement with clients' traumatic events. Continuous exposure to graphic accounts of human cruelty, trauma, and suffering, as well as the empathetic relationship between the client and health care provider, may leave the provider open to emotional and spiritual consequences. A number of factors contribute to the onset of vicarious traumatization: individual characteristics such as previous personal trauma, lack of coping strategies, and unrealistic self-expectations; social and community context; physical, organizational, structural, and contextual work environment; and work-related attitudes such as the need to fulfill all the needs of the clients.

The effects of vicarious traumatization resemble those of PTSD, including recurring feelings of horror, fear, and helplessness. These effects can disrupt and alter the health care provider's sense of self. While few studies have investigated this phenomenon and its associated symptoms with regard to nurses, it would seem reasonable to suggest that health care workers who provide continuous care for victims of violent crimes may experience similar effects, particularly if caring work is delivered in a work environment that is incongruent with the philosophy of their health care profession. Health care providers may experience intrusive images, alterations in the ability to trust, loss of independence, decreased capacity for intimacy, and loss of control, as well as increased arousal, including anxiety, unexplained anger, and irritability. The effects are argued to be cumulative and permanent, and these may overlap both the personal and professional life of an individual.

Burnout

Burnout occurs when a person is unable to relieve the physical and mental symptoms associated with unrelenting stress. Anyone can feel burnout, although certain commonalities occur. It is a psychological experience that manifests itself in individuals as part of their working practice. Burnout is a negative experience that results from interaction between environment and individual and is thus a response to chronic occupational stress. Some providers who work with forensic mental health clients (typically mentally ill offenders) have been identified as at risk of suffering from occupational stress and possibly developing burnout syndrome. The main stressors on these professionals are identified as interprofessional conflicts, workload, and lack of involvement in decision making.

SIGNS OF STRESS

Stress overload can challenge the health care provider's ability to provide effective services and maintain personal and professional therapeutic relationships. It can also cause stress-related disorders. Stress-related disorders encompass a broad array of conditions, including psychological disorders (depression, anxiety, PTSD), emotional distress (job dissatisfaction, fatigue, tension), maladaptive behaviors (aggression, substance abuse), and cognitive impairment (concentration and memory problems). These conditions can lead to poor work performance or even injury, as well as various biological reactions that may lead ultimately to compromised health, such as cardiovascular disease. Stress is also expensive. High levels of stress are associated with substantial increases in health service utilization, longer disability periods for occupational injuries and illnesses, and major turnover in organizations.

Chronic stress leads to feelings of being "stressed out" or "burned out." Stress may not be easy to recognize because it often affects the body, leading the stressed person to believe that they are ill rather than stressed. Signs of chronic stress include:

- Headaches, backaches, chest pain, stomachaches, indigestion, nausea or diarrhea
- Rashes
- Overeating or undereating
- Sleep disturbances (too much sleep, restless sleep, difficulty falling asleep, difficulty staying asleep, waking up early)
- Fatigue
- Disillusionment
- Sexual dysfunction
- Workaholic behavior and/or continuously thinking about work
- Twitching
- Having trouble concentrating or with school work
- Breakdown of personal relationships
- Feeling anxious or worried
- Feeling inadequate, frustrated, helpless, or overwhelmed
- Feeling bored or dissatisfied
- Feeling pressured, tense, irritable, angry, or hostile
- Aggressive behavior
- Substance abuse
- Excessive or inappropriate crying
- Avoiding others
- Mood swings
- Inability to organize or make decisions
- Blocked creativity or judgment

- Poor memory/forgetfulness
- Difficulty concentrating

MANAGING STRESS

The effects of stress disorders can be devastating; however, health care professionals can actively work to avoid these pitfalls, especially compassion fatigue, vicarious victimization, and burnout. Stress should be minimized at both the individual and institutional level, even if the "institution" is a small private practice.

Individual Stress Management

Stress overload can impair overall functioning. Do not make major life decisions (job changes, divorce, relocations) while stressed, and do not make major purchases, which may cause temporary relief but long-term stress if you cannot afford them. Do not blame others for job-related problems; instead, work together to find solutions.

- Practice what you preach.
- Maintain professional boundaries, including those between work and home lives.
- Take time for yourself with time-outs and leisure activities.
- Make time for family and friends.
- Use humor—laughter is the best medicine.
- Eat right, exercise regularly, and get enough sleep.
- Discontinue or minimize your use of caffeine.
- Use time management techniques.

  - Keep a calendar.
  - Do not overcommit yourself.
  - Prioritize.

- Try meditation or relaxation exercises.
- Delegate—rely on teamwork and do not do it all.
- Stop being a perfectionist.
- Debrief—develop a professional group to discuss your caseload.

The Center for Sex Offender Management (CSOM, n.d.) suggests an ABC approach to decreasing one's risk of secondary trauma: awareness, balance, and connection (with modifications for health care professionals):

Awareness

- Be aware of your own "trauma map." Acknowledge your past and be aware that it can affect how you view and perform with victims and offenders.
- Inventory your current lifestyle choices and make necessary changes—are you eating, sleeping, and exercising adequately?
- Take care of yourself. Make a self-care list and post it prominently in your home or office. Include some of the following:

  - Be creative.
  - Get away.
  - Get outside and appreciate the weather.
  - Enjoy other environments.
  - Have fun.
  - Socialize with people who aren't criminal!

Balance

- Allow yourself to fully experience emotional reactions. Do not keep your emotions bottled up.
- Avoid working overtime and do not spend all of your free time socializing only with coworkers, discussing the negative factors of your job.
- Know your limits and accept them. Set realistic goals.
- Practice time management skills to help achieve a sense of balance in both your professional and personal lives.
- Seek out a new leisure activity unrelated to your job.
- Recognize negative coping skills and avoid them, and substitute these coping skills with more positive coping skills.

Connection

- Listen to feedback from colleagues, friends, and family members, and encourage at least one of them to conduct periodic "pulse checks."
- Avoid professional isolation and remain connected with and supported by your coworkers on the job. Just don't spend all your time with them.

- Debrief after difficult cases.
- Develop support systems with an informal peer support group, or seek out or become a mentor.
- Obtain continuing education to improve job skills and capacity. Get certified in forensics if possible.
- Nurture your spiritual side.

Institutional Stress Management

Institutions benefit greatly when they keep stress levels to a minimum; employees are more productive and clients are more satisfied. Administrators can start by being positive role models, managing their own stress at home and work. Administrators can also:

- Educate health care professionals about job stress, compassion fatigue, and vicarious trauma.
- Minimize stressors, including work overload, inadequate work space, insufficient resources, and unsafe equipment and situations.
- Hold regular staff meetings; keep the lines of communication open and provide support.
- Provide regular debriefing meetings.
- Maintain an organized and efficient workplace.
- Take action on legitimate complaints.
- Provide readily available counseling.

Employers can also establish programs that address workplace stress, such as Employee Assistance Programs (EAP). EAPs can improve the ability of workers to cope with difficult work situations. Stress management programs teach workers about the nature and sources of stress, the effects of stress on health, and personal skills to reduce it.

RESOURCES

Compassion Fatigue Awareness Project: http://www.compassionfatigue.org
National Institute for Occupational Safety and Health: http://www.cdc.gov/niosh
Occupational Safety and Health Administration: http://www.osha.gov

REFERENCES

Center for Sex Offender Management (CSOM). (n.d.). *Secondary trauma and the management of sex offenders.* Retrieved from http://www.csom.org/train/index.html

Collins, S., & Long, A. (2003). Working with the psychological effects of trauma: Consequences for mental health-care workers—a literature review. *Journal of Psychiatric and Mental Health Nursing, 10,* 417–424.

National Institute of Occupational Safety and Health: Center for Disease Prevention and Control. (2008). *Workplace stress.* Retrieved from http://www.cdc.gov/niosh/blog/nsb120307_stress.html

Office for Victims of Crime. (n.d.). *Victim assistance training.* Retrieved from http://www.ovcttac.gov/VATOnline_Course

Pfifferling, J., & Gilley, K. (2000). Overcoming compassion fatigue. *Family Practice Management.* Retrieved from http://www.aafp.org/fpm/20000400/39over.html

Sabo, B. (2008). Adverse psychosocial consequences: Compassion fatigue, burnout and vicarious traumatization: Are nurses who provide palliative and hematological cancer care vulnerable? *Indian Journal of Palliative Care, 14*(1), 23–29.

Tehrani, N. (2007). The cost of caring—The impact of secondary trauma on assumptions, values and beliefs. *Counselling Psychology Quarterly, 20*(4), 325–339.

U.S. Department of Labor: Occupational Safety and Health Administration (OSHA). (n.d.). *Stress.* Retrieved from http://www.osha.gov/SLTC/etools/hospital/hazards/stress/stress.html

Adults and Older Adults as Victims

10 Effects of Victimization on Adults and Older Adults

DESCRIPTION

A violent crime may only last seconds, but its effects can last a lifetime. In one study by Draper and associates (2008), 1,458 (6.7%) and 1,429 (6.5%) out of 21,000 participants reported childhood physical and sexual abuse, respectively. Multivariate models indicated that participants who had experienced either childhood sexual or physical abuse had a greater risk of poor physical and mental health. Older adults who reported both childhood sexual and physical abuse also had a higher risk of poor physical and mental health.

Victimization can have significant and long-lasting effects on victims and their families. Victims may suffer physical, psychological, social, and/or financial trauma that can leave them devastated if they do not get proper intervention. Numerous studies have examined the long-term consequences of relationship violence during childhood. These studies have suggested that physical and sexual abuse in early life can lead to problems in adulthood, including poor mental and physical health, as well as higher rates of substance abuse. However, few studies have examined the long-term consequences of relationship violence in adulthood. Those that exist, however, have suggested that women who experience relationship violence in adulthood have poor health trajectories, including depressive symptoms, functional impairment, and alcohol consumption. Levine (2008) showed that past-year abuse was independently associated with increased hospital admissions, and that psychological effects of recent abuse combined with depression may particularly increase rates of medical/surgical hospitalizations.

Effect of Violence Against Adult Males

The effect of victimization on adult males is still woefully understudied, and thus most of this chapter focuses on females. However, the National Center for Victims of Crime (http://www.ncvc.org) notes that men experience many of the same psychological reactions to violence as women, including guilt, shame, and humiliation; anger and anxiety; depression; and withdrawal from relationships. In male-perpetrated assaults, male victims are more likely to be strangled, beaten with closed fists, and threatened with weapons, while in female-perpetrated assaults, male victims are more likely to be kicked, slapped, or have objects thrown at them. Males also can experience significant physical consequences from extrafamilial violence, including gang violence.

Effects of Violence on Older Adults

Abuse has a significant impact on people at any age, but older adults are especially vulnerable and are twice as likely to suffer serious injury and require hospitalization as any other age group. Older adults have less physical strength and resilience than younger persons, and some older adults may be very frail, or already have disabilities or impairments that leave them particularly vulnerable. They often suffer more financial harm than younger adults, since many elders live on a low or fixed income and often cannot afford the professional services and products that could help them in the aftermath of a crime. Violence and neglect can have serious long-term effects on the health and well-being of older adults. The stress alone may trigger chest pain or angina and may be a factor in other serious heart problems. Panic attacks, high blood pressure, respiratory problems, and gastrointestinal disturbances are common stress-related symptoms among abused elders. Older bones break more easily and take longer to heal. An injury or accumulation of injuries over time can lead to serious harm or death.

Many abused elders are isolated, and their abusers often threaten, harass, or intimidate them. As a result of abuse, older adults often experience worry, depression, or anxiety. These signs may be mistaken for memory loss or illness, when really they are the effects of stress or worry. An older adult may also feel shame, guilt, or embarrassment that someone in the family or someone close has harmed them. Some abused older adults may start to eat less, use more medications, or abuse alcohol to help them cope with the emotional and physical hurt. They may have difficulty sleeping or sleep too much. Some abused elders may lose interest in life or become withdrawn. Some may develop suicidal ideation.

PHYSICAL EFFECTS OF VIOLENCE

The physical effects of abuse vary according to the type of abuse perpetrated and may stem from physical or sexual abuse or from neglect. Some effects may be short-term, such as bruising or a minor fracture, while others are permanent. Victims may suffer from brain damage from head injury or functional disabilities from spinal cord injuries.

Physical Effects of Intimate Partner Violence on Women

Victims of intimate partner violence (IPV) may experience traumatic injuries (lacerations, bruises, broken bones, head injuries, internal bleeding), chronic pelvic pain, abdominal and gastrointestinal complaints, frequent vaginal and urinary tract infections, sexually transmitted diseases, and HIV. Many of the physical injuries sustained by women from intimate partner violence seem to cause chronic health problems as women age. Women have anecdotally identified arthritis, hypertension, and heart disease as being caused by or aggravated by IPV early in their adult lives. Disorders such as diabetes mellitus or hypertension may be aggravated in victims of IPV, because the abuser may not allow them access to medications or adequate medical care.

Campbell (2002) suggests that abused women may experience chronic pain such as headaches or back pain, or recurring central nervous system symptoms including fainting and seizures. Many report choking (incomplete strangulation) and blows to the head resulting in loss of consciousness, both of which can lead to serious medical problems, including neurological sequelae. Gastrointestinal symptoms (loss of appetite, eating disorders) and functional gastrointestinal disorders (chronic irritable bowel syndrome) are associated with chronic stress, and these may begin during a violent relationship, be related to child sexual abuse, or both. Campbell further notes that gynecological problems are the most consistent, persistent, and largest physical health difference between battered and non-battered women. They include sexually transmitted diseases, vaginal bleeding or infection, fibroids, decreased sexual desire, genital irritation, pain on intercourse, chronic pelvic pain, and urinary-tract infections. Forced sex may explain the higher prevalence of gynecological problems, although few studies have measured forced sex separately.

A study of 157 abused women by Woods, Hall, Campbell, and Angott (2008) showed that all types of IPV experienced by women (physical, emotional, and sexual abuse; threats of violence; and risk of homicide) are significantly associated with increased reports of physical health problems and PTSD. A substantial proportion of these women reported neuromuscular, stress, sleep, and gynecologic symptoms. It is important to know that these physical symptoms tend to be vague or nonspecific and include low back pain, fatigue, muscle weakness, pounding or racing heart, lightheadedness, stomach cramps, and sleep difficulties. Many of the women also report a large number of symptoms that cross diagnostic boundaries.

Physical Effects on Fetal Development

In a study of 2,562 women, Alio, Nana, and Silohu (2009) showed that those exposed to spousal violence ($n = 1,307$) were 50% more likely to experience a single or repeated stillbirth or spontaneous abortion. In this group, physical violence was most common (39%), followed by emotional abuse, defined as verbal or physical public humiliation or verbal threatening of the woman or her family (31%), and sexual abuse (15%). Physical assault during pregnancy can result in placental separation; antepartum hemorrhage; fetal fractures; rupture of the uterus, liver, or spleen; preterm labor; low birth-weight babies; and risk for urinary tract infections, sexually transmitted diseases, and poor prenatal care. Research also suggests an association between intimate partner violence and preterm labor, premature delivery, and miscarriage. Abusive partners may also pressure their pregnant wives or girlfriends not to gain weight, or abuse could cause stress, which has in turn been associated with smoking, low weight gain, and consequent low birth weight.

Physical Effects of Sexual Assault

According to Stop Violence Against Women (http://www.stopvaw.org), the physical consequences of sexual assault can be quite severe. Forced sexual contact can result in genital injuries and gynecological complications, such as bleeding, infection, chronic pelvic pain, pelvic inflammatory disease, and urinary tract infections. Sexual violence can put women at risk of sexually transmitted infections, including HIV/AIDS, and unwanted pregnancies. The unwanted pregnancies may lead to unsafe abortions or to injuries sustained during an abortion. Women can also suffer injuries resulting from physical abuse that may accompany the sexual assault.

PSYCHOLOGICAL EFFECTS OF VIOLENCE

Victims can experience long-term psychological effects from violence. Depression remains the most common response, and battered women are at greater risk for suicide attempts. Victims may also experience acute or posttraumatic stress disorder (PTSD), and/or Stockholm syndrome.

Acute Stress Disorder

Data on acute stress disorder (ASD) is limited, since it was only formally recognized in 1994. However, the main cause of acute stress disorder is exposure to severe trauma. The impact of trauma is influenced by several factors, particularly the severity of the event, the duration of the event, the proximity to the event (whether the event was directly experienced or witnessed), the type of the event, and the intent (whether the event was planned or accidental). Human acts of violence, especially those that are particularly cruel, create a greater risk for this disorder than natural events. Individuals with ASD develop dissociative responses and may experience decreased emotional responsiveness, often finding it difficult to experience pleasure and frequently feeling guilty. Symptoms appear during or immediately after the trauma, last for at least two days, and resolve within four weeks after the conclusion of the traumatic event or when the diagnosis is changed. Symptoms lasting more than four weeks may warrant a diagnosis of PTSD, provided the full criteria for that disorder are met.

The criteria for ASD per the *Diagnostic and Statistical Manual of Mental Disorders* (4th ed., text revision) (*DSM-IV-TR*) are the following: (a) the person was exposed to a traumatic event in which the person experienced, witnessed, or was confronted with an event(s) that involved actual or threatened death or serious injury to themselves or others, and the person's response involved intense fear, helplessness, or horror; (b) while experiencing or after experiencing the distressing event, the individual has three (or more) of the following dissociative symptoms: a subjective sense of numbing, detachment, or absence of emotional responsiveness; a reduction in awareness of his or her surroundings; derealization; depersonalization; or dissociative amnesia; (c) the traumatic event is persistently reexperienced in at least one of the following ways: recurrent images, thoughts, dreams, illusions, flashbacks, a sense of reliving the experience, or distress on exposure to reminders of the traumatic event; (d) there is marked avoidance of stimuli that cause recollections of the trauma; (e) there are marked symptoms of anxiety or increased arousal, such as difficulty sleeping, poor concentration, hypervigilance, or exaggerated startle response; (f) the disturbance causes clinically significant distress or impairment in social, occupational, or other important areas of functioning; (g) the disturbance lasts for a minimum of 2 days, a maximum of 4 weeks, and occurs within 4 weeks of the traumatic event; and (h) the disturbance is not due to substance abuse or a general medical condition is not better accounted for by brief psychotic disorder, and is not merely an exacerbation of a preexisting psychiatric disorder.

ASD is a relatively new diagnosis, and thus there are few well-established and empirically validated measures to assess it. Tools with strong psychometric properties are:

- The Acute Stress Disorder Interview (ASDI): This structured clinical interview has been validated against *DSM-IV* criteria for ASD and appears to meet standard criteria for internal consistency, test-retest reliability, and construct validity. It was validated through a comparison with independent diagnostic decisions made by clinicians with experience in diagnosing both ASD and PTSD.
- The Acute Stress Disorder Scale (ASDS): This self-report measure of ASD symptoms correlates highly with symptom clusters on the ASDI, and it has good internal consistency, test-retest reliability, and constructs validity.

Both tools are available in Bryant and Harvey (2000).

Posttraumatic Stress Disorder

Posttraumatic stress disorder (PTSD) often presents in primary and community care but goes unrecognized. Failure to identify and treat PTSD has adverse effects on client health, since PTSD is associated with increased health complaints, health services utilization, morbidity, and mortality. Persons with PTSD have persistent frightening thoughts and memories of the traumatic incident and feel emotionally numb, especially with people they were once close to. They may experience sleep disturbances, feel numb or detached, or be easily startled.

In 2000 the American Psychiatric Association revised the diagnostic criteria for PTSD in the *DSM-IV-TR*. The criteria now include a history of exposure to a traumatic event that meets two stressor criteria and symptoms from each of three symptom clusters: intrusive recollections, avoidant or numbing symptoms, and hyperarousal symptoms. Additional criteria address symptom duration and functioning. As part of the stressor criteria, the person must have experienced, witnessed, or faced an event that involved actual or perceived threatened death or serious harm to himself/herself or others that evoked intense fear, horror, or helplessness. The person must manifest at least one intrusive recollection criterion, such as recurrent and intrusive images, thoughts, or perceptions of the event, flashbacks, or the sensation of reliving the event. The person must manifest at least three avoidant or numbing criteria, such as efforts to avoid conversations associated with the trauma, inability to remember critical aspects about the trauma, significantly decreased participation in important activities, feeling detached from others, or a sense of a shortened future. The person must also manifest at least two hyperarousal criteria, such as hypervigilance, difficulty sleeping, outbursts of anger or irritability, difficulty concentrating, or an exaggerated startle response. Symptoms need to last more than one month and must cause significant distress or impairment in social, occupational, or other important areas of functioning. PTSD often presents with comorbid disorders, including depression, substance abuse, and other anxiety disorders. Thus health care providers need to consider other symptoms not specific to PTSD as they may indicate an additional psychiatric disorder.

The National Center for PTSD provides links to a number of PTSD screening tools (http://www.ptsd.va.gov/professional /pages/assessments/list-screening-instruments.asp). This site includes training resources as well as information on multiple assessment instruments used to measure trauma exposure and PTSD. The information for each measure includes descriptions, references, contacts, and sample items. There are also charts that list the instruments by category to help compare various measures and select the one most suitable for your practice (see Table 10.1).

Table 10.1

SCREENING TOOLS FOR PTSD

SCREENING TOOL	RESOURCE FOR OBTAINING
Primary Care PTSD Screen (PC-PTSD)	This screening tool may be found at: Prins, A., Ouimette, P., Kimerling, R., Cameron, R. P., Hugelshofer, D. S., Shaw-Hegwer, J., Thrailkill, A., Gusman, F.D., & Sheikh, J. I. (2003). The primary care PTSD screen (PC–PTSD): Development and operating characteristics. Primary Care Psychiatry, 9, 9–14. http://www.ptsd.va.gov/professional/articles/article-pdf/id26676.pdf
Trauma Screening Questionnaire (TSQ)	This screening tool is available from: Brewin, C. R., Rose, S., Andrews, B., Green, J., Tata, P., McEvedy, C., Turner, S., & Foa, E. B. (2002). Brief screening instrument for post-traumatic stress disorder. The British Journal of Psychiatry, 181, 158–162. http://bjp.rcpsych.org/cgi/content/full/181/2/158
Short Screening Scale for PTSD	Breslau, N., Peterson, E. .L., Kessler, R. C., & Schultz, L.R. (1999). Short screening scale for DSM-IV post-traumatic stress disorder. American Journal of Psychiatry, 156, 908–911. http://ajp.psychiatryonline.org/cgi/content/full/156/6/908

Screening tools include:

■ Primary Care PTSD Screen (PC-PTSD): The PC-PTSD is a four-item screen designed for use in primary care and other medical settings. It is currently used to screen for PTSD in veterans at the Veterans Administration (VA). The screen includes an introductory sentence to cue respondents to traumatic events, and, in most circumstances, its results should be considered positive if a client answers "yes" to any three items. Those screening positive should then be assessed with a structured interview for PTSD.

■ Trauma Screening Questionnaire (TSQ): The TSQ is a 10-item symptom screen that was designed for use with survivors of all types of traumatic stress. The TSQ is based on items from the PTSD Symptom Scale—Self Report and has five reexperiencing items and five arousal items. Respondents are asked to endorse those items that they have experienced at least twice in the past week. The screen is considered positive when at least six items were endorsed, but is recommended to be conducted 3 to 4 weeks post-trauma to allow for normal recovery processes to take place. Those screening positive should then be assessed with a structured interview for PTSD.

- Short Screening Scale for PTSD: The Short Screening Scale for PTSD is a seven-item screen designed for all trauma survivors, but it was empirically derived in the context of an epidemiological study of PTSD in an urban area of the United States. The screen was designed to be administered after an assessment of trauma exposure and consists of five avoidance items and two hyperarousal items. The screen is scored by adding the number of "yes" responses, and the suggested cutoff is four. Those screening positive should then be assessed with a structured interview for PTSD.

Stockholm Syndrome

Stockholm syndrome is a psychological state in which victims identify with their offenders. The term was originally used in cases of kidnapping and hostage situations but has been extended to other forms of violence, including intimate partner violence and child abuse. There is no universally accepted definition of Stockholm syndrome, but it has been suggested that it is present if one or more of the following is observed: positive feelings by the captive toward his or her captor; negative feelings by the captive toward the police or authorities trying to win his or her release; and positive feelings by the captor toward his or her captive. These conditions must be met for Stockholm syndrome to occur:

1. A perceived threat to survival and a belief that the captor is willing to carry out that threat
2. A perception by the captive of some small kindness from the captor within the context of terror
3. Isolation from perspectives other than those of the captor
4. Perceived inability to escape

Suggested treatment for Stockholm syndrome includes:

1. Recovery from isolation: Help the client identify sources of supportive intervention, using self-help groups or group therapy

(group needs to be homogeneous to needs), as well as hotlines, crisis centers, shelters, and friends.

2. Recovery from violence: As victims in abusive relationships minimize the abuse, or are in denial, it may be necessary to ask directly about the different types of violent behavior. Many women (and children) are confused about acceptable male (or parental/ authority) behavior and how to distinguish between acceptable and unacceptable behavior. Journal keeping, autobiographical writing, reading of firsthand accounts, or viewing and discussing films that deal with abuse may be helpful in providing clients with a more concrete understanding of how to define these parameters.

3. Recovery from perceived kindness (provided by captor): Encourage the client to develop alternative sources of nurturance and caring, particularly family members and friends. Assist victims in rediscovering simple acts of kindness, such as a friend offering to drive the client to the store or the client's child drawing a picture to help the client feel batter.

4. Validating both love and terror—Helping the client integrate both disassociated sides of the abuser will assist the client in giving up the dream that the relationship will become what she or he had hoped it would be.

SOCIAL EFFECTS OF VIOLENCE

IPV has also been found to cause negative attitudes toward pregnancy, to change relationships with extended family members and friends, and to decrease the possibility of being employed or attending school. The World Health Association (2009) notes that the social and economic costs of violence against women are enormous and have ripple effects throughout society. Women may suffer isolation, inability to work, loss of wages, lack of participation in regular activities, and limited ability to care for themselves and their children. Wisner, Gilmer, Saltzman, and Zink (1999) noted that women who were victims of intimate partner violence cost health plans approximately 92% more than a random sample of general female enrollees. Findings are significantly higher for mental health services, as well.

INTERVENTIONS AND VICTIM RIGHTS

Physical interventions are found throughout this text in the crime-specific chapters, such as chapter 17, "Female Victims of Sexual Assault." The following list of victim rights provides basic interventions for all victims, as well as those with psychological, safety, and financial problems. Health care providers should also be aware of victim rights and needs, as well as victim safety, including how to direct victims to obtain orders of protection.

Victim Rights

The majority of states have amended their constitutions to guarantee certain rights for crime victims. Typically, these include the following fundamental rights:

- The right to notification of all court proceedings related to the offense
- The right to be reasonably protected from the accused offender
- The right to have input at sentencing (in the form of a victim impact statement)
- The right to information about the conviction, sentencing, imprisonment, and release of the offender
- The right to an order of restitution from the convicted offender
- The right to notice of these rights
- The right to enforcement of these rights

Victim Needs

The Office for Victims of Crime (OVC) states that there are three critical needs for all victims:

1. Victims need to feel safe: People usually feel helpless, vulnerable, and frightened by victimization. When working with victims, be sure to follow these guidelines:
    - Introduce yourself by name and title and briefly explain your role.
    - Ensure privacy during your interview. Assure confidentiality when possible (extent of confidentiality depends n your role).

■ Reassure victims of their safety. Pay attention to your own words, posture, mannerisms, and tone of voice. Use body language to show concern, such as nodding your head, using natural eye contact, placing yourself at the victim's level, keeping an open stance, and speaking in a calm, sympathetic voice. Tell victims that they are safe and that you are there for them.

■ Ask victims to tell you in just a sentence or two what happened, and ask if they have any physical injuries. Tend to medical needs first.

■ Offer to contact a family member, friend, victim advocate, or crisis counselor.

■ Ask simple questions to allow victims to make decisions, assert themselves, and regain control over their lives, such as "How would you like me to address you?"

■ Ask victims if they have any special concerns or needs.

■ Develop a safety plan before leaving them. Pull together personal or professional support for the victims. Give victims a pamphlet listing resources available for help or information, including contact information for local crisis intervention centers and support groups, the prosecutor's office and the victim-witness assistance office, the state victim compensation/assistance office, and other nationwide services, including toll-free hotlines and Web addresses.

■ Give them, in writing, your name and information on how to reach you. Encourage them to contact you if they have any questions or if you can be of further help.

2. Victims need to express their emotions: Victims need to express their emotions and tell their story after the trauma. They need to have their feelings accepted and have their story heard by a nonjudgmental listener. They may feel fear, self-blame, anger, shame, sadness, or denial, and most will say, "I don't believe this happened to me." Some may have a reaction formation and act opposite to how they feel, such as laughter instead of crying. Some feel rage at the sudden, unpredictable, and uncontrollable threat to their safety or lives, and this rage can even be directed at the professionals who are trying to help them. When working with victims, be sure to follow these guidelines:

■ Listen. Show that you are actively listening to victims through your facial expressions, body language, and comments such as

"Take your time; I'm listening," and "We can take a break if you like. I'm in no hurry."

■ Notice victims' body language, to help you understand and respond to what they are feeling as well as what they are saying.

■ Assure victims that their emotional reactions are not uncommon. Sympathize with the victims by saying things such as: "You've been through something very frightening. I'm sorry."

■ Counter self-blame by victims by saying things such as, "You didn't do anything wrong. This was not your fault."

■ Ask open-ended questions.

■ Avoid interrupting victims while they are telling their story.

■ Repeat or rephrase what you think you heard the victims say for validation.

3. Victims need to know "what comes next" after their victimization: Victims usually have concerns about their role in the criminal investigation and legal proceedings. They may also be concerned about payment for health care or property damage. You can help relieve some of their anxiety by telling victims what to expect in the aftermath of the crime and by preparing them for upcoming stressful events and changes in their lives. When working with victims, be sure to follow these guidelines:

■ Refer the victim to a victim's advocate who will assist the victim through the investigative and legal proceedings.

■ Tell victims about subsequent law enforcement interviews or other kinds of interviews they can expect.

■ Discuss the general nature of medical forensic examinations the victim will be asked to undergo and the importance of these examinations for the legal proceedings.

■ Counsel victims that lapses of concentration, memory losses, depression, and physical ailments are normal reactions for crime victims. Encourage them to reestablish their normal routines as quickly as possible to help speed their recovery.

■ Give victims a listing of resources that are available for help and information.

■ Ask victims whether they have any questions. Encourage victims to contact you if you can be of further assistance.

Treatment of Acute and Posttraumatic Stress Disorders

The American Psychiatric Association (APA) revised its Practice Guideline for the Treatment of Patients with Acute Stress Disorder and Posttraumatic Stress Disorder in March 2009. They noted that increasing research attention has been focused on the assessment and treatment of PTSD since the publication of their 2004 guideline, and that much work remains to be done. The treatment of these disorders is beyond the scope of this book; however, health care providers can refer to the APA guidelines at http://www.psychiatryonline.com/content.aspx?aID=156502.

ORDERS OF PROTECTION

Victims may fear for their lives, and in some cases—especially those of intimate partner violence—victims may be in danger of being killed. Offenders may not yet have been caught or may be out on bail, probation, or parole.

An order of protection is a legally binding court order that restrains an individual who has committed an act of violence against a person from further acts against that person. Protective orders vary state by state and are called by various names (restraining orders, protection from abuse orders [PFAs], etc.). Most are used to protect against family/intimate partner violence; some jurisdictions use them for strangers. There are different types of protective orders, demonstrated by the three stages of protection from abuse (PFA) orders issued in Pennsylvania:

- Emergency orders issued by the district justice when the Court of Common Pleas is closed. It is in effect until the next business day at the Court of Common Pleas.
- Temporary order issued on a daily basis by the Court of Common Pleas and is in effect until the hearing for a permanent PFA is held.
- Permanent order issued for up to 18 months at a hearing before the Court of Common Pleas. The hearing date is scheduled when the temporary PFA is received.

Health care providers can contact the police, district attorney's office, or victim advocate center to learn how victims may obtain protective orders in their areas. However, it is best that they do this before a situation occurs and keep the information readily available for emergent purposes.

The protection order can prohibit the abuser from committing acts of violence; exclude the abuser from the residence shared by the petitioner and abuser; prohibit the abuser from harassing or contacting the petitioner by mail, telephone, or in person; award temporary custody of minor children; establish temporary visitation and restrain the abuser from interfering with custody; prohibit the abuser from removing the children from the jurisdiction of the court; and order the abuser to participate in treatment or counseling. Some states, including New York, include pets in the protective orders. Although seemingly powerful, protective orders are nothing more than pieces of paper—they are not bulletproof. They seem to work best on those offenders who have something to lose if they disobey them, and in some cases, they may aggravate the situation. Therefore, victims still need to take precautions to keep themselves safe.

VICTIM COMPENSATION

Many victims lose their jobs because of absenteeism due to injury or illness related to the violence. Absences from court appearances can occur, which can also jeopardize victim livelihood. Victims of IPV and stalking may have to move many times to avoid violence. This is costly and can interfere with continuity of employment. Victims may also have had to forgo financial security during divorce proceedings to avoid further abuse, and many become impoverished as they grow older.

The financial effects on society are staggering. A study by Corso, Mercy, Simon, Finkelstein, and Miller (2007) of several nationally representative data sets showed that the total costs associated with nonfatal injuries and deaths due to violence in 2000 were more than $70 billion. Most of this cost ($64.4 billion or 92%) was due to lost productivity. However, an estimated $5.6 billion was spent on medical care for the more than 2.5 million injuries due to interpersonal and self-directed violence. Victims of violence cost health plans more than those persons who have not been victimized. Violence-related injuries, including suicide, adversely affect all Americans through premature death, disability, medical costs, and lost productivity.

Crime victims often incur a significant number of expenses when victimized, yet most health care professionals are unaware of compensation mechanisms. Conviction of the offender is not required, and victims of crime under state, federal, military, and tribal jurisdiction are eligible to apply for compensation. Eligible crime victims include those who have been physically injured and/or who suffer emotional injury as a result of violence or attempted violence, even though no physical injury resulted. Some states also include family members of deceased victims and other individuals who pay for expenses resulting from a victim's injury or death.

According to the National Association of Crime Victim Compensation Boards, each state's eligibility requirements vary slightly, but victims are generally required to:

- Report the crime promptly to law enforcement, usually within 72 hours
- File a timely application with the compensation program in the state where the crime occurred, and provide any information requested
- Cooperate in the investigation and prosecution of the crime
- Be innocent of any criminal activity or misconduct leading to the victim's injury or death

Many states require that the application be filed within one year from the date of the crime, but some states have shorter or longer periods. Applications can be obtained from the state compensation program, police, prosecutors, or victim service agencies. Most state programs have brochures describing their benefits, requirements, and procedures. Health care providers can refer victims to victim service programs for assistance in completing the application. The application should be submitted to the compensation program as soon as possible, where it will be reviewed to determine eligibility and to decide what costs can be paid. The program will notify the applicant of its decision.

Depending on the state, expenses may be covered if they are not paid for by insurance or by another public benefit program, and if they result directly from the crime. These include: medical and hospital care, and dental work to repair injury to teeth; mental health counseling; lost earnings due to crime-related injuries; loss of support for dependents of a deceased victim; and funeral and burial expenses. Expenses that are not covered usually include: property loss, theft, and damage (unless damage is to eyeglasses, hearing aids, or other medically necessary devices), and expenses paid by other sources, such as any type of public or private health insurance, automobile insurance, disability insurance, or workers compensation. A few states may pay limited amounts for the loss of essential personal property during a violent crime and for cleaning up the crime scene.

RESOURCES

Court Order of Protection (U.S. Department of Health & Human Services): http://www.womenshealth.gov/violence/prevent/civil.cfm
National Association of Crime Victim Compensation Boards (NACVCB): http://www.nacvcb.org
National Center for PTSD: http://www.ptsd.va.gov
Office for Victims of Crime: http://ovc.gov/

REFERENCES

Alio, A., Nana, P., & Salihu, H. (2009). Spousal violence and potentially preventable single and recurrent spontaneous fetal loss in an African setting: Cross-sectional study. *Lancet, 373,* 318–324. Retrieved from http://health.usf.edu/nocms/publicaffairs/now/pdfs/Lancet_SpousalViolence_1_24_09.pdf

Bain, P., & Spencer, C. (2009). *Abuse of older adults: Signs and effects.* Yukon Health and Social Services. Federal/provincial/territorial ministers responsible for seniors in Canada. Retrieved from http://www.hss.gov.yk.ca/pdf/elder_fact4.pdf

Bryant, R. A., & Harvey, A. G. (2000). *Acute stress disorder: A handbook of theory, assessment, and treatment.* Washington, DC: American Psychological Association.

Campbell, J. (2002). Health consequences of intimate partner violence. *The Lancet, 359,* 1331–1336.

Corso, P., Mercy, J., Simon, T., Miller, T., & Finkelstein, E. (2007). Medical costs and productivity losses due to interpersonal and self-directed violence in the United States. *American Journal of Preventive Medicine, 32*(6), 474–482.

Draper, B., Pfaff, J., Pirkis, J., Snowdon, J., Lautenschlager, N., Wilson, I., et al. (2008). Long-term effects of childhood abuse on the quality of life and health of older people: Results from the Depression and Early Prevention of Suicide in General Practice Project. *Journal of the American Geriatrics Society, 56*(2), 262–271.

Duffy, F. F., Craig, T., Moscicki, E. K., West, J. C., & Fochtmann, L. J. (2009). Performance in practice: Clinical tools to improve the care of patients with posttraumatic stress disorder. *Focus: The Journal of Lifelong Learning in Psychiatry, 7,* 186–203.

Hill, T., Schroeder, R., Bradley, C., Kaplan, L., & Angel, R. (2009). The long-term health consequences of relationship violence in adulthood: An examination of low-income women from Boston, Chicago, and San Antonio. *American Journal of Public Health, 99*(9), 1645–1650.

Levine, J. (2008). Major depression and recent physical or sexual abuse increase readmissions among high-utilizing primary care patients. *Mental Health in Family Medicine, 5,* 23–28.

Morland, L., Leskin, G., Block, C., Campbell, J., & Freidman, M. (2008). Intimate partner violence and miscarriage: Examination of the role of physical and psychological abuse and posttraumatic stress disorder. *Journal of Interpersonal Violence, 23,* 652–669.

Wisner, C., Gilmer, T., Saltzman, L., & Zink, T. (1999). Intimate partner violence against women: Do victims cost health plans more? *Journal of Family Practice, 48*(6), 439–443.

Woods, S., Hall, R., Campbell, J., & Angott, D. (2008). Physical health and posttraumatic stress disorder symptoms in women experiencing intimate partner violence. *Journal of Midwifery & Women's Health, 53*(6), 538–546.

World Health Organization. (2009). *Violence against women.* Retrieved from http://www.who.int/mediacentre/factsheets/fs239/en

11

Victimization of Adults and Older Adults With Disabilities

DEFINITION

The American Disabilities Act describes a person with disabilities as a person who: has a physical or mental impairment that substantially limits one or more major life activities; has a record of such impairment; or is regarded as having such impairment. The World Health Organization (WHO) defines a disability as lack (resulting from an impairment) of ability or any restriction to perform an activity in the manner or within the range considered normal for a human being. The term covers a wide range of abilities, including: mobility, agility, hearing, vision, speech, and others such as mental disabilities, cognitive disabilities, and learning disabilities. Persons may have one or more disabilities, and disabilities vary in severity.

PREVALENCE

According to the U.S. Census Bureau's 2000 Census, approximately one in five Americans has a disability. Many in this population become victims of crime during their lifetimes. Unfortunately, acts of physical aggression, domestic violence, sexual assault, and other crimes against persons with disabilities often go unreported, making it difficult to document and respond to the true scope of this abuse and victimization. Even when professionals are able to intervene in the aftermath of a crime, many professionals lack experience working with persons with disabilities. Thus they may not understand how best to guide and support them through the processes of reporting an incident and navigating the criminal justice system.

A recent survey of women with physical disabilities showed that more than half of all respondents (56%) reported being abused: 87% reported physical abuse; 66% reported sexual abuse; 35% were refused help with a physical need; 19% were prevented from using an assistive device they required; and 74% reported ongoing victimization. Yet only 33% of women with physical disabilities sought help with their situation, and they had "mixed reactions" as to whether getting assistance had been a positive experience.

Other statistics show that:

- People with developmental disabilities are 4 to10 times more likely to be victims of crime than other people.
- Children with disabilities are more than three times more likely to be abused or victimized than children without disabilities.
- As many as 50% of patients who are long-term residents of hospitals and specialized rehabilitation centers are there due to crime-related injuries.
- It is estimated that criminal acts cause at least six million serious injuries each year, resulting in either a temporary or permanent disability.

ETIOLOGY

Perpetrators of crimes against people with disabilities frequently know or have access to their victims through a personal or service relationship. One study estimated that more than half of all abuse of people with disabilities is perpetrated by family members or peers. The literature also reveals that persons working in disability-related fields (caregivers, doctors, nurses, and other professionals) also abuse persons with disabilities. When the abuser is an intimate partner or someone involved in the victim's well-being, seeking help or justice can be extremely complicated for the victim.

ASSESSMENT

General Principles

Health care professionals are well versed in the general issues of persons with disabilities. But they should also be aware of the obstacles faced by those who have been victimized.

Isolation: Society often segregates persons with disabilities through physical and social isolation, with institutionalization representing the extreme. Pervasive isolation can cause people with disabilities to be unaware of available services and resources, as well as the rights they have by law. This is especially true for people with severe disabling conditions, older people with disabilities, and younger people with developmental disabilities. Many people who are chronically victimized do not even know that society condemns such predatory conduct and that there is help to address this wrongdoing.

Limited Access: Access can be minimized due to physical or attitudinal inaccessibility.

- Physical accessibility: Crime victims with disabilities may not have physical access to services, due to architectural barriers in buildings and public transportation systems, despite the Americans with Disabilities Act of 1990 (ADA). Titles II and III of the ADA pertain to the criminal justice and victim assistance fields.
- Attitudinal accessibility: Program staff must be welcoming toward people with disabilities and demonstrate in the quality of their programs that they sincerely want to work collaboratively to serve the community.

Underreporting of the Crime: Crime may go unreported for many reasons: mobility or communication barriers, the social or physical isolation of the victim, a victim's normal feelings of shame and self-blame, ignorance of the justice system, or the fact that the perpetrator is a family member or primary caregiver. In crimes against a victim with a disability, one or more of these factors may prevent the crime from ever being reported.

Limited Advocacy: Despite progress by disability rights activists, advocacy remains limited. Just as with many crime victims, a person who wants to access criminal justice decision-making processes may be unable to do so without adequate tools to enable full participation.

Criminal victimization of a person with a disability frequently compounds existing problems caused by a lack of accessibility to basic social services, poverty, institutionalization, and other barriers to equal rights. A crime that would be damaging to an able-bodied person is frequently a devastating blow to a person with a disability. For many, it is the criminal assault itself that results in a disability. Many persons with disabilities are especially vulnerable to victimization because of their real or perceived inability to fight or flee, or to notify others and testify about the victimization. Offenders are motivated by a desire to obtain control over the victim and measure their potential prey for vulnerabilities.

Most crime victims experience a sense of shock, disbelief, or denial that the crime occurred, often followed by powerful emotions including fear, anger, confusion, guilt, humiliation, and grief. People with disabilities may have intensified reactions. because they may already feel stigmatized and often have low self-esteem due to societal attitudes. The sense of self-blame, vulnerability, confusion, and loss of trust may be exaggerated, as may be an ambivalence or negativity related to their perception of their own bodies. Denial and avoidance of the need to cope with the aftermath may complicate the identification of crime victims with a disability. Some victims, particularly those with developmental disabilities, will need services designed to enhance a feeling of safety and security regarding future victimization.

History and Physical Assessment, Diagnostic Testing

These processes should be based on type of disability and injuries. Treat all victims with respect.

INTERVENTION

Any intervention should be appropriate to the type of individual disability and the injuries sustained. Victims with developmental disabilities experience the full affective range of the effects of trauma and may benefit from a variety of interventions. Psychotherapeutic and psychoeducational interventions should be adapted so that emotions, resultant actions, and ongoing concerns can be effectively expressed and addressed.

While assessments and interventions are similar to those persons who do not have disabilities, health care providers will benefit from tips on victims with disabilities provided for first responders by the Office for Victims of Crime (2002).

Tips on Responding to Crime Victims Who Have Alzheimer's Disease

- Approach victims from the front and establish and maintain eye contact. Introduce yourself and explain that you are there to help. Due to their impaired short-term memory, victims may repeatedly ask who you are; therefore, you may need to reintroduce yourself several times.
- Ask for identification and observe for a Safe Return bracelet, necklace, lapel pin, key chain, or label inside their clothing collar. (Safe Return identification provides the person's first name, indicates that he or she has memory impairment, and gives the 24-hour toll-free number for the Alzheimer's Association's Safe Return Program. The program provides the full name of the registrant, a photograph, identifying characteristics, medical information, and emergency contact information. Call the program's crisis number at (800) 572–1122, and a Safe Return clinician will contact the registrant's caregivers.)
- Remove victims from crowds and noisy environments. These can cause restlessness, pacing, agitation, and panic in people with Alzheimer's.
- Talk in a low-pitched, reassuring tone, while maintaining eye contact. Alzheimer's shortens attention span and increases suspicion, and calm support can make victims less agitated and panicked.
- Speak slowly and clearly, using short, simple sentences with familiar words. Repeat yourself and accompany your words with gestures when this can aid in communication. But avoid sudden movements.
- Explain your actions before proceeding. If victims are agitated or panicked, avoid physical contact that could seem restraining.
- Do not assume victims understand you or are capable of answering your questions and complying with your instructions.
- Give simple, step-by-step instructions and, whenever possible, use a single instruction.
- Ask one question at a time and use closed-ended questions ("yes" and "no" questions). Victim answers may be confusing and may keep changing. If victims' words are unintelligible, ask them to point, gesture, or otherwise physically communicate their answer.
- Do not argue with victims or challenge their reasoning.

- Do not leave victims alone; they may wander away.
- Find emergency shelter for victims with the help of a local Alzheimer's Association chapter if caregivers can be found.

Tips on Responding to Crime Victims
Who Have Mental Illness

- Approach victims in a calm, nonthreatening, and reassuring manner. They may be overwhelmed by delusions, paranoia, or hallucinations and may feel threatened by you.
- Immediately contact their family member, guardian, or mental health service provider who helps them with daily living.
- Victims may experience a psychiatric crisis. Contact the local mental health crisis center immediately if victims are extremely agitated, distracted, uncommunicative, or displaying inappropriate emotional responses.
- Ask victims about their medications. Make sure victims have access to water, food, and toilet facilities, because side effects of the medications may include thirst, urinary frequency, nausea, constipation, and diarrhea.
- Keep your interview simple, brief, and free of distractions. Understand that rational discussion may not be possible on some or all topics.
- Be aware that victims experiencing delusions, paranoia, or hallucinations may still be able to accurately provide information outside their false system of thoughts, including details related to their victimization and informed consent to medical treatment and forensic exams.
- Avoid the following:

  - Circling, surrounding, closing in on, or standing too close.
  - Sudden movements or rapid instructions and questioning.
  - Whispering, joking, or laughing in their presence.
  - Direct continuous eye contact, forced conversation, or signs of impatience.
  - Any touching.
  - Challenges to or agreement with their delusions, paranoia, or hallucinations.
  - Inappropriate language, such as "crazy," "psycho," and "nuts."

- Allow victims time to calm down before intervening if they are acting manic or dangerous and there is no immediate threat to anyone's safety. Outbursts are usually of short duration.
- Break the speech pattern of victims who talk nonstop by interrupting them with simple questions, such as their birth date or full name, to bring compulsive talking under control.
- Do not assume that victims who are unresponsive cannot hear you. Be sensitive to all types of response, including a victim's body language.
- Understand that hallucinations are frighteningly real to victims. Never try to convince victims that their hallucinations do not exist. Rather, reassure victims that the hallucinations will not harm them and may disappear as their stress lessens.
- Acknowledge paranoia and delusions by empathizing with victims' feelings, but neither agree nor agitate victims by disagreeing with their statements.
- Recognize also that victims who state that others are trying to harm them may be the victims of stalking or other crimes.
- Continually assess victims' emotional state for any indications that they may be a danger to themselves or others.
- Be honest; deception will only increase their fear and suspicion of you.
- Provide for victims' care by a family member, guardian, or mental health service provider before leaving them.

Tips on Responding to Crime Victims Who Have Developmental Disabilities

- Avoid using the words "retardation" or "retarded" in front of victims. Instead, use terms like "person with disability" if you need to refer to a victim's impairment.
- Ask victims if there is anyone they would like you to contact to be with them during your interview. But use caution, as family members, service providers, and others can have a vested interest in the interview. They could be the offenders or try to protect the offenders.
- Treat adult victims as adults, not children.
- Do not assume that victims are incapable of understanding or communicating with you. Most people who have mental retardation

live independently or semi-independently in the community, so a fairly normal conversation is possible.

- Create a safe atmosphere, establish a trusting rapport, and limit distractions before and while interviewing victims.
- Be mindful of the issue of a victim's competency to give or withhold consent to medical treatment and forensic exams, notification of next of kin, and other services, but do not assume victims are incompetent. (See chapter 7 on competency for more information.)
- Explain written information to victims and offer to help them fill out paperwork.
- Allot adequate time for your interview and take a break every 15 minutes.
- Speak directly and slowly to victims, keeping your sentences short and words simple. Listen to how victims talk, and match your speech to their vocabulary, tempo, and sentence structure. Do not raise your voice when you speak.
- Deconstruct complex information into smaller parts and use gestures and other visual props to get your meaning across. But do not overload victims with too much information.
- Wait patiently at least 30 seconds for victims to respond to an instruction or question. If victims do not respond or if they reply inappropriately, calmly repeat yourself, using different words.
- Get feedback by having victims state in their words what they understood.
- Recognize that victims may be eager to please or be easily influenced by you. They may say what they think you want to hear, so do not ask leading questions. Use open-ended questions such as "Tell me what happened." This allows the victims to lead the interview as they disclose information.
- Help victims understand your questions by giving points of reference, such as, "What color was the man's hair?"
- Repeat the last phrase of victims' responses in question form to help them stay focused during your interview and to transition victims through a sequence of events.
- Minimize questions that require victims to do much reasoning or that can confuse them.
- If you need assistance in working with a victim with a developmental disability, contact your local United Way or local chapter

of The Arc, or call The Arc of the United States at (800) 433-5255 for help on how best to serve victims who have developmental disabilities.

Tips on Responding to Crime Victims Who Are Blind or Visually Impaired

- Introduce yourself immediately when you approach victims and have others who are present introduce themselves. These introductions let the victim know who is present and where they are situated, and also help the victim recognize voices during subsequent interviews.
- Tell victims your name, credentials, and the telephone number of your office/agency when responding to victims who are alone, and support them in verifying your identity.
- Speak in a normal tone. Most people who are blind or visually impaired hear well.
- Identify other person(s) to whom you are speaking when conversing in a group because it may not be apparent to victims.
- Let victims know when you or someone with you steps away during a conversation.
- If you need a moment of silence during the interview, such as when writing, explain it to the victim beforehand.
- Express attentiveness, concern, and compassion through your voice and word choice, because victims cannot see your facial expressions or body language to know if you are listening to them and interested.
- Offer to fill out forms and read aloud written information for victims. Explain what printed materials you are providing and make those materials available—as is legally required, with few exceptions, by ADA and Section 504—in alternative format, including large print, audiotape, computer diskette, and Braille, on request. Contact the National Federation for the Blind for assistance, if needed (http://www.nfb.org).
- Respect guide dogs. They are working animals and should not be distracted. Do not pet or talk to them without the owner's permission.
- Offer your arm, instead of holding the arm of victims, if they want you to guide them in moving around. Let victims take your arm

from behind, just above the elbow. In this position, they can follow the motion of your body. Walk in a relaxed manner and expect victims to keep a half-step behind you so they can anticipate curbs and steps.

- Orient victims to their surroundings and provide cues as to what lies ahead when guiding them. Close partially opened doors to cabinets, rooms, and cars that obstruct their path. When possible, remove hazardous objects from the victim's path. Do not move objects at a crime scene (a hospital room is a crime scene if a person is victimized there).

- Warn victims of hazardous objects around them. And be sure to make your warnings and directions specific, such as "straight in front of you," "two steps going up," and "directly to your left."

Tips on Responding to Crime Victims Who Are Deaf or Hearing Impaired

- Do not assume that victims are unable to speak or use their voices. Deaf people have the ability to use their voices but may prefer not to speak because of the quality of their speech.
- Never use the words "deaf mute" or "deaf and dumb."
- Signal your presence to victims by waving your hand or gently touching victims on the arm or shoulder if victims do not notice you.
- Determine how victims desire to communicate by initially communicating through writing in situations where victims are unable to hear you, or if they do not speech- or lip-read and a sign language interpreter is not present.
- Avoid shouting or speaking very slowly to make yourself heard and understood. This distorts your speech, lip movements, and facial expressions, which can make you seem upset.
- Never speak directly into a victim's ear.
- Realize that victims may not be literate in written English but may know American Sign Language (ASL).
- Do not use a child to communicate with adult victims.
- Do not assume that because victims are wearing hearing aids they can hear or understand you. The degree and type of a person's hearing loss may render hearing aids of limited assistance with the tones of speech.
- Keep in mind that deaf and hard of hearing people are visually oriented.

- Realize that not all people who are deaf or hard of hearing can speech- or lip-read and that only about 20% of words are readable from the lips; the rest is guessing.
- Use gestures and pantomime to better communicate. For example, you can motion toward a chair to offer victims a seat; touch your clothing, or hair, when interviewing victims for a description of the offender; and mimic drinking from a glass to ask victims if they are thirsty.
- Observe victims' facial expressions and other physical gestures closely, as deaf and hard of hearing people communicate a lot of information visually through their body language.
- Include victims in all conversations and describe any commotion.
- If you look away from victims to overhear another conversation, if you are distracted because of a noise or disturbance, or if you turn from victims to converse with someone else, explain to victims exactly what you are doing or what is happening.
- When interviewing victims who are hard of hearing, or victims who desire to communicate by speech- or lip-reading, select a location free of distractions and interference, and:

    - Face victims so your eyes and mouth are clearly visible.
    - Do not block your mouth with your hands or speak while looking away from victims or looking down at your notes.
    - Stand or sit at a distance between 3 and 6 feet from victims in a well-lit and glare- and shadow-free area. Avoid unnecessary gesturing and body movement because it is difficult for victims to speech- or lip-read if you are not physically still.
    - Begin speaking after you have the victim's attention and have established eye contact.
    - Make your questions and instructions short and simple.
    - Speak clearly, distinctly, and slightly slower than usual but not unnaturally slow, and do not exaggerate your pronunciation of words.
    - If necessary, talk slightly louder than usual, but never shout. Extremely loud tones are not transmitted as well as normal tones by hearing aids, and shouting distorts lip movements.
    - Be prepared to repeat yourself. Use different words to restate your questions and instructions. The victim may have only missed a word or two initially and repetition will clarify what was missed.

- Use open-ended questions to prevent misunderstandings.

- Honor victims' request for a sign language interpreter as is legally required (with few exceptions) by ADA and Section 504. The national Registry of Interpreters for the Deaf, at (703) 838-0030, has affiliate chapters in all 50 states that can help you locate an interpreter.
- When communicating through an interpreter, remember the interpreter is present solely to transmit information back and forth between you and the victim, not to explain information or give opinions. Thus, when using an interpreter, you should

  - Stand or sit across from victims, in a glare- and shadow-free area, with the interpreter beside you so that victims can easily shift their gaze between you and the interpreter.
  - Speak at a normal volume and pace and directly to victims, not to the interpreter.
  - Ask victims, not the interpreter, to repeat or clarify an answer if you do not understand it.
  - Take breaks. Interpreting (signing) and receiving information visually can be tiring for both interpreters and victims.

- Recognize that a Deaf culture exists. This culture has a language, ASL, and experiences, practices, and beliefs about itself and its connection to the larger hearing society.
- Crime victims who identify with the Deaf culture may live more isolated from the hearing society and be less comfortable with that society, including you, than victims for whom their hearing loss is merely a physical condition.

PREVENTION/PATIENT TEACHING

Primary Prevention

Since offenders are most often those who care for the disabled, consider the following.

1. Minimize caregiver stress by promoting respite care for the caregivers. Respite care is short-term or temporary care of the sick or disabled for a few hours or weeks to provide relief, or respite, to the regular caregiver, usually a family member. Contact the local

social service agency or the National Respite Locator: http://chtop.org/ARCH.html.

2. Assure that providers who care for or volunteer for persons with disabilities have been carefully screened for past histories of abuse or criminal activity. The state police may help with this service.

Secondary Prevention

Screen all persons with disabilities for abuse. Make sure that they know help is available to them.

Tertiary Prevention

Assure that victims with disabilities get the physical, psychological and financial assistance they require. Chapter 10, on the effects of victimization, discusses these options.

RESOURCES

Americans with Disabilities Act: http://www.ada.gov
Americans with Disabilities Act Information Line: (800) 514–0301; (800) 514–0383, TTY; http://www.usdoj.gov/crt/ada/adahom1.htm
Disabilities Resources.org: http://www.disabilityresources.org
Fact Sheet on Respite Care: http://www.archrespite.org/docs/FRIENDSfactsheet14-Respite.pdf
Serving Crime Victims with Disabilities: http://www.ovc.gov/pdftxt/188515.pdf
Victims of Crime With Disabilities Resource Guide: http://wind.uwyo.edu/resource guide

REFERENCES

Focht-New, G., Barol, B., Clements, P., & Milliken, T. (2008). Persons with developmental disability exposed to interpersonal violence and crime: Approaches for intervention. *Perspectives in Psychiatric Care, 44*(2), 89–98.
National Organization for Victim Assistance (NOVA). Retrieved from http://www.trynova.org
Office for Victims of Crime. (n.d.). Serving crime victims with disabilities. Retrieved from http://www.ovc.gov/publications/infores/ServingVictimsWithDisabilities_bulletin/welcome.html
Office for Victims of Crime. (2002). First response to victims of crime who have disability (NCJ 195500). Retrieved from http://www.ojp.usdoj.gov/ovc/publications/infores/firstrep/2002/NCJ195500.pdf

Sullivan, P., & Knutson, J. (2000). Maltreatment and disabilities: A population-based epidemiological study. *Child Abuse & Neglect, 24*(10), 1257–1273.

Tyiska, C. (1998; updated 2008). *Working with victims of crime with disabilities.* National Organization for Victim Assistance. Retrieved from http://www.ojp.usdoj.gov/ovc/publications/factshts/disable.htm

Wayne State University. (2004). *Michigan study on women with physical disabilities.* Washington, DC: U.S. Department of Justice, National Institute of Justice.

12

Intimate Partner Violence in Adults

DEFINITION

There is no universally accepted definition of intimate partner violence (IPV), formerly known as domestic violence. However, the Centers for Disease Control and Prevention (CDC, 2006) define IPV as abuse that occurs between two people in a close relationship. Thus, violence by a domestic partner from whom a person has separated and moved away is a form of IPV. The term "intimate partner" includes current and former spouses and dating partners, and the violence exists along a continuum from a single episode of violence to ongoing battering. The scope of IPV includes the following:

- Physical abuse occurs when the perpetrator hurts or tries to hurt a partner by hitting, kicking, choking, pushing, punching, choking, pushing, punching, burning, or other physical force.

- Verbal abuse can take the form of constant criticism, making humiliating remarks, using abusive language, mocking, name-calling, yelling, swearing, and interrupting.

- Threats include the use of words, gestures, weapons, or other means to communicate the intent to cause harm.

- Sexual abuse is forcing a partner to take part in a sex act when the partner does not consent.

- Emotional abuse includes disrespect, minimizing, denying, blaming, and isolating.

- Stalking generally describes a pattern of overtly criminal and/or apparently innocent behaviors whereby an individual inflicts repeated, unwanted communications and intrusions upon another. Stalking has also been referred to as a pattern of behavior directed at a specific person that would cause a reasonable person to feel fear. It can be distinguished from other crimes in two ways: stalking involves repeated victimization, and it is partly defined by its impact on the victim.

- Financial abuse includes the perpetrator's not paying bills, refusing to give the partner money, hiding or withholding financial resources, not letting the partner work or interfering with the partner's job, and refusing to work and support the family.

- Coercion consists of making the partner feel guilty, manipulating the children and other family members, and making up impossible rules and punishing the partner for breaking them.

- Animal cruelty consists of harming or threatening to harm the family pets to control the partner.

- Property destruction occurs when the perpetrator destroys furniture, punches walls/doors, throws things, breaks dishes, or causes other destruction of the victim's or joint property.

Children Exposed to Intimate Partner Violence

Parents may think that their children are shielded from exposure to intimate partner violence; however, research findings indicate otherwise. Research suggests that children frequently observe or hear the abuse as well as its aftermath (e.g., crying or injuries). In a sizable percentage of cases the children are actually physically involved in their parent's partner violence and may be injured themselves.

Children exposed to intimate partner violence experience the risk of exposure to traumatic events, the risk of neglect, the risk of being abused, and the risk of losing one or both of their parents. These traumas can lead to negative outcomes for children and may affect their well-being, safety, and stability. Childhood problems associated with exposure to domestic violence fall into three primary categories.

Psychological: Fear, anxiety, low self-esteem, withdrawal, and depression; problematic relationships; higher levels of aggression, anger, hostility, oppositional behavior, and disobedience

Cognitive: Lower cognitive functioning, poor school performance, lack of conflict resolution skills, limited problem-solving skills, pro-violence attitudes, and belief in rigid gender stereotypes and male dominance

Long-term: Higher levels of depression and trauma symptoms, increased tolerance for and use of violence in relationships during adulthood.

Reaction and risk exist on a continuum. Some children demonstrate resiliency, while others show signs of maladaptive adjustment. Protective factors can help shield children from the adverse affects of exposure to domestic violence. These include: social competence, intelligence, high self-esteem, outgoing temperament, strong sibling and peer relationships, and a supportive relationship with an adult.

PREVALENCE

Domestic or intimate partner violence within one's home is the most commonly reported crime in America. Anywhere in America, domestic violence is the most common crime to which law enforcement must respond. Law enforcement defines domestic violence or intimate partner violence as physical violence. Law enforcement is called when a victim, someone else in the household, or a neighbor has called police because of physical violence or a perceived threat of physical violence.

Each year, women experience about 4.8 million intimate-partner-related physical assaults and rapes, while men are the victims of about 2.9 million intimate-partner-related physical assaults. Women aged 16–24 years are more likely than other women to be victims of IPV, and 20% to 30% of university women report violence during a date. Half of homeless women and children are fleeing domestic violence. According to the Bureau of Justice Statistics (2007), between 2001 and 2005, nonfatal intimate partner victimizations represented 22% of nonfatal violent victimizations against females age 12 or older, and 4% of nonfatal violent victimizations against males age 12 or older. Regarding fatal IPV, 30% of all homicides were female victims of IPVs and 5% of all homicides were male victims of IPV. Spousal homicide rates for all groups peak in the 15- to 24-year-old age category, and as the age differential between husband and wife increases, so does the risk of spouse homicide. Like many other types of violence, the actual incidence of IPV is unknown. Many victims do not report IPV to police, friends, or family because they fear that people will not believe them. Other do not report because they think that no one can help them.

Very little is known about the number of men who are abused or treated violently by women within a relationship. However, it is estimated that, every year in the U.S., about 3.2 million men are the victims of an assault by an intimate partner.

ETIOLOGY

Violence within a relationship is usually analyzed by academics in a context of one person victimizing another. This certainly may be true, but it is also possible that violence is a way of life in some families, and it is difficult to determine, at a superficial glance, who is the victim and who is the offender. Both parties may be physically violent and emotionally abusive. At the moment when health care or law enforcement becomes aware of a violent episode, identifying who is the victim and who is the offender may or may not be easy to discern. It is possible that for some people, violence is a common response to frustration in both men and women in a domestic or interpersonal relationship.

In families in which one partner or the other or both display violent behavior, it is not unusual for the children of such a relationship to be exposed to violence as well. Health care providers should be aware that detection of one type of violence within a home should lead to careful evaluation as to other sources of violence and other victims of violence, including partners, elders, children, and pets.

The cycle of violence is descriptive of the pattern of abuse and consists of the cycle's three components:

1. Tension building
2. Explosive, acute battering
3. Absence of tension, also called loving respite, reconciliation, or the "honeymoon phase"

Health care providers should understand the three components of the cycle of violence to fully grasp the nature of domestic violence, its clinical presentation, and appropriate intervention. During the tension-building phase, the victim frequently actively tries to avoid violence. Despite these efforts, the abuser still becomes angry with increasing frequency and intensity. Sometimes the victim may be so terrified during the tension-building phase that she or he attempts to precipitate abuse, just to get through the episode. When battering occurs, it frequently is followed by a period during which the batterer is contrite and demonstrates loving behavior.

Victims do not leave their abusive partners for a number of reasons. Some do not want to lose their partner's perceived love; some hope the partner will change; and many are dependent on the partner for financial reasons. Some women fear for the safety of their children and or pets. However, one of the most significant reasons why battered partners do not leave is fear. The most dangerous time for a battered woman is when she attempts to leave her batterer. Women who are separated from their husbands have a risk of violence about three times more than the risk of divorced women and approximately 25 times more than that of married women. Almost 75% of domestic assaults reported to law enforcement occur after separation of the couple, with women most likely to be murdered when reporting abuse or attempting to leave an abusive relationship.

ASSESSMENT

General Principles

IPV increases mortality and morbidity, decreases general health, and increases chronic pain, substance abuse, reproductive disorders, poor pregnancy outcomes, and overuse of health services. Victims of IPV have many unmet needs for services; however, they may be resistant to obtaining these services. Those performing assessment and intervention should consider the cycle of violence and reasons for not leaving. This will help them to understand clients' willingness to accept help and take steps to extricate themselves from the domestic violence. The client may be more amenable to intervention during the tension-building and battering phases. However, during the reconciliation phase, the battered person typically is showered with expressions of love and apology and with assurances that the abuse will never happen again. The dynamics of this stage usually make it less likely that a client will be willing to seek or receive help.

Careful detection of injury and referral for medical intervention is essential. Btoush and Campbell (2009) reviewed 111 Emergency Department (ED) charts that contained a code for IPV. The information for the study was retrieved from a national survey of emergency departments (12 visits for IPV per 100,000 ED visits). Review of the data revealed that 86% of the time, the victim of IPV presented to the ED with a complaint of pain. Fifty percent presented with a complaint of physical or sexual violence. Thirty-eight percent reported with a complaint of injuries to the body. The most common ED interventions were radiologic testing, wound care, and pain management. The most common disposition of the patients was referral to a physician or clinic (42%). Return to the ED was the disposition in 20% of the cases and referral to supportive services including social work services was 14%.

The most critical part of the assessment is ascertaining the safety of the victim, the children, other family members living in the home, and the family pets.

History

Health care providers should realize that the batterer often accompanies the patient to the emergency department (ED). The batterer may refuse to leave the patient alone, may insist on answering questions for the patient, and may display hostility or anger directed at the patient or medical staff. The victim may seem afraid or reluctant to disagree with her companion's explanation of what occurred and may even not attempt to speak for herself. These factors should raise suspicions and reinforce the necessity for taking the history in private.

In incidences of mandatory reporting, inform the client about limited confidentiality. As of 2009, six states (California, Colorado, Kentucky, New Hampshire, New Mexico, and Rhode Island) have mandatory reporting laws for IPV, whereby suspicions must be reported to a law-enforcement agency, even over the protests of the victim involved. If a translator is needed, do not use someone from the client or suspected abuser's family. Ask simple but direct questions, such as "Has your partner ever punched or kicked you?" instead of asking the client if she was "battered." When questioning the family, be careful, because the batterer may be among them. Use open-ended questions, such as "Jennifer seems upset today. What have you noticed about her?"

The following may indicate IPV:

History inconsistent with the type of injury

Time delay between injuries and presentation

An "accident-prone" history for the victim

Vague complaints of sexual problems, depression, or anxiety

Acute pain with no visible injuries

Chronic pain (especially if evidence of tissue damage cannot be found)

Repetitive complaints inconsistent with organic disease

History of multiple prior visits to the ED (traumatic and non-traumatic)

Noncompliance with treatment regimens and/or missed appointments

Problem pregnancies, preterm bleeding, and/or miscarriage, or self-induced abortion

Injuries during pregnancy

Repetitive psychosomatic complaints

History of being restrained or locked in or out of shared domiciles

Depression and suicidal ideation/gestures/attempts (Clients with psychiatric complaints should always be questioned about current or past domestic violence.)

Anxiety, panic attacks, other anxiety symptoms, and posttraumatic stress disorder (PTSD)

Fatigue and chronic headaches

Abuse of alcohol and other drugs

Palpitations, dyspnea, atypical chest pain, abdominal or other GI complaints, dizziness, and paresthesias

Current or past self-mutilation

Injuries sustained in a single-vehicle crash, either as driver or passenger

Physical Assessment

Health care providers should refer to chapters 3 and 4 for more detailed information in forensic assessment and evidence collection. Pay special attention to:

Bilateral injuries, especially to the extremities

Multiple injuries

Fingernail markings

Signs of manual or ligature strangulation

Cigarette or rope burns

Patterned injuries

Signs of blunt force trauma

Subconjunctival hemorrhages

Injuries of the face, neck, throat, and genitals

Signs of sexual assault (labial or vaginal hematomas, small vaginal lacerations, or rectovaginal foreign bodies)

Defensive injuries, including fractures, dislocations, sprains, and/or contusions of the wrists or forearms

Violence during pregnancy

Diagnostic Testing

Diagnostic testing is recommended as per agency protocols, including diagnostic radiology and laboratory analysis. Any diagnostic testing done in a medical context may enhance the law enforcement investigation of intimate partner violence. Diagnostic testing may detect any old untreated injuries. These older injuries may be important to health care as well as to law enforcement. Diagnostic testing may also be important for evaluating the severity of injury, including head injury.

The Family Violence Prevention Fund (http://www.endabuse.org) has several tools for the assessment of IPV, many of which are online and/or downloadable to MP4 players.

INTERVENTION

The Joint Commission on Accreditation of Healthcare Organizations (JCAHO) requires hospitals to have policies for the identification, evaluation, management, and referral of adult victims of domestic violence, including the following:

1. The hospital is responsible for safeguarding information and evidentiary material(s) that could be used in future actions as part of the legal process.
2. Hospitals must have policies and procedures that define their responsibility for collecting these materials and must define these activities and specify who is responsible for their implementation.

Elements to be documented in the patient's medical record include consents from the patient, parent, or legal guardian, or compliance with other applicable laws; evidentiary material released by the patient; legally required notifications and releases of information to authorities; and referrals made to community agencies for victims of abuse.

The health care provider should:

- Provide a safe environment, which may include referral to a shelter. The safety plan must include a safe place for the children and the family pets. Some shelters do not allow male children over age 12; few accept pets. Therefore, health care providers should contact social services to assist in the placement of older male children and the local animal shelter or animal control for pets.
- Report suspected child abuse to legal authorities (this is mandated). Health care providers are not mandated to report animal cruelty; however, felony animal cruelty may warrant psychiatric treatment in some states and may create an avenue of treatment for the batterer.
- Treat physical injuries and other medical or surgical problems. If client has been sexually assaulted, see chapters 17 (females) or 18 (males).
- Acknowledge the abuse and reassure the client that she or he is not to blame for it.
- Counsel the patient that violence may escalate.

- Discuss the possible physiologic and psychological reactions of trauma syndromes (see chapter 10).
- Refer the victim to counseling and/or a victim advocacy center. The latter usually provides counseling, as well as assistance with legal issues and obtaining shelter.
- Refer those who wish to stay in the relationship to counseling agencies that also provide interventions for the batterers. Many victims choose to stay in relationships that have been violent. The victim may choose therapy for the identified violent individual in the family.
- Determine the need for legal intervention and report abuse when appropriate or mandated.
- Suggest a civil order of protection (see chapter 10) to a victim of intimate partner violence. According to Logan and Walker (2009), protection orders are effective three out of five times they are issued.
- Help the victim create a safety plan. The plan should include safety at home and at work, a plan to leave the batterer, and what to do after leaving. There are several plans available; however, the National Center for Victims of Crime has a plan that can be printed free of charge directly from the Internet at http://www.ncvc.org/ncvc/main.aspx?dbName=DocumentViewer&DocumentID=41374.
- Develop a follow-up plan that includes follow-up phone contact and appointments.

PREVENTION/PATIENT TEACHING

Primary Prevention

Primary prevention for intimate partner violence includes interventions such as teaching nonviolent methods for resolving conflict. Programs initiated by education systems, social work programs, or advocacy groups include teaching nonviolent methods for resolving issues, via schools and churches and community centers.

Secondary Prevention

The U.S. Preventive Services Task Force states that it cannot determine the balance between the benefits and the harms of screening for family and intimate partner violence among children, women, and older adults at this time. However, given the statistics on IPV, and its significant mortality and morbidity, screening seems prudent. Several tools are available for screening, and no one screening tool is used universally. The mnemonic SAFE, developed by Sebastian (1996), directs inquiry into domestic violence.

S = stress/safety: What stress do you experience in your relationships? Do you feel safe in your relationship? Should I be concerned for your safety?

A = afraid/abused: What happens when you and your partner disagree? Do any situations exist in your relationships that cause you to feel afraid? Has your partner ever threatened or abused you or your children (or your pets)? Have you been physically hurt by your partner? Has your partner forced you to have unwanted sexual relations?

F = friends/family: If you have been hurt, are your friends or family aware of it? Do you think you could tell them if it did happen? Would they be able to give you support?

E = emergency plan: Do you have a safe place to go and the resources you (and your children and pets) need in an emergency? If you are in danger now, would you like help in locating a shelter? Do you have a plan for escape? Would you like to talk with a social worker, counselor, or health care professional to develop an emergency plan?

Abuse Assessment Screen (AAS): The AAS is a validated tool that contains five simple questions, using a checklist and body map for easy and efficient documentation (http://www.ucdmc.ucdavis.edu/medtrng/pdf/Abuse_Assessment_english.pdf).

Abuse Assessment Screen-Disability (AAS-D): The AAS-D is a four-question screening tool developed specifically for women with disabilities. Standard screening tools may not expose abuse common to women with disabilities, such as withholding assistance or treatment (http://www.rnao.org/pda/wabuse/page14.html).

HITS Domestic Violence Screening Tool: The HITS scale shows good construct validity in its ability to differentiate family practice patients from abuse victims. HITS also differentiates between male victimized respondents and nonvictims in clinical settings (http://www.orchd.com/CommunityViolence/DomesticScreenTool.pdf).

Tertiary Prevention

According to Btoush and Campbell (2009), only 14% of victims of IPV seen in EDs were referred to social services. The public health nature of this issue requires referral for all victims of IPV into appropriate support services. A referral to support services should be made in every case of identified IPV. According to Kothari and Rhodes (2006), of 964 female victims of IPV, surveyed via the prosecutor's office, 81.7% of the victims generated 4,456 ED visits. ED visits may not be an appropriate venue for health care interventions for many victims of IPV.

RESOURCES

Domestic Violence: Medline Plus: http://www.nlm.nih.gov/medlineplus/domesticviolence. html
National Coalition Against Domestic Violence: http://www.ncadv.org
National Domestic Violence Hotline: http://www.ndvh.org

REFERENCES

Bell, K. M., & Naugle, A. E. (2008). Intimate partner violence theoretical considerations: Moving towards a contextual framework. *Clinical Psychological Review, 28*(7), 1096–1107.
Btoush, R., Campbell, J. C., & Gebbie, K. M. (2009). Care provided in visits coded for intimate partner violence in a national survey of emergency departments. *Women's Health Issues, 19*(4), 253–262.
Burnett, L., & Alder, J. (2009). Domestic violence. *Emedicine.* Retrieved from http://emedicine.medscape.com/article/805546-overview
Bureau of Justice Statistics. (2007). Retrieved from http://www.ojp.gov.bjs
Centers for Disease Control and Prevention. (2006). *Understanding intimate partner violence: Fact sheet.* Retrieved from http://www.cdc.gov/violenceprevention/pdf/IPV-FactSheet.pdf
Daugherty, J. D., & Houry, D. E. (2008). Interpersonal violence screening in the emergency department. *Journal of Postgraduate Medicine, 54*(4), 301–305.
Gunter, J. (2007). Interpersonal violence. *Clinics of North America, 34*(3), 367–388.
Horner, G. (2005). Domestic violence and children. *Journal of Pediatric Health Care, 19,* 206–212.
Koenen, K., Moffitt, T., Caspi, A., Taylor, A., & Purcell, S. (2003). Domestic violence is associated with environmental suppression of IQ in young children. *Development and Psychopathology, 15*(2), 297–311.
Kothari, C. L., & Rhodes, K. V. (2006). Missed opportunities: Emergency department visits by police identified victims of intimate partner violence. *Annals of Emergency Medicine, 47*(2), 190–199.
Kropp, P. R. (2008). Intimate partner violence risk, assessment and management. *Violence and Victims, 23*(2), 202–220.

Logan, T., & Walker, R. (2009). Protection order outcomes: Violations and perceptions of effectiveness. *Journal of Interpersonal Violence, 24*(4), 675–692.

McHugh, M. C., & Friez, I. H. (2006). Interpersonal violence: New directions. *Annals of the New York Academy of Science, 1087*, 121–141.

Osofsky, J. (1999). The impact of violence on children. *The Future of Children: Domestic Violence and Children, 9*(3), 35–49.

Plichta, S. B. (2004). Interpersonal violence and physical health consequences: Policy and practice implications. *Journal of Interpersonal Violence, 19*(1), 1296–1323.

Robin, R. E., Rubin, R., Jennings, J., Campbell, J., & Bair-Merritt, M. (2009). Intimate partner violence screening tools: A systemic review. *American Journal of Preventative Medicine, 35*(5), 439–445.

Rothman, E., Meade, J., & Decker, M. (2009). Email use among a sample of IPV shelter residents. *Violence Against Women, 15*(6), 736–744.

Salber, P., & Taliafrro, E. (2006). *The physician's guide to intimate partner violence and abuse: A reference for all health care professionals* (2nd ed.). Volcano, CA: Volcano Press.

Swan, S. (2008). Review of research on women's use of violence with male intimate partners. *Violence and Victims, 23*(3), 301–314.

Thomas, I. (2009). Against the mandatory reporting of intimate partner violence. *Virtual Mentor, 11*(2), 137–140.

13 Intimate Partner Violence in Older Adults

DEFINITION

The National Clearinghouse on Abuse in Later Life defines later life intimate partner violence (IPV) as violence that occurs when older individuals, those aged 50 and older, are physically, sexually, or emotionally abused, exploited, or neglected by someone with whom they have an ongoing relationship. The abuser intentionally uses coercive tactics, such as isolation, threats, intimidation, manipulation, and violence to gain and maintain control over the victim.

PREVALENCE

The prevalence of IPV in elder relationships is unknown. However, as baby boomers (those born between 1946 and 1964) age, it is likely that the numbers will increase. Bonomi et al. (2007) randomly sampled a total of 370 English-speaking women (65 years of age and older) in a cross-sectional telephone interview. The researchers used 5 questions from the Behavioral Risk Factor Surveillance System (BRFSS) and 10 questions from the Women's Experience with Battering (WEB) Scale to assess the women's exposure to partner violence. Their results showed that

131

lifetime partner violence prevalence was 26.5%; 18.4% of women experienced physical or sexual violence and 21.9% experienced nonphysical violence (threats or controlling behavior). Past-5-year violence prevalence was 3.5%, and past-year violence prevalence was 2.2%. Many abused women reported more than 20 episodes of violence in their lifetime, with the median duration ranging from 3 years (forced sexual contact) to 10 years (controlling behavior). The proportion of abused women rating their abuse as severe ranged from 39.1% (forced sex or sexual contact) to 70.7% (threats). The researchers concluded that the high lifetime partner violence occurrence, frequency, duration, and severity of partner violence suggest a need for increased efforts to address partner violence in older women.

ETIOLOGY

Intimate partner violence can persist for many years. If the victim of the intimate partner violence does not report the violent living situation to others, no intervention may take place for many years. Women or men may choose to stay in interpersonal violence situations for many reasons, including fear, lack of financial security, lack of family support, and/or the belief that children need both parents regardless of the home situation.

IPV can also begin later in life. Dementia can create an interpersonal violence situation that is new to the relationship. In these cases, the afflicted individual may be either the victim or offender. Later life substance abuse may also underlie IPV, as can the change in lifestyle that comes with retirement, declining physical and mental health, and reduced sexual ability.

There are many reasons why victims maintain contact with abusers or feel they cannot leave an abusive relationship; some are the same as for younger victims and some are different. Some stay because they love or care about the abuser; some want to keep the family together for many reasons, including religious and cultural beliefs. Other victims fear that they will be seriously hurt or killed if they leave their abusers, while still others do not have the financial resources and/or housing they need to leave. Many older victims also have medical conditions and disabilities that may make living on their own difficult or impossible, or the abusive individual may need the victim's care.

ASSESSMENT

General Principles

Health care providers often struggle to believe that domestic violence happens to women beyond the age of 45. They also struggle to accept that older adults can be in intimate relationships or that they can be violent. Thus, health care providers must first accept the fact that elder IPV exists.

Abuse of an elder within a relationship is similar and yet different from other types of family violence. Older people can experience abuse from their partner throughout their lives. Whereas children and younger victims of domestic violence are healthy and not expected to die, older people may be suffering from additional health problems and are more vulnerable to dying from abuse. Victims of abuse share similar characteristics such as fear of retaliation, fear of stigmatization, a desire not to leave home, a desire to protect the abuser, and emotional distress. In cases of elders and IPV, dementia or diminished capacity makes communication of the abuse difficult.

History and Physical Assessment

Health care providers should refer to chapter 12 for information on IPV in adults. They should also consider the following factors that are specific to older adults. In general, studies indicate that injured elderly persons differ from the younger population in terms of cause of injury, response to injury, and outcome.

- Skin and mucous membranes—As a person ages, the skin becomes thin, loose, and transparent, and its vascularity decreases. The skin of the elderly is atrophic, making it more fragile. The lighter the skin of the elder, the more it tends to look pale and more opaque with age. The elder IPV victim has more skin and mucous membrane injury than the younger victims of abuse due to the fragility of the skin and mucous membranes. Fragility of the vessels in and under the skin creates bruising in the elderly. Elderly people bruise under force or pressure that would not create bruising in younger people. In a recent report published by the Department of Justice, bruising in elders who have been abused was located 40% of the time on the head, neck, and torso. This report also stated that inflicted bruises are larger than bruises occurring in an accidental circumstance.

- Abrasions—The elder's body should be examined for abrasions. If the elderly victim is pulled or dragged across a surface, the skin will abrade, or be rubbed off. This can be seen when an elder victim is dragged across pavement or grass, but it can also be seen, because of the fragility of the skin on elder victims, on those who have been dragged across a sheet or a carpet. If a pillow or similar object is held over the elderly victim's face, injury to the skin on the face is likely to occur.
- Cutting and lacerations—Cutting can occur if a knife or similar weapon is utilized in the commission of the crime. Lacerations from blunt force trauma are much more common in abuse and may occur from splitting of the skin due to force applied. If the elderly victim is punched, pulled, or restrained, the fragile skin will often tear, creating a laceration.

Diagnostic Testing

Diagnostic testing is recommended as per agency protocols, including diagnostic radiology and laboratory analysis. Any diagnostic testing done in a medical context may enhance the law enforcement investigation of intimate partner violence. Importantly, diagnostic testing may detect older, untreated injuries. These older injuries may be important to health care as well as to law enforcement. Diagnostic testing may also be important for evaluating the severity of injury, including head injury.

The Family Violence Prevention Fund (http://www.endabuse.org) has several tools for the assessment of IPV, many of which are online and/or downloadable to MP4 players.

INTERVENTION

The social situation of an elder is very different from that of children and younger women. Elders, even the most frail, have lived a long life, and even though they may be in need of protective services, they should not be infantilized. Policies and services are in place that are specific to elders. However, older women who are victims of IPV fall between the cracks because they may be overlooked by both domestic violence advocacy and by service resources designed for older persons. IPV programs generally serve women under the age of 50, while adult protective services focus on the frail and most vulnerable older adults.

Although health care providers would expect that domestic violence research and elder abuse research would include this population, researchers often exclude them. The domestic violence movement grew out of feminist organizations, and the movement to identify and treat elder abuse grew out of professionals' concern for frail and dependant older adults. Research does not support caregiver stress or dependence as primary causes of IPV in the elderly. In fact, the dynamics of power and control appear to be similar to cases of IPV in younger women.

Intervention, as in all cases of IPV, is extremely complex. Leaving the partner may not be an option for older women. Older women may not find support groups that include younger women helpful, and shelters filled with young women and children are not adapted for older women. Health care providers should approach the elder victim of IPV in a respectful and humanistic manner. Referrals to help resources must be individualized to the older person.

Not all situations of elder IPV require emergency intervention, but it is important to establish and move toward implementing a plan that will ensure the person's safety when it is suitable to the situation. Safety plans include: knowing a safe place to go if one needs to leave; altering one's routine to avoid using the same routes and behaviors repeatedly; carrying a cell phone; creating a kit with important documents such as bank account statements, birth certificates, medical records, insurance records, health care–related items including medications; saving extra money; and filling a bag with clothes and other essentials. If the elder has pets, they should be assisted in locating a shelter or rescue group that can harbor the pet in times of crisis. (A general safety plan checklist can be found at http://www.womenshealth.gov/violence/planning.) Health care providers must remember that elders have the capacity to refuse an intervention and do have the right to remain in the abusive situation.

Mandatory reporting and adult protection programs are linked. Most jurisdictions require professionals to report elder abuse, including elder IPV. A report of suspected abuse triggers an assessment and possible intervention by adult protective services. When an elder is abused and agrees to intervention, safety plans and alternative living arrangements can be arranged by adult protective services from any living arrangement, including nursing homes, personal care facilities, and assisted living facilities. If an elder refuses an intervention, an assessment must be made as to the elder's capacity to refuse. A determination must be made via adult protective services that the elder has the ability to understand the information presented to her or him and has the ability to apply the information as it is relevant to his or her situation. The elder must also be able to appreciate the consequences of a decision or lack of decision.

Mental capacity is specific to the situation at hand. The underlying question related to capacity is capacity to do exactly what. A blanket capacity statement does not exist. An elder may have capacity to consent to certain types of interventions but may not have capacity to consent to certain interventions. A delicate balance must be found for elders concerning their civil rights and self-determination, and interventions to prevent further IPV (see chapter 7 for more information). A sample safety plan for older adult victims of IPV can be found at http://www.ncall.us/docs/SafetyPlanExample10-06.pdf.

PREVENTION/PATIENT TEACHING

Primary Prevention

Education about elder IPV is an example of primary prevention. Increased knowledge for service providers and community members will result in early detection of elder IPV. In New York City, a program is in place in which education about elder abuse is distributed to public housing projects. This program, after its initiation, saw an increase in reporting of suspected elder abuse, including IPV. Increased appreciation for the fact that intimate partner violence can occur and be undetected for many years enhances the nursing care of elderly populations. The realization that IPV exists in the elder population will place intimate partner violence on the radar screen of nurses who care for elderly individuals. Primary screening for intimate partner violence should occur at all ages, including the elderly population. Asking the elder population about their safety and security in their home may reveal long-term interpersonal violence.

Secondary Prevention

Community nursing and day treatment programs for elders with physical deficits and/or dementia are examples of secondary prevention of elder abuse. The theory is that increased services will decrease stress for the people who are living with the elder. Increased understanding of the symptoms of dementia enhances the health care provider's ability to care for elderly clients. The domestic partners of people diagnosed with dementia should include screening for violence.

Tertiary Prevention

Tertiary prevention includes services provided to abused elders to prevent further violence. Providing alternative housing arrangements of an abused elder is one example. Diagnosing and treating elder abuse is fundamental to ensuring the protection of this vulnerable population. Recognizing intimate partner violence in the elderly population is important for all health care providers who work with elder populations in any clinical context. Recognizing the problem via history and physical examination and making appropriate referrals can prevent future violence between domestic partners.

RESOURCES

National Clearing House on Abuse in Later Life: http://www.ncall.us
Protocol for Older Domestic Violence Victims and Victims with Disabilities: http://www.daytonmunicipalcourt.com/pdf/PROTOCOL%20Addendum.pdf

REFERENCES

Abuse of power: A look into domestic violence among older people. (2008, October 27). *Nursing Times Net.* Retrieved from http://www.nursingtimes.net/abuse-of-power-a-look-into-domestic-violence-among-older-people/1907535.article
Bobb, J. (1995). Trauma in the elderly. *Journal of Gerontologic Nursing, 13,* 8–15.
Bonomi, A., Anderson, M., Reid, E., Carrell, D., Fishman, P., Rivara, F., et al. (2007). Intimate partner violence in older women. *The Gerontologist, 47,* 34–41.
Centers for Disease Control and Prevention. (n.d.). *Elder maltreatment.* Retrieved from http://www.cdc.gov/ViolencePrevention/eldermaltreatment/index.html
National Association of State Units on Aging. (2006). *Domestic violence in later life: A guide to the aging network for domestic violence and victim service programs.* Issue Brief, National Center on Elder Abuse. Retrieved from http://www.ncea.aoa.gov/ncearoot/Main_Site/pdf/publication/nceaissuebrief.agingnetworkguideDV.pdf

14 Lesbian, Gay, Bisexual, and Transgender Intimate Partner Violence

DEFINITION

Intimate partner violence is not confined to heterosexual relationships. Intimate partner violence can and does occur between lesbian couples, gay couples, bisexual couples, and couples in which one or both partners is transgendered. It is a common myth among the American public, including health care providers, that only heterosexual males perpetrate violence against their domestic partners.

Lesbians and gay men are individuals who develop intimate and/or sexual connections with members of the same sex. Bisexuals are individuals who develop intimate and sexual connections with others regardless of the other person's gender. Transgender individuals are individuals who feel that their gender is not congruent with their biological sex. Transgender does not imply sexual orientation.

PREVALENCE

Statistics on this crime are not collected by state and federal agencies; however, it is estimated that IPV occurs in approximately 30% to 40% of lesbian, gay, bisexual, and transgender (LGBT) relationships, which is the incidence of violence in heterosexual relationships. Bartholomew, Regan, White, and Oram (2008) reported that in interviews of 284 gay males who reported intimate partner violence, one-third of the victims were physically abused. All victims reported psychological abuse, and 10% of the victims reported sexual abuse.

The National Coalition of Anti-Violence Programs (NCAVP) reported that there were 3,319 reported incidents of intimate partner violence affecting LGBT individuals in 2007, a decrease (of 13%) versus the 3,839 incidents reported by NCAVP members in 2006. These results were from community-based antiviolence organizations in 14 regions throughout the United States. The regions include Tucson, Arizona; San Francisco; Los Angeles; Colorado; Chicago; Boston; Kansas City, Missouri; New York; Columbus, Ohio; Philadelphia; Houston, Texas; Virginia; Seattle, Washington; and Milwaukee, Wisconsin. Three regions reported murders attributable to LGBT intimate partner violence for a total of five IPV-related deaths in 2007, reported by New York (2), Illinois (2), and Pennsylvania (1). *Healthy People 2010,* a prevention agenda designed to identify significant preventable health threats in the United States, notes that it is important to realize that IPV does occur in lesbian, gay, bisexual, and transgender (LGBT) relationships and that there is a lack of research specific to IPV and LGBT communities (Gay and Lesbian Medical Association and LGBT Health Experts, 2001).

ETIOLOGY

IPV is always about power and control. One partner *intentionally* gains more and more power over his or her partner. Tactics can include physical, emotional, or verbal abuse; isolation; threats; intimidation; minimizing; denying; blaming; coercion; financial abuse; or using children or pets to control behavior. The etiology of intimate partner violence does not vary according to the sexual orientation of the victim. Bartholomew et al. (2008) note that many of the same background issues seen in heterosexual IPV relationships are present in LGBT IPV relationships. The similar variables noted are: income, education, substance abuse, attachment, and connection to a violent family of origin.

While the incidence, types, purpose, and cycle of abuse are similar to that of the heterosexual population, the Gay Men's Domestic Violence Project (http://www.gmdvp.org) points out that there are some key differences related to LGBT intimate partner violence:

1. There are very limited services for LGBT people affected by IPV, and in many areas there are no specific services for this population. Most mainstream domestic violence programs do not serve men, and most do not overtly indicate that they are LGBT-friendly.

2. Homophobia is still a huge problem in U.S. culture, as is as bi- and transphobia. This can cause LGBT IPV victims to be reluctant to seek service from mainstream organizations, including the police, courts, and health care, for fear of being abused by the system, which can range from discounting or minimizing their abuse, to inappropriate service, to refusal of service.

3. Most heterosexual professionals know little about LGBT people and less about domestic violence amongst LGBT people. This lack of knowledge hampers providing services for people affected by LGBT partner abuse, whether the support is informal from family and heterosexual friends or formal, through service providers such as mental health professionals or law enforcement.

4. Seeking services and support often means that an individual has to *come out*. This adds to the reluctance to use formal support services. The abuser may also use threats of outing the partner's sexual orientation or gender identity as another abusive means to control him or her.

5. Courts sometimes take away or withhold custody rights for children because of the parent's sexual orientation. Fear of losing custody of children creates yet another barrier to seeking formal services, and the abuser can also use this fear as another abusive control tactic.

6. Many LGBT people who are abused do not realize that they are being abused or do not label their experience as abuse, because they know too little about domestic violence. Even when they do understand they are being abused, they may not know what to do or where to go for help and support.

ASSESSMENT

General Principles

Recognizing the LGBT victim/survivor is an important first step to help referral resources. Health care providers should also recognize and appreciate how difficult it is for the victim to report this crime.

The Gay Men's Domestic Violence Project (http://www.gmdvp.org) suggests that service providers take the following steps to enhance their work with this population:

- Be knowledgeable about LGBT partner abuse, and be aware that anyone can be abused, men as well as women.

- Create a workplace environment in which individuals feel comfortable to talk about their abuse. This is especially true for LGBT people who need to know it is safe to talk about being LGBT and about their abuse. It is helpful to have LGBT-specific intimate partner violence posters and brochures, or better yet, gender-neutral posters and brochures.

- Routinely include questions about partner abuse in appropriate procedures, such as wellness assessments, health history, physical exams, and emergency room protocols.

- Screen for abuse during significant change events, such as when an individual is first seen by a provider, during a visit for a significant new complaint, and after every new intimate partner relationship begins, as well as 6 to 12 months after the relationship has begun.

- Be aware that it is not always obvious which partner is the abuser and which is the abused. Like other abusers, LGBT abusers sometimes portray themselves as the abused party.

- Know at least basic information about lesbians, gay men, bisexual men and women, and transgender individuals. This knowledge helps demonstrate that you are a "safe place" for LGBT people and that you understand the issues of abuse as they relate to LGBT people.

History and Physical Assessment

Flinck and Paavilainen (2008) report that gay male victims of intimate partner violence desire respect and human dignity when they report the crime. As with any victim of IPV, the interview must be conducted without the abusive partner present. Using open-ended questions and taking a nonjudgmental approach will assist the victim in reporting.

While many aspects of LGBT domestic violence are similar to those experienced by heterosexual victims, the National Coalition of Anti-Violence Programs (2007) notes that it is not in all ways the same. Perpetrators frequently use racism, homophobia, transphobia, classism, ableism, immigration, HIV status, and even the batterers' own vulnerabilities, to inflict harm.

Perpetrators often use highly specific forms of abuse based on identity and community dynamics. Perpetrators may:

- "Out" or threaten to out their partner's sexual orientation or gender identity to the partner's family, employer, police, religious institution, or community, or in child custody disputes and other situations where this information may pose a threat.
- Reinforce fears that no one will believe and/or help the partner because of the partner's sexual orientation, or that the partner deserves the abuse because of their sexual orientation.
- Justify abuse by stating that the partner is not "really" lesbian, gay, bisexual, or transgender.
- Tell the partner that abusive behavior is a normal part of LGBT relationships, or that it cannot be domestic violence because it is occurring between LGBT individuals.
- Monopolize support resources through the perpetrator's manipulation of friends and family supports and generating sympathy and trust in order to cut off these resources to the partner. This is major problem for those who live in small insular communities, where there are few community-specific resources, neighborhoods, or social outlets.
- Portray the violence as mutual and even consensual, especially if the partner attempts to defend against it, or portray it as an expression of masculinity or some other "desirable" trait.
- Depict the abuse as part of sado-masochistic (S/M) activity. Domestic violence is not an S/M activity, and nonconsensual violent or abusive acts that take place outside of a prearranged scene or in violation of predetermined safe words or boundaries are not to be considered part of, or justified as, a normal S/M relationship.

Diagnostic Testing

For more information on diagnostic testing, see chapter 12.

INTERVENTION

Detection and treatment of injury must occur for any victim of violence. Either partner in an LGBT relationship may be injured. According to

Meiz and Shaekelford (2008) women are more physically violent than men. Referrals are necessary, as with any form of interpersonal violence. As with any other adult victim/survivor of interpersonal violence, referral to help resources by nursing is critical to the health and well-being of the victim. When the victim is LGBT, resources for referral for counseling must be carefully considered. Resources within the LGBT population should be the first consideration for referral. See chapter 12 for further interventions.

PREVENTION/PATIENT TEACHING

Primary and Secondary Prevention

For more information on primary and secondary prevention, see chapter 12.

Tertiary Prevention

Weisz (2009) reports that heavy alcohol use, smoking, and obesity can result from untreated intimate partner violence in lesbian and bisexual women. Bartholomew et al. (2008) reported that in gay male relationships, intimate partner violence has parallels to heterosexual intimate partner violence in terms of the victim staying in the relationship for reasons of income, education, and attachment to the abusive partner. Substance abuse as a reaction in gay males is also noted by Bartholomew. Referrals to appropriate counseling for victims of this crime is essential.

RESOURCES

American Academy of Family Physicians Gay, Lesbian, Bisexual and Transgender Resources: http://www.aafp.org/online/en/home/membership/specialconst/patientpopulations/glbt.html

Gay, Lesbian, Bisexual and Transgendered Domestic Violence: http://www.rainbowdomesticviolence.itgo.com

Gay Men's Domestic Violence Project: http://www.gmdvp.org

National Center on Domestic and Sexual Violence: http://www.ncdsv.org/publications_lgbti.html

National Coalition of Anti-Violence Programs: http://www.ncavp.org

REFERENCES

Bartholomew, K., Regan, K., & White, M. (2008). Correlates of partner abuse in male same sex relationships. *Violence and Victims, 23*(3), 344–360.

Feldman, M. (2007). Interpersonal violence and HIV sexual risk behavior among Latino gay and bisexual men: The role of situation factors. *Journal of LGBT Research, 3*(4), 75–87. Retrieved from http://www.ncvc.org/ncvc/main.aspx?dbName=DocumentViewer&DocumentID=32369

Flinck, A., & Paavilainen, E. (2008). Violent behavior of men in intimate relationships, as they experience it. *American Journal of Men's Health, 2*(3), 244–253.

Gay and Lesbian Medical Association and LGBT Health Experts. (2001). *Healthy people 2010 companion document for lesbian, gay, bisexual, and transgender (LGBT) health.* San Francisco, CA: Gay and Lesbian Medical Association. Retrieved from http://www.lgbthealth.net/downloads/hp2010doc.pdf

Meiz, K., & Shaekelford, T. (2008). Interpersonal violence homicide methods in homosexuals, gays and lesbians. *Violence and Victims, 23*(1), 98–111.

National Coalition of Anti-Violence Programs. (2005). *Domestic violence.* Retrieved from httpa://www.ncavp.org/issues/DomesticViolence.aspx

National Coalition of Anti-Violence Programs. (2007). Lesbian, gay, bisexual and transgender domestic violence in the US. Retrieved from http://www.ncavp.org/common/document_files/Reports/2007%20NCAVP%20DV%20REPORT.pdf

Weisz, V. (2009). Social justice considerations: Lesbian and bisexual women in health care. *Journal of Obstetric, Gynecologic, & Neonatal Nursing, 38*(1), 81–87.

15 Elders Abused by Family Members

DEFINITION

The term *elder* is usually used to refer to persons over the age of 65. The legal definition of abuse includes the element of intentionality. It is required by law that the person who committed the abusive act(s) be aware that the behavior or absence of behavior is abusive. This definition excludes behavior that is accidental. The law also includes in the definition of the perpetrator of abuse a person who has responsibility or duty to protect and does so in an abusive manner.

There are six types of elder abuse:

- Physical abuse is the intentional use of physical force that may result in bodily injury and/or pain
- Neglect and self-neglect, the most common form of elder abuse, is the refusal of a caretaker or family member to provide the elder with adequate food, water, clothing, and medical attention. Self-neglect occurs when an elder adversely affects his or her own health and safety, usually by denying himself or herself food, water, shelter, clothing, and medical attention.
- Psychological abuse is the emotional abuse of an elder through the infliction of verbal actions, including insults and humiliation.

- Financial exploitation is the illegal or improper use of an elder's property or funds.
- Sexual abuse is nonconsensual sexual contact.
- Abandonment is the desertion of an elder by a caregiver or family member who has custody of the elder.

PREVALENCE

There are an estimated one to two million cases of elder abuse and neglect in the United States every year. Family members, adult children, or spouses are implicated in 90% of the cases of elder abuse, and those affected are usually elders who are cognitively or physically frail, physically disabled, depressed, lonely, lacking social support, and/or who lack familiarity with financial matters or have suffered recent losses. Both sexes can be abused, but females are more commonly victims.

Mortality rates in physically abused elders are significantly higher than for younger adults. Even with correction for severity of injury, elders are five to six times more likely to die of similar injuries than younger people. Elders who are victims of abuse, caregiver neglect, or self-neglect have triple the mortality of those never abused.

ETIOLOGY

As with other forms of violence, there is no single answer to explain behavior in an abusive relationship; many psychosocial and cultural factors are involved. However, several theories exist that explain elder abuse, and these can be divided into four major categories: physical and mental impairment of the patient, caregiver stress, transgenerational violence, and psychopathology in the abuser.

Recent studies failed to show direct correlation between elder frailty and abuse, even though this has been assumed to be a risk factor for abuse. Nevertheless, physical and mental impairment appear to play an indirect role in elder abuse, decreasing seniors' ability to defend themselves or to escape. The effect of stress factors—both stress caused by the elder (incontinence, wandering) and stressors in the caregiver's life (substance abuse, job loss)—may culminate in caregivers' expressions of anger or antagonism toward the elderly person, resulting in abuse. However, many caregivers endure multiple stressors without becoming abusive, and stressors may be more triggers than cause.

Transgenerational violence theory states that family violence is a learned behavior passed down from generation to generation. Thus the abused child continues the cycle of violence when he becomes caretaker to the parent. Psychopathology in the abuser theory focuses on a psychological deficiency in the development of the abuser, such as substance abuse, personality disorders, mental retardation, dementia, and other conditions. Unfortunately, family members with such conditions are most likely to be primary caretakers for elderly relatives, because they are the individuals typically at home due to lack of employment. Other risk factors are shared living arrangements between the elder person and the abuser, dependence of the abuser on the victim, and social isolation of the elder person.

ASSESSMENT

A red flag for elder abuse or neglect is withdrawal from necessary health care. Additional risk factors for elder abuse are advanced age, physical and or psychological impairment, incontinence, mental illness of the family member, and financial problems with the caregiver.

History and Physical Assessment

Routinely asking elders about safety and security as to living circumstances is recommended. When a family member of the elder is the perpetrator of neglect and/or abuse it is difficult for an elder to report the behavior. A shift in power does not change the affection a parent has for a child. It is very difficult for any parent to implicate a child in abuse or neglect. Rationalizations are commonplace in elder abuse/neglect situations when the perpetrator is a family member. The elder who is now in a dependant position needs a family member to care for him or her and is unlikely to implicate the family member in abuse. Implicating the family member may result in the elder being placed in a facility for care, and few elders desire such a placement. Acquiring a history from an elder regarding abuse requires that the elder be interviewed alone without family members present. (See chapter 13 for more information on elder assessment.)

It is suggested that health care professionals perform a Mini-Mental Status Examination (MMSE) to screen for cognitive dysfunction.

Cognitive dysfunction does not rule out abuse. On the contrary, it increases the elder's risk of abuse and may be the result of abuse (neglect, overmedication, head trauma, etc.).

When examining the elder person, assess the following areas for signs of abuse:

1. *Interactions between elder and caregiver*

Some "red flag" signs of elder abuse include the following behaviors of the caregiver:

- Caregiver constantly speaking for the elder when the elder is capable of speaking for her/himself
- Caregiver belittles, threatens, and uses other power and control techniques
- Strained or tense relationships, frequent arguments between the caregiver and elder
- Caregiver's refusal to allow you to see the elder alone

2. *General historical assessments and clinical observations of the elder*

Any of the following behaviors can be signs of any abuse, especially emotional abuse:

- Emotional distress such as crying, depression, or despair
- Nightmares or difficulty sleeping
- Sudden loss of appetite that is unrelated to a medical condition
- Confusion and disorientation (this may be the result of malnutrition)
- Emotional numbness, withdrawal, or detachment
- Regressive behavior
- Self-destructive behavior
- Fear toward the caregiver
- Unrealistic expectations about their care (e.g., claiming that their care is adequate when it is not)
- Significant weight loss or gain that is not attributed to other causes
- Stress-related conditions, including elevated blood pressure

- Behavior usually attributed to dementia (e.g., sucking, biting, rocking)

3. *Signs of physical abuse*

Be especially sensitive to the following when taking the elder's history and physical assessment:

History

- Unexplained injuries
- Implausible explanations for injuries (do not "fit" with the injuries observed)
- Discrepancies in injury history among family members
- History of similar injuries, and/or numerous or suspicious hospitalizations
- Elder brought to different medical facilities for treatment to prevent medical practitioners from observing a pattern of abuse
- Delay between onset of injury and seeking medical care

Physical Examination

- Unexplained signs of injury, especially if they appear symmetrically on two side of the body
- Signs of drug overdose or apparent failure to take medication regularly
- Broken eyeglasses or frames
- Sprains, dislocations, fractures, or broken bones
- Burns from cigarettes, appliances, or hot water
- Abrasions on arms, legs, or torso that resemble rope or strap marks
- Internal injuries (evidenced by pain and tenderness, difficulty with normal organ functioning, and bleeding from body orifices)
- Bruises, which are rarely accidental
- Signs of traumatic hair and tooth loss
- Bilateral bruising to the arms (may indicate that the elder has been shaken, grabbed, or restrained)
- Bilateral bruising of the inner thighs (may indicate sexual abuse)
- "Wrap around" bruises that encircle an older person's arms, legs, or torso (may indicate that the person has been mechanically restrained)

- Multicolored bruises (indicating that they were sustained over time)
- Injuries healing through "secondary intention" (indicating that they did not receive appropriate care)

4. *Signs of sexual abuse*

Some signals that sexual abuse has occurred include:

- Unexplained vaginal or anal bleeding
- Torn, stained, or bloody underclothing
- Genital or anal pain, irritation, or bleeding
- Bruises on external genitalia or inner thighs
- Difficulty walking or sitting
- Torn, stained, or bloody underclothing
- Unexplained sexually transmitted infections
- Inappropriate sex-role relationship between victim and suspect
- Inappropriate, unusual, or aggressive sexual behavior

5. *Signs of neglect by caregivers or self-neglect*

The assessment of the elder should include a focus on signs of possible neglect including:

Home

- Lack of necessities including food, water, heat
- Inadequate living environment evidenced by lack of utilities, sufficient space, and ventilation
- Animal or insect infestations and/or animal excrement
- Signs of medication mismanagement (empty or unmarked bottles, outdated prescriptions, too many or too few pills since date of dispensing)
- Unsafe housing (significant disrepair, faulty wiring, inadequate sanitation, substandard cleanliness, or architectural barriers

Person

- Unusual weight loss, malnutrition, dehydration
- Unsuitable clothing or covering for the weather

- Desertion of the elder at a public place
- Poor personal hygiene including soiled clothing, dirty nails and skin, matted or lice-infested hair, odors, and the presence of feces or urine
- Unclothed, or improperly clothed for weather
- Untreated physical problems, including decubiti
- Skin rashes
- Dehydration
- Untreated medical or mental health conditions
- Lack of needed dentures, eyeglasses, hearing aids, walkers, wheelchairs, braces, or commodes
- Exacerbation of chronic diseases despite a care plan
- Worsening dementia

6. *Signs of financial exploitation*

The assessment of the elder patient should be sensitive to the possibility of financial abuse or exploitation, including:

- Sudden changes in the elder's financial condition
- Items or cash missing from the elder's household
- Unusual changes in wills, power of attorney, titles, and policies
- Addition of names to the elder's signature card
- Unpaid bills or lack of medical care, although the elder has enough money to pay for them
- Financial activity the elder could not have done, such as an ATM withdrawal when the elder is bedridden
- Unnecessary services, goods, or subscriptions
- Unpaid bills, eviction notices, or notices to discontinue utilities
- Withdrawals from bank accounts or transfers between accounts that the older person cannot explain
- Bank statements and canceled checks no longer come to the elder's home
- Sudden appearance of new "best friends"
- Legal documents, which the elder did not understand at the time he or she signed them
- Unusual activity in the elder's bank accounts, including large withdrawals
- Care of the elder not commensurate with the size of his or her estate

- Caregiver expresses excessive interest in the amount of money being spent on the older person
- Missing belongings or property
- Suspicious signatures on checks or other documents
- Absence of documentation about financial arrangements
- Implausible explanations given about the elder's finances by the elder or the caregiver
- The elder is unaware of or does not understand financial arrangements that have been made for him or her

Differential Diagnosis

The diagnosis of elder abuse can be impeded by preexisting medical or psychiatric disorders, which may include:

Apathy

Drug and alcohol abuse

Depression

Dementia

Dehydration

Falls

Gait disturbances

Pathologic fractures

Coagulation disorders or medications

Diagnostic Testing

Health care providers should evaluate abused elders for evidence of infection, dehydration, electrolyte abnormalities, malnutrition, improper medication administration, and substance abuse. Laboratory tests may include: CBC, Chem-7 or Chemistry profile, calcium, magnesium, phosphorous, coagulation studies, medication levels, ethanol level and urine for drug screen. Imaging studies can include radiographs of relevant body parts to detect fractures; head CT to detect bleeding from trauma or rule out medical problems, such as hydrocephalus; and forensic sexual assault examination, if sexual assault is suspected (see chapter 19).

INTERVENTION

Once elder abuse is suspected, it should be reported to adult protective services per state statute and agency protocol. Mandatory reporting of elder abuse varies per state. For your state law, refer to http://www.rainn.org/public-policy/legal-resources/mandatory-reporting-database.

As with all abuse, the priority is to assure the elder is safe and that his or her emergent medical needs are attended. Safety may warrant hospital admission and obtaining an order of protection (see chapter 10). Referrals to social and mental health services are also warranted. A psychiatric evaluation can determine if the elder is capable of meeting his or her own basic needs, making decisions about services, offering testimony, and protecting him or herself against abuse. Counseling can help the elder assess their options, plan for their safety, resolve conflicts, and overcome trauma.

Many abused elders require legal assistance, which is provided by private attorneys, programs operated by local or state bar associations, or subsidized legal aid programs. The Older American's Act established a network of free legal services for persons over 60, and members of the American Association of Retired Persons (AARP) may be able to get legal assistance through AARP. Abused elders may need legal services for: orders of protection, lawsuits to recover their property or assets, annulments of trick marriages, guardianship (see chapter 7), or assistance with obtaining restitution.

PREVENTION/PATIENT TEACHING

Primary Prevention

Primary care focuses on strengthening or increasing exposure to factors that promote healthy aging and protect against sources of risk.

Secondary Prevention

The University of Iowa Department of Family Medicine Elder Mistreatment/Elder Abuse has several screening tools for elder abuse (http://www.uihealthcare.com/depts/med/familymedicine/research/eldermistreatment/screeninginstruments/index.html):

Actual Abuse Tool is a "first decision point that asks whether there has been a reliable report of abuse or violence."

Brief Abuse Screen for the Elderly (BASE) is designed to help practitioners assess the likelihood of abuse.

Caregiver Abuse Screen (CASE) screens for abuse through multiple sources (caregivers, care receivers, and/or abuse interveners) and is designed for community use.

Elder Assessment Instrument (EAI) is a comprehensive approach for screening suspected elder abuse victims in all clinical settings.

Health, Attitudes Toward Aging, Living Arrangements, and Finances (HALF) identifies elders at risk in a health service setting.

Hwalek-Sengstock Elder Abuse Screening Test (H-S/EAST) identifies elders at high risk of the need for protective services.

Indicators of Abuse (IOA) Screen screens for abuse and neglect at the client's home.

Risk of Abuse Tool identifies common risk factors associated with cases of elder abuse and/or domestic violence.

Tertiary Prevention

Post-discharge follow-up is needed to assure that the elder returns to a place of safety and not to the abuser, unless interventions have taken place to assure that the abuser will no longer harm the elder. Utilization of a case management or home nursing program can help assure that follow-up care is received.

RESOURCES

Administration on Aging: http://www.aoa.gov
Elder Abuse Medline Plus: http://www.nlm.nih.gov/medlineplus/elderabuse.html
National Center on Elder Abuse: http://www.ncea.aoa.gov
National Committee for the Prevention of Elder Abuse (NCPEA): http://www.prevent
    elderabuse.org
Office for Victims of Crime on Elder Abuse: http://www.ojp.usdoj.gov/ovc/help/ea.htm
State Resources on Elder Abuse Prevention: http://www.ncea.aoa.gov/NCEAroot/Main_
    Site/Find_Help/State_Resources.aspx

REFERENCES

Bird, P., Harrington, D., & Barillo, D. (1998). Elder abuse: Call to action. *Journal of Burn Care Rehabilitation, 19*(6), 522–527.

Brown, K., Streubert, G., & Burgess, A. (2004). Effectively detect and manage elder abuse. *Nurse Practitioner, 29*(8), 22–33.

Lachs, M., & Pillemer, K. (1995). Abuse and neglect of elderly persons. *New England Journal of Medicine, 332*(7), 437–443.

National Committee for the Prevention of Elder Abuse. Retrieved from http://www.preventelderabuse.org/index.html

Pearsall, C. (2005). Forensic biomarkers of elder abuse: What clinicians need to know. *Journal of Forensic Nursing, 1*(4), 182–186.

Sellas, M., & Krouse, L. (2009). Elder abuse. *Emedicine.* Retrieved from http://emedicine.medscape.com/article/805727-overview

United States Department of Justice. (2009). National Incidence Study on Elder Abuse. Retrieved from http://www.aoa.gov/AoARoot/AoA_Programs/Elder_Rights/Elder_Abuse/docs/ABuseReport_Full.pdf

Wiglesworth, A., Austin, R., Corona, M., Schneider, D, Laio, S., Gibbs, L., et al. (2009). Bruising as a forensic marker of physical elder abuse. *Journal of American Geriatric Society, 57*(7), 1191–1196.

16 Elders Abused by Health Care Workers

DEFINITION

As people age and become more fragile, they are less able to stand up for themselves or fight back if attacked. They may have mental, visual, and/ or auditory impairments that leave them more vulnerable to unscrupulous people who take advantage of them, including health care professionals whose very job is to care for them. Nursing home abuse is abuse perpetrated by health care providers against residents of a residential care facility, such as a nursing home or long-term care (LTC) facility. As with abuse by family members, categories include physical, emotional, sexual, and financial abuse, as well as neglect. Specific types of residential abuse include:

Inappropriate use of physical or chemical restraints

Deprivation of food or water

Giving too much medication or not giving prescribed medication

Forcing an older person to stay in a room

Disregard for the necessities of daily living

Lack of care for existing medical problems

Failure to prevent dehydration, malnutrition, and bed sores

Failure to assist in personal hygiene, or in the provision of food, clothing, or shelter

Failure to protect from health and safety hazards

Poor access to medical services

Resident on resident abuse (failure to protect by health care staff)

Harassment

Assault

Battery

Sexual Assault

Homicide (including serial homicide as seen in killings by so-called Angels of Death)

PREVALENCE

Unfortunately, few data are available on the numbers of elders abused in residential facilities. However, in 2003, state long-term care ombudsman programs nationally investigated 20,673 complaints of abuse, gross neglect, and exploitation on behalf of nursing home and board and care residents. Physical abuse was the most common type reported among seven types of abuse categories.

ETIOLOGY

Federal and state statutes mandate minimal care requirements in elder residential facilities. Those who do not comply with these guidelines and who abuse their elder clients do so for a number of various reasons: lack of training, inadequate staffing, substance abuse, mental illness, criminality, greed, and other factors.

Mercy and hero homicides are committed against the elderly. The mercy killer believes she or he is relieving the victim's suffering, while the hero killer creates a life-threatening condition for the victim and then unsuccessfully attempts to save the victim to gain notoriety. Both these types of murderers ("Angels of Death") tend to have multiple victims before detection.

ASSESSMENT

The assessment section in chapter 15 applies to these victims. However, health care professionals also need to be cognizant of other signs within facilities. Lindbloom and colleagues 2005) examined coroners' reports of elderly nursing home residents in Arkansas over a 1-year period. Although a majority of the coroner investigations did not raise suspicions of mistreatment, the researchers identified four categories of forensic markers that often led to referral for further investigation:

1. Physical condition of the patient: documented but untreated injuries; undocumented injuries and fractures; multiple, untreated, and/or undocumented pressure sores; medical orders not followed; poor oral care, poor hygiene, and lack of cleanliness of residents; malnourished residents who have no documentation for low weight; bruising on nonambulatory residents; bruising in unusual locations; statements from family concerning adequacy of care; and observations about the level of care for residents with nonattentive family members.
2. Facility characteristics in which the elder resides: unchanged linens; strong odors (urine, feces); trash cans that have not been emptied; food issues (unclean cafeteria); and documented problems in the past.
3. Inconsistencies within the facility: inconsistencies between the medical records, statements made by staff members, and/or observations of investigators; inconsistencies in statements among groups interviewed; and inconsistencies between the reported time of death and the condition of the body.
4. Specific markers for elder abuse in facilities: staff members who follow an investigator too closely; lack of knowledge and/or concern about a resident; unintended or purposeful verbal or nonverbal evasiveness; and a facility's unwillingness to release medical records.

The National Institute of Justice (2008) provides specific characteristics identified by researchers in Arkansas within four categories of markers that can be used to determine whether elder mistreatment is occurring or has occurred. These include:

1. Physical condition and quality of care

    Documented but untreated injuries
    Undocumented injuries and fractures
    Multiple, untreated, or undocumented pressure sores
    Medical orders not followed
    Poor oral care, poor hygiene, and lack of cleanliness of residents (e.g., unchanged adult diapers, untrimmed finger- and toenails)
    Malnourished residents that have no documentation for low weight
    Bruising on nonambulatory residents; bruising in unusual locations
    Family statements and facts concerning poor care
    Level of care for residents with nonattentive family members

2. Facility characteristics

    Unchanged linens
    Strong odors (urine, feces)
    Trash cans that have not been emptied
    Food issues (cafeteria smells at all hours; food left on trays)
    Past problems

3. Inconsistencies between—

    Medical records, statements made by staff members, or what is viewed by investigator
    Statements given by different groups
    The reported time of death and condition of the body

4. Staff behaviors

    Staff members who follow the investigator too closely
    Lack of knowledge or concern about a resident
    Evasiveness, unintended and purposeful, verbal and nonverbal
    Facility's unwillingness to release medical records

INTERVENTION

Medical and nursing records are critical in case building regarding elderly victimization by caregivers. Emphasis on an interdisciplinary approach to this form of elder abuse cannot be over-emphasized. No single person or agency can effectively meet the needs of an elder abused by a caregiver. Statements made by the elder, detection and documentation of injury, and caregiver statements must be documented via writing, traumagrams, and photography (see chapters 3 and 4). Proper documentation enhances investigation and actually decreases the possibility that the health care provider will be called to court in a criminal or civil action.

Suspected elder abuse via caregivers should be reported to Adult Protective Services (APS). The role of APS, in addition to taking reports, is to conduct investigations and arrange for services for the abused elder. Many states have hotlines for reporting, as well as laws requiring a report by health care professionals. Elder abuse is a crime. If the health care provider suspects elder abuse, APS and law enforcement should be notified. APS and law enforcement will investigate the case together. APS will determine the elder's functional capacity as well as his or her capacity to refuse interventions. Competent elders have the right to refuse APS services. If the victim agrees to accept services, a wide range of support can be given via APS, including safe living arrangements, meals, and financial management. Law enforcement will conduct an investigation to identify the perpetrator of abuse and hold the offender accountable for his or her behavior.

PREVENTION/PATIENT TEACHING

Primary Prevention

Teach families how to choose a quality facility. Choosing a long term care facility (LTC) is as important as choosing child care services. Once in a LTC facility, the elder is under the complete care of those who work there, and family members may not know something is wrong until something serious happens. These suggestions may make it easier for families to choose wisely:

- While this is not always possible, do not wait until the last minute to choose a facility. The best way to make the choice is to let the elder chose when that elder is still competent.
- Talk to family, friends, and health care providers to get recommendations on facilities.
- Know your rights. When hospitals want to hurriedly discharge elders to LTC facilities, families can demand time to investigate the facilities.

- Use the AARP Nursing Home Evaluation Checklist (http://assets. aarp.org/www.aarp.org_/promotions/text/life/NursingHome Checklist.pdf) when you evaluate each home. This helps you make a complete assessment and gives you an easy method of comparing different facilities.
- Begin your search with the Eldercare Locator (800-677-1116), which will connect you with your local Area Agency on Aging. They will give you a list of nursing homes in your area, as well as contact information for the local long-term care ombudsman. Your ombudsman cannot recommend one facility over another but will answer specific questions about staffing, continuing problems, and administration turnover.
- Visit the ones nearest to you. If you are a regular visitor, there are less likely to be problems.
- Visit unannounced, at different times of day to get a good sense of staffing. You will want to choose a facility with adequate staffing. Ask to have someone in charge, preferably the administrator, give you a tour.
- When touring, ask to see client rooms, dining areas, treatment areas, and socialization areas. Check for cleanliness, the courtesy of staff, and the staff–resident interactions. If the staff is disinterested in the residents, choose another facility.
- Note the activity level of the residents. Are they restrained? Subdued? Or are they interacting with each other and staff and engaged in fun or purposeful activities? Do they appear happy, well nourished, and clean?
- Ask for the weekly resident activity schedule and observe the activities scheduled for the time you are there to make sure the activities actually exist.
- Ask to sample a meal and ask for the weekly menu. Check to see if residents have drinking water available at their bedsides.
- Use the public restroom. Check it for cleanliness, adequacy of supplies including hand soap, and hot water temperature.
- If your family member likes pets, ask if they utilize animal-assisted activities (such as pet therapy) and if your family member can have his or her pet visit or stay with them.
- Ask your attorney to find out if there have been any citations or other negative reports on the facility.
- Once your family member is admitted, visit often and repeat the steps above to assure that all is still well.

Rigorous background checks of staff and volunteers can help minimize the numbers of potential elder abusers in health care facilities. Background checks can be obtained via the Federal Bureau of Investigation (FBI, 2007), state police, and state child/elder abuse reporting agencies. An FBI Identification Record (also called Criminal History Record or Rap Sheet) contains information taken from fingerprint submissions retained by the FBI in connection with arrests and, in some instances, federal employment, naturalization, or military service. If the fingerprints are related to an arrest, the Identification Record includes the name of the agency that submitted the fingerprints to the FBI, the date of arrest, the arrest charge, and the disposition of the arrest, if known to the FBI. All arrest data included in an Identification Record is obtained from fingerprint submissions, disposition reports, and other reports submitted by agencies having criminal justice responsibilities.

Staff should be well educated on the care of elder clients, including issues such as dementia, incontinence, sensory deprivation, and mobility. Staffing should be adequate for both the number and acuity/chronicity of the clients.

Secondary Prevention

Staff supervision should include monitoring for inappropriate staff behaviors, as well as signs of elder abuse. Early identification and intervention are critical to prevent further abuse to the affected elder as well as other elders.

Tertiary Prevention

If elder abuse is detected in a facility, investigation must follow to ensure that other residents of the facility are not being abused as well. Protecting the identified elder from future abuse via APS and law enforcement is critical.

Development of an accurate standard evaluation of functional capacity would assist in providing abused elders with more protection. The mini-mental status test often performed by APS workers is inadequate for determining functional capacity.

RESOURCES

Administration on Aging: http://www.aoa.gov
Elder Abuse: report elder abuse, nursing home neglect and financial exploitation: http://www.elder-abuseca.com/index.html

Federal Requirements for States and Long-Term Care Facilities: http://ecfr.gpoaccess. gov/cgi/t/text/text-idx?c=ecfr&sid=a16fe15dcc122a3dc4248181e6e4172c&rgn=div5 &view=text&node=42:5.0.1.1.2&idno=42

Long Term Care Ombudsman Resource Center: http://www.ltcombudsman.org

The National Consumer Voice for Quality Long-Term Care: http://nccnhr.org

Reporting Nursing Home Abuse: http://www.ncea.aoa.gov/ncearoot/Main_Site/Find_ Help/Help_Hotline.aspx

Stop Abuse for Everyone (SAFE): http://www.safe4all.org/help

REFERENCES

Bartholomew, M. (2010). Elder abuse and neglect. In R. Riviello (Ed.), *Forensic emergency medicine: A guide for clinicians* (pp. 165–170). Boston: Jones and Bartlett.

Dyer, C., Sanchez, L., Kim, J., Burnett, S., Mitchell, B., Reilley, S., et al. (2008). Factors that impact the determination by medical examiners of elder mistreatment as a cause of death in older people. *Final report to the Office for Victims of Crime.* Retrieved from http://www.ncjrs.gov/pdffiles1/nij/grants/223288.pdf

Federal Bureau of Investigation (FBI). (2007). Federal Bureau of Investigation record request. Retrieved from http://www.fbi.gov/hq/cjisd/fprequest.htm

Lindbloom, E., Brandt, J., Hawes, C., Phillips C., Zimmerman, D., Robinson J., et al. (2005). Role of forensic science in identification of mistreatment deaths in long-term care facilities. *Final report to the National Institute of Justice.* Retrieved from http://www.ncjrs.gov/pdffiles1/nij/grants/209334.pdf

MacNamee, C., & Murphy, M. (2006). Elder abuse in the United States. *NIJ Journal, 255.* Retrieved from http://www.ojp.usdoj.gov/nij/journals/255/elder_abuse.html

Mosqueda, L., Burnight, K., & Liao, S. (2006). Bruising in the geriatric population. Final report to the National Institute of Justice (NCJ 214649). Retrieved from http://www.ncjrs.gov/pdffiles1/nij/grants/214649.pdf

National Center on Elder Abuse. (2005). Fact sheet on elder abuse. Retrieved from http://www.ncea.aoa.gov/NCEAroot/Main_Site/pdf/publication/FinalStatistics050331.pdf

National Institute of Justice. (2008). Potential markers for elder mistreatment. Retrieved from http://www.ojp.usdoj.gov/nij/topics/crime/elder-abuse/potential-markers.htm

Otto, J. (2008, Summer). Fitting elder abuse into the family violence continuum. *Family and Intimate Partner Violence Quarterly, 1,* 89–95.

Reyes, K. (2007). Choosing a nursing home. *AARP Magazine.* Retrieved from http://www.aarpmagazine.org/health/embedded_sb.html

United States Department of Justice. (2000). *National incidence study on elder abuse.* Retrieved from http://www.aoa.gov/AoARoot/AoA_Programs/Elder_Rights/Elder_Abuse/docs/ABuseReport_Full.pdf

Wiglesworth, A., Austin, R., Corona, M., & Mosqueda, L. (2009). Bruising as a forensic marker of physical elder abuse. *Final Report to the National Institute of Justice.* Retrieved from: www.ncjrs.gov/pdffiles1/nij/grants/226457.pdf

17 Female Victims of Sexual Assault

DEFINITION

The World Health Organization (WHO, 1997) defines sexual violence as "Any sexual act, attempt to obtain a sexual act, unwanted sexual comments or advances, or acts to traffic, or otherwise directed against a person's sexuality using coercion, by any person regardless of their relationship to the victim, in any setting, included but not limited to home and work."

Health care and legal terminologies for sexual violence tend to differ, as they do for many other issues. "Rape" is a legal term that usually denotes unlawful sexual intercourse. Statutory rape is sexual penetration by an adult of a person who is legally incapable of consenting to sex, usually a minor under a specific age (not all states use age 18). Forced oral or anal intercourse may be labeled involuntary deviant sexual intercourse or sodomy in some jurisdictions.

The National Center for Victims of Crime notes that a sexual assault typically occurs when someone touches any part of another person's body in a sexual way, even through clothes, without that person's consent. Examples of sexual acts that fall under the category of sexual assault include forced sexual intercourse (rape), sodomy (oral or anal sexual acts), child molestation, incest, fondling, and attempted rape. All forms of sexual assault can be devastating to the victim. Perpetrators can be strangers, acquaintances, friends, or family members, and they commit sexual assault by way of violence, threats, coercion, manipulation, pressure, or tricks. Regardless of the circumstances, no one asks or deserves to be sexually assaulted.

Most jurisdictions have replaced the term *rape* with *sexual assault* in the state statutes. This term is more gender-neutral and covers more specific types of sexual victimization and various levels of coercion. For example, some state codes define Sexual Assault in the First Degree or Aggravated Sexual Assault as physically or psychologically forced vaginal, anal, or oral penetration (previously termed rape). Sexual Abuse, Sexual Misconduct, Sodomy, Involuntary Deviant Sexual Intercourse, Lascivious Acts, Indecent Contact, Indecent Assault and Indecent Exposure are all examples of sexual assault charges in various jurisdictions. Essentially, almost any sexual behavior a person has not consented to and that causes that person to feel uncomfortable, frightened, or intimidated is included in the sexual assault category.

The National Center for Victims of Crime notes that the law usually assumes that a person does not consent to sexual conduct if he or she is forced or threatened or is unconscious, drugged, a minor, developmentally disabled, chronically mentally ill, or believes they are undergoing a medical procedure. Some examples of sexual assault include:

- A person putting his finger, tongue, mouth, penis, or an object in or on a victim's vagina, penis, or anus without consent
- A person touching, fondling, kissing, or making any unwanted physical contact
- A person forcing a victim to perform oral sex or forcing the victim to receive oral sex
- A person forcing a victim to masturbate, or forcing the victim to masturbate them
- A person forcing a victim to look at sexually explicit material or forcing the victim to pose for sexually explicit pictures
- A health care professional giving a victim an unnecessary internal examination, or touching the victim's sexual organs in an unprofessional, unwarranted, and inappropriate manner.

Sexual assault victims deserve competent and compassionate care, and thus, those health care providers who perform sexual assault forensic examinations should receive adequate educational preparation and practicum prior to performing these exams. The *National Protocol for Sexual*

Assault Medical Forensic Examinations (http://www.ncjrs.gov/pdffiles1/ovw/206554.pdf) provides detailed guidelines for criminal justice and health care practitioners in responding to the immediate needs of sexual assault victims. Effective collection of evidence is of paramount importance to successfully prosecuting sex offenders, as is performing sexual assault forensic exams in a sensitive, dignified, and victim-centered manner. For individuals who experience this horrendous crime, having a positive experience with the criminal justice and health care systems can contribute greatly to their overall healing.

Several factors influence a victim's response to, and recovery from, sexual assault:

- Age and developmental maturity of the victim

- Frequency, severity, and duration of the assault(s)

- Setting of the attack

- Level of violence and injury inflicted

- Response by the criminal justice system

- Community attitudes and values

- Victim's relationship to the offender

- Meaning attributed to the traumatic event by the sexual assault survivor

- Response to the attack by police, medical personnel, and victim advocates

- Response to the attack by the victim's loved ones

- Social support network available to the victim

Some sexual assault survivors find they can recover relatively quickly, while others feel the lasting effects of their victimization throughout their lifetime.

PREVALENCE

Tjaden and Thoennes (2000) reported that 17.6% of women in then National Violence Against Women Survey (NVAWS) were raped at some time in their lives. In the United States the prevalence of rape is equal to one in every six women. Because some victims were raped more than one time, Tjaden and Thoennes (2000) estimated that 17.7 million women were forcibly raped at some time in their lives, with more than 300,000 women forcibly raped in the year prior to the survey.

Rape is much more extensive than what is reported and the majority of rapists are never arrested. In 2007, there were 90,427 incidents of rape reported to law enforcement and 23,307 arrests. More than one-half of all victims of sex crimes, including rape and sexual assault, are women younger than 25 years of age (Federal Bureau of Investigation, 2008).

ETIOLOGY

The etiology of sexual assault lies with the perpetrator (chapter 33). However, health care providers should understand why some women do not want to report this crime. A comparison of rape and sexual assault law enforcement statistics reveals that rape and sexual assault are very underreported crimes. The victim must perceive that a rape or sexual assault has occurred. The victim must decide that the act was illegal. The victim must also decide whether or not to disclose the assault. If the assault is reported to police, the police must decide whether or not the report meets the definition of an illegal act.

Guilt, fear of retribution, humiliation, and lack of knowledge and trust in the legal system and medical system are all important as to whether or not a person reports a sexual assault. It is not at all unusual, according to survey statistics, that denial that a crime occurred is a victim response. Women who perceived the assault to be violent were more likely to report the crime. Women may fear the response of the legal system to a report of rape or sexual assault. Campbell and colleagues (2001) found that only 25% of sexual assaults reported to the legal system were prosecuted. Of the 25% that were prosecuted, 10% were tried but the suspect was not convicted, 10% were convicted at trial, and 50% were resolved via a plea agreement.

Fear of retaliation was reported by some victims via analysis of survey data. Self-blame is a recurring theme for victims in cases of sexual assault. Self-blame is reinforced by friends and family who question the victim's behavior with questions such as: why were you there, why did you invite him, and why were you drinking.

The relationship between the victim and the offender can influence reporting and other victim responses to sexual assault. Bureau of Justice Statistics reported that the closer the relationship between the victim and the offender, the greater the likelihood that the victim will not report a crime.

ASSESSMENT

General Principles

Rape can produce psychological trauma in women. In a classic study, conducted by Burgess and Holstrom (1974), this trauma was noted immediately after the assault and for a period of time after the assault. Female victims in this study described flashbacks, intrusive thoughts, fear, anxiety, nightmares, daymares, and the development of phobias. In the immediate phase, the psychological response completely disrupts the woman's life. In the long-term phase, the victim reorganizes her disrupted lifestyle.

There is no one typology or profile that describes all sex offenders. Clinical experience, both with victims and offenders of reported sex crimes, makes it clear that three components are present in the offender: anger, power, and sexuality. The hierarchy and interrelationship among these factors is in the complete control of the offender. The victim's experience is dependent upon her particular offender's interrelationship with these factors. All victims suffer psychologically from a nonconsensual sexual experience. The degree of psychological trauma varies dependent upon many victim variables, such as age, education, and life skills, as well as the nature of the crime itself.

Physical injuries can and do occur in cases of sexual assault. The type and location of physical injury is related to what happens before, during, and after the assault. The offender must gain control of the victim in order for the crime to occur. The method of obtaining control may include drugs and/or alcohol, physical strategies, psychological strategies, or any combination of these strategies, and the victim may be injured due to restraint. Victims may also be injured deliberately by the perpetrator, who may be angry, sadistic, or trying to kill the victim to avoid having a witness. Injuries can be extensive. Before commencing, make sure to obtain written informed consent and to have all forms and equipment ready. Also make sure to inform the client about limited confidentiality.

History

The interview of the victim/survivor of sexual assault guides physical examination and evidence collection. If the victim/survivor is able to give information about what happened during the assault, this facilitates the location of injury and the location and nature of evidence.

The interview is affected by the psychological trauma the victim experiences post–sexual assault. Victims may have difficulty recalling details of the assault due to psychological trauma. Victims also have difficulty describing details related to the sexual components of the crime.

The history may take place with law enforcement present to minimize repetition and repeated trauma, as well as a victim advocate for support. Specific questions vary per jurisdiction, as do documentation forms; however, the following information should be sought routinely from clients, as per the *National Protocol for Sexual Assault Medical Forensic Examination*:

1. Date and time of the sexual assault(s): It is essential to know how much time has elapsed between the assault and the collection of evidence. Collection and interpretation of both the physical exam and evidence analysis may be influenced by the time interval between the assault and the exam.

2. Pertinent client medical history: The interpretation of physical forensic findings may be affected by medical data related to menstruation, recent anal-genital injuries, surgeries or diagnostic procedures, blood-clotting history, and other pertinent medical conditions or treatment.

3. Recent consensual sexual activity: DNA analysis makes it important to gather information about recent consensual intercourse, whether it was anal, vaginal, and/or oral, and whether a condom was used. Trace amounts of semen or other bodily fluid may be identified and may not be associated with the crime. It may need to be associated with a consensual partner and thus may be used for elimination purposes to aid in interpreting evidence.

4. Post-assault activities of clients: The quality of evidence is affected both by actions taken by clients, such as urinating, defecating, wiping genitals or the body, douching, removing/inserting tampons/sanitary pads/diaphragm, using oral rinse/gargling, bathing, brushing teeth, eating, drinking, smoking, using drugs, or changing clothing.

5. Assault-related client history: Information regarding memory loss, lapse of consciousness, vomiting, nongenital injury, pain and/ or bleeding, and anal-genital injury, pain, and/or bleeding can direct evidence collection and medical care. Toxicology samples are recommended if there was either loss of memory or lapse of consciousness, according to jurisdictional policy.

6. Suspect information (if known): Forensic scientists seek evidence on cross-transfer of evidence among clients, suspects, and crime scenes (Locard's principle, chapter 4). Knowing the gender and number of suspects may provide guidance to the types and amounts of foreign materials that might be found on clients' bodies and clothing. Suspect information should be limited to that which will guide the exam and forensic evidence collection, as detailed questions about suspects are asked during the investigative interview.

7. Nature of the physical assault(s): Information about the physical surroundings of the assault(s) (indoors/outdoors, car, alley, room, rug, dirt, mud, or grass) and methods employed by suspects is crucial to the detection, collection, and analysis of physical evidence. Methods are numerous and may include use of weapons (threatened and/or injuries inflicted), physical blows, grabbing, holding, pinching, biting, using physical restraints, strangulation, burns (thermal and/or chemical), threat(s) of harm, and involuntary ingestion of alcohol/drugs. Knowing whether suspects may have been injured during the assault may be useful when recovering evidence from clients or from suspects (e.g., bruising, fingernail marks, or bite marks).

8. Description of the sexual assault(s): An accurate but brief description is crucial to detecting, collecting, and analyzing physical evidence. The description should include any:

Penetration of genitalia, however slight
Penetration of the anal orifice, however slight
Oral contact with genitals (of clients by suspects or of suspects by clients)
Other contact with genitals (of clients by suspects or of suspects by clients, such as suspect rubbing genitals on victim's breasts)
Oral contact with the anus (of clients by suspects or of suspects by clients)
Nongenital act(s) (e.g., licking, kissing, suction injury, and biting)

Other act(s) including use of objects (such as penetration of vagina with soda bottle)

Whether ejaculation occurred and location(s) of ejaculation (e.g., mouth, vagina, genitals, anus/rectum, body surface, on clothing, on bedding, or other)

Use of contraception or lubricants

These questions may be difficult for clients to answer. Health care providers should explain that these questions are asked during every sexual assault medical forensic exam, and they should also explain why each question is being asked. It may help to show the client the documentation form so that she can see it is asked of everyone and that she is not being singled out.

Physical Assessment

Careful observation for injury is a priority for nursing as it relates to victims of sexual assault. Physical injuries related to the crime must be identified and treated. Any injury that requires medical intervention requires quick and accurate identification and rapid entry into necessary medical care. Any injury, whether it requires medical intervention or not, should be identified and documented. Documentation of any injury can be used by law enforcement and prosecution as evidence of the force aspect of hands-on sex crimes.

The *National Protocol for Sexual Assault Medical Forensic Examination* recommends the following for health care providers to facilitate the exam and evidence collection:

Recognize that the forensic purpose of the exam is to document physical findings and facilitate the collection of evidence from patients.

Strive to collect as much evidence from the victim as possible, guided by the scope of informed consent, the medical forensic history, examination findings, and evidence-collection kit instructions.

Be aware of evidence that may be pertinent to the issue of whether the patient consented to the sexual contact with the suspect.

Understand how biological evidence is tested.

Prevent exposure to infectious materials and contamination of evidence.

Understand the implications of the presence or absence of seminal evidence.

Modify the exam and evidence collection to address the specific needs and concerns of patients.

Explain exam and evidence collection procedures to patients.

Conduct the general physical and anogenital exam and document findings on body diagram forms.

Collect evidence to submit to the crime lab for analysis, according to jurisdictional policy.

Collect blood and/or urine for toxicology screening if applicable.

Keep medical specimens separate from forensic specimens collected during the exam.

According to one study, the prevalence of genital injury can range from 5% via direct visualization to 87% when a colposcope is utilized for detection. Staining with toluidine blue may increase the possibility of injury detection. The most common locations for injury, according to Sommers (2007), are:

posterior fourchette (tense band of tissue that connects the two labia minora), labia minora (two inner folds of skin within the vestibule of the vulva), hymen (thin membrane composed of connective tissue just inside the entrance to the vagina), fossa navicularis (shallow depression located on the lower portion of the vestibule and inferior to the vaginal opening).

Many health care providers use the TEARS pneumonic to describe the different types of genital injuries. This mnemonic device describes:

T = tears, any break in tissue integrity

E = ecchymosis, any discoloration of skin or mucous membranes; also called bruising

A = abrasion, skin excoriations caused by the removal of the most superficial layer of skin

R = redness, erythemous skin that is abnormally inflamed because of irritation

S = swelling, edematous or transient engorgement of tissues

This simple mnemonic device helps the health care provider search for different types of injuries that may occur to the genital area after rape or sexual assault.

In addition to genital injuries, the patient may experience injuries anywhere else on the body. These injuries may or may not require medical intervention. Injury to the body is common in sexual assault. In one survey of victims, one in five rape victims reported at least one nongenital injury. This survey, performed by Amar and Gennaro (2005), found that physical injury was detected in one-third of sexual assault victims who presented to a health care setting. Most of the injuries noted by health care personnel did not require medical intervention; however, 17% reported more serious injuries, including lacerations, broken bones, dislocated joints, head or spinal cord injuries, chipped or broken teeth, or internal injuries.

Diagnostic Testing

Cultures for sexually transmitted infections (STIs) may be performed post–sexual assault; however, the health care provider must appreciate that cultures taken in the immediate aftermath of sexual assault are not testing for infections transmitted during the assault. Many providers choose to give prophylactic medication to prevent STIs post-assault in lieu of cultures. That being said, if the victim/survivor presents to health care post-assault with an infection, cultures may be a necessary part of the treatment protocol. It should be noted that if the victim is tested for STIs during the forensic evaluation, the results become part of the medical record and will be available to the assailant's attorney if the case goes to trial. Positive results can be used to discredit the victim, and thus the victim may chose to not be tested for STIs during the forensic exam.

Female victims should be offered a blood or urine pregnancy test. A positive test within five days after sexual assault may indicate that the woman was pregnant at the time of the assault. However, it does not indicate if the woman will become pregnant as a result of the assault.

Alcohol and illicit drugs are frequently a part of the crime of sexual assault. Alcohol and or drugs may be given to the victim/survivor of sexual assault by the offender, but more commonly the victim/survivor consumes drugs and alcohol prior to the assault. The offender may encourage the victim to consume but rarely administers the alcohol or drugs himself. When the victim/survivor appears to be intoxicated or drugged or both post-assault, a forensic toxicology screening is advised. Forensic toxicology screening is different from clinical toxicology screening. Clinical screening is performed via a hospital laboratory, with the expectation that the results will guide clinical management. Forensic toxicology is designed to identify alcohol and/or drugs consumed and quantify the amount of these substances. Forensic toxicological screening is performed by a forensic science laboratory. The level of impairment at the time of the assault may be important to the investigative process.

INTERVENTION

Sexual assault of an adult by another adult does not generally fall into the category of a mandated report by health care personnel. The intent of mandatory reporting is not to force competent adults to report sexual assault. Mandated reporting laws are designed to protect vulnerable populations. Every state has mandatory reporting laws that must be examined by the health care practitioner working in that state for details on reporting. In many states there is a requirement for the mandated reporting of sexual assault in certain circumstances, such as serious injury or use of a weapon in the assault. If the victim of sexual assault is not seriously injured and the health care provider determines that the victim is competent to make a decision about reporting, the decision to report to law enforcement is left to the victim/survivor. The victim has the ability to refuse to report the crime. If the victim understands the implications to her situation if she does not report, she may refuse any police intervention.

Evidence collection in cases of rape and sexual assault focuses on the collection of DNA via the collection of semen and saliva. Careful and meticulous examination of the patient, seeking trace evidence that has transferred from the suspect to the victim, is the primary concern of evidence collection. Common areas of the body where semen and saliva from the suspect may be retrieved are: the mouth, breasts, thighs, external genitalia, vagina, and rectal/anal area. Areas of the body that are moist by nature do not require moistened swabs for evidence collection. Skin that is dry requires evidence collection via swabs moistened by sterile water.

Evidence collection aimed at retrieval of DNA, in the immediate aftermath of an assault, can be focused utilizing an evidence collection kit. However, a kit is not necessary for evidence collection. If a kit cannot be located when the health practitioner suspects rape or sexual assault has occurred recently (within three to five days), evidence can be collected without a kit.

Each area of the body where retrieval of evidence may be possible (guided by interview) is swabbed separately. Cross-contamination of evidence from one area of the body with evidence from another area of the body is not advised. Swabs are dried at room temperature and packaged in envelopes marked with the location from which the specimens were derived. Envelopes must be retained by the health care provider and handed to law enforcement for processing to maintain the chain of custody (see chapter 4). *Do not refer to the sexual assault evidence collection kit as a "rape kit." Rape kits are what rapists keep in the trunks of their car.*

Collection of evidence should occur only if the sexual assault happened in the previous three to five days (see chapter 3 on forensic assessment and chapter 4 on evidence). Documentation of injury is completed via writing on the patient's chart, drawing on a body diagram, and photography. If the victim is reporting a sexual assault that happened more than 5 days before the health care visit, evidence collection is not attempted. However, evaluation for medication to prevent sexually transmitted infections should be offered, emergency contraception may be offered, and injuries must be treated.

The role of the health care provider during the immediate aftermath of sexual assault is not limited to forensic evidence collection. The health care provider is in a unique position to provide psychological support for females who are victims of sex crimes. Health care providers are also in a unique position to refer victims/survivors of sexual assault to help resources such as rape care advocacy, counseling, and law enforcement.

Victims have a 26% chance of receiving an STI, especially Neisseria gonorrhoeae, Trichomonas vaginalis, and Chlamydia trachomatis. The Centers for Disease Control and Prevention publishes a guide for the prevention of sexually transmitted diseases post-rape/sexual assault (CDC, 2006). This guide provides detailed suggestions for medications to be given post–sexual assault. The CDC does not recommend testing of or prophylaxis for HIV. However, many health care providers offer diagnosis and treatment of HIV post–sexual assault. Health care providers strongly suggest HIV prophylaxis in sexual assault cases in which the suspect is known to have HIV, the suspect is an IV drug abuser, the victim was assaulted by more than one offender, and in cases in which the victim has sustained serious bodily injury.

Victims who were not previously immunized with the hepatitis B vaccine should receive one dose immediately, followed by additional doses one and six months later. Preventive treatment for hepatitis B may not be needed for victims who were previously immunized with the full series of three hepatitis B vaccines.

All victims who were exposed to blood or bodily fluids during the attack should be advised to use a condom with any sexual activity. Condoms reduce —but do not completely eliminate—the chance of transmitting hepatitis and HIV infection to others. Female victims should avoid becoming pregnant for three months, and all victims should refrain from donating blood, plasma, organs, tissue, or semen during the first three months after the assault.

Follow-up care is crucial. Clients should be evaluated two weeks after the initial exam to assess their emotional state and treatment status. Testing for gonorrhea, chlamydia, trichomonas, and bacterial vaginosis may be recommended if preventive treatments were not taken at the initial evaluation. It is also recommended for clients who develop symptoms of an infection or who would like to be tested. Pregnancy testing is recommended four weeks after the initial examination if the woman took an emergency contraceptive pill and/or if she did not have her menstrual period on time. Testing for HIV is usually repeated at six weeks, three months, and six months after the assault, because it takes up to six months for the blood test to become positive.

PREVENTION/CLIENT TEACHING

Primary Prevention

Primary prevention efforts include preventing the offender from assaulting, and changing societal norms to decrease rape-supportive attitudes. Prevention efforts include school-based programs, public education media campaigns, and rape deterrence by threat of criminal sanction.

Victims are not responsible for being assaulted. However, it is still prudent to teach safety precautions, particularly those related to "date rape." Date or acquaintance rape is the use of force to have sex with someone against that person's will by someone the victim knows or is dating. One factor in its occurrence appears to be the double standard about appropriate sexual behavior for men and women that causes a commonly held cultural myth: nice women do not say yes to sex, even when they want it, and real men do not take no for an answer.

To help prevent date rape, females should be counseled to: avoid going to parties alone; stay sober at parties; double date and/or use their own transportation with new acquaintances; avoid going into their date's room unless they know them very well; and learn to say no assertively. Males should be taught to be aware of social pressure and that it is permissible to not "score." They should learn to understand what "no" means, and not assume that sexy dress and flirtatious behavior are invitations to sexual activity. Both males and females need to know that alcohol and drugs interfere with clear communications regarding sex.

Secondary Prevention

Secondary prevention focuses on early identification of risk factors. Clients at higher risk for sexual assault, including those with mental health or developmental disabilities, should be given extra teaching to prevent assaults.

Tertiary Prevention

Throughout the United States there is a movement toward caring for female victims of sexual assault via sexual assault nurse examiners (SANE) and sexual assault response teams (SART). All programs are designed to provide comprehensive and expert care for sexual assault survivors. Policies and procedures do vary from program to program. Collection of evidence is at the core of each SANE and SART program. The utilization of SANE and SART programs promotes tertiary prevention by helping to decrease the effects of sexual assault and by aiding in the arrest and conviction of offenders who may otherwise assault again.

The most common risk factor for adult women who are sexually assaulted is previous victimization. A woman with a history of victimization as a child, as an adolescent, or as an adult is part of a subpopulation of persons most likely to be victimized. Targeting the population of victimized girls and women with effective interventions prevents future victimizations.

RESOURCES

National Alliance to End Sexual Violence: http://www.naesv.org
National Center for Victims of Crime: http://www.ncvc.org
National Sexual Violence Resource Center: http://www.nsvrc.org
Office on Violence Against Women: http://www.ovw.usdoj.gov/index.html
State Sexual Assault Coalitions: http://www.ovw.usdoj.gov/statesexual.htm
Understanding the Needs of the Victims of Sexual Assault in the Deaf Community: http://
    www.ncjrs.gov/pdffiles1/nij/grants/212867.pdf

REFERENCES

Amar, A., & Gennaro, S. (2005). Dating violence in college women: Associated physical injury, healthcare usage and mental health symptoms. *Nursing Research, 54*(4), 235–242.

Bachman, R. (1998). The factors related to rape reporting behavior and arrest: New evidence from the National Crime Survey. *Criminal Justice and Behavior, 25*, 8–29.

Bachman, R., & Paternoster, R. (1993). A contemporary look at the effects of rape law reform: How far have we really come? *Journal of Criminal Law and Criminology, 84*, 554–574.

Bates, C., & O'Connor, A. (2008). *Patient information: Care after sexual assault.* Up-To-Date for Patients. Retrieved from http://www.uptodate.com/patients/content/topic. do?topicKey=~iiHZInAOnqVE5#9

Bondurant, B. (2001). University women's acknowledgment of rape: Individual, situational, and social factors. *Violence Against Women, 7*, 294–314.

Burgess, A. W., Fehder, W. P., & Hartman, C. R. (1995). Delayed reporting of the rape victim. *Journal of Psychosocial Nursing and Mental Health Services, 33*(9), 21–29.

Burgess, A. W., & Holmstrom, L. L. (1974). Rape trauma syndrome. *American Journal of Psychiatry, 131*, 981–986.

Campbell, R., Sefl, T., Barnes, H. E., Ahrens, C. E., Wasco, S. M., & Zaragoza-Diesfeld, Y. (1999). Community services for rape survivors: Enhancing psychological well-being or increasing trauma? *Journal of Consulting and Clinical Psychology, 67*, 847–858.

Campbell, R., Wasco, S., Ahrens, C., Sefl, T., & Barnes H. (2001). Preventing the "second rape": Rape survivors' experiences with community service providers. *Journal of Interpersonal Violence, 16*, 1239–1260.

Catalano, S. M. (2006). *Criminal victimization, 2005* (NCJ214644). Washington, DC: Bureau of Justice Statistics, Office of Justice Programs, U.S. Department of Justice. Retrieved from http://www.ojp.usdoj.gov/bjs/abstract/cv05.htm

Centers for Disease Control and Prevention. (2006). *Sexually transmitted diseases treatment guide: Sexual assault and STDs.* Retrieved from http://www.cdc.gov/STD/treatment/2006/sexual-assault.htm

Clay-Warner, J., & Burt, C. H. (2005). Rape reporting after reforms: Have times really changed? *Violence Against Women, 11*, 150–176.

Douglas, J. E., Burgess, A. W., Burgess, A. G., & Ressler, R. K. (2006). *Crime classification manual.* San Francisco: Jossey-Bass.

DuMont, J., Miller, K. L., & Myhr, T. (2003). The role of "real rape" and "real victim" stereotypes in the police reporting practices of sexually assaulted women. *Violence Against Women, 9*(4), 466–486.

Federal Bureau of Investigation. (2008). *Crime in the United States, 2007.* Retrieved March 14, 2009, from http://www.fbi.gov/ucr/cius2007/about/index.html

Fisher, B., Daigle, L., Cullen, F., & Turner, M. (2000). *The sexual victimization of college women.* Washington, DC: U.S. Department of Justice, National Institute of Justice, and Bureau of Justice Statistics. Retrieved from http://www.ncjrs.gov/pdffiles1/nij/182369.pdf

Groth, A. N., Burgess, A. W., & Holmstrom, L. L. (1977). Rape: Power, anger, and sexuality. *American Journal of Psychiatry, 134*, 1239–1243.

Sommers, M. (2007). Defining patterns of genital injury from sexual assault: A review. *Trauma, Violence, & Abuse, 8*(3), 270–280.

Straight, J., & Heaton, P. (2007). Emergency department crime for victims of sexual offenses. *American Journal of Health System Pharmacy, 64*(17), 1845–1850.

Tjaden, P., & Thoennes, N. (2000). *Full report of the prevalence, incidence, and consequences of violence against women: Findings from the National Violence Against Women survey* (NCJ183781). Washington, DC: National Institute of Justice, Office of Justice Programs, U.S. Department of Justice. Retrieved from http://www.ncjrs.gov/pdffiles1/nij/183781.pdf

Tjaden, P., & Thoennes, N. (2006). *Special report on the extent, nature, and consequences of rape victimization: Findings from the National Violence Against Women Survey.* Retrieved from http://www.ncjrs.gov/pdffiles1/nij/210346.pdf

U.S. Department of Justice. (2004). *National protocol for sexual assault medical forensic examinations* (NCJ 206554). Retrieved from http://www.ncjrs.gov/pdffiles1/ovw/206554.pdf

World Health Organization. (1997). *Violence against women fact sheets.* Retrieved from http://www.who.int/en

18   Male Victims of Sexual Assault

DEFINITION

Most jurisdictions have replaced the term *rape* with *sexual assault* in the state statutes. This term is more gender-neutral and covers more specific types of sexual victimization and various levels of coercion. As noted in the previous chapter, legal definitions of sexual assault can vary from state to state.

PREVALENCE

Tjaden and Thoennes (2006) found that approximately 3% of American men have experienced sexual assault at some point in their lifetime. Because some people reported being raped more than once, the survey estimated that 2.8 million men were forcibly raped at some time in their lives and more than 92,000 men were forcibly raped in the year prior to the survey. Seventy-one percent of male victims were first raped before their 18th birthday, 16.6% were 18–24 years old, and 12.3% were 25 or older.

    According to a report by Beck and Harrison (2007), 4.5% of male prison inmates reported an incident of sexual victimization by either another inmate or by staff. More than 7.3 million Americans are confined in correctional facilities or supervised in the community, at a cost of more than $68 billion annually. Given this enormous investment in corrections, these environments should be as safe and productive as they can be. Sexual abuse undermines both safety and productivity, making correctional environments more dangerous for staff as well as prisoners, consuming scarce resources, and undermining rehabilitation. Sexual abuse can also devastate the lives of victims.

The actual numbers are probably significantly higher, since males are the least likely to report a sexual assault, though it is estimated that they make up 10% of all victims. Some experts believe that sexual assault on men is significantly underreported, even more so than female sexual assault. Possible reasons for the underreporting of male sexual assault are:

- Abundance of myths about male sexual abuse, such as

  - Men cannot be raped.
  - Only homosexual males are sexually assaulted.
  - Only homosexual men assault other men.
  - Men should not express emotions.
  - Men should be able to fight off attackers.
  - Men like all sex, so they must have enjoyed the assault.
  - Male survivors are more likely to become sexual predators.
  - Sexual assaults against males are committed only within prisons.
  - Males are less affected by sexual assault than females.

- Denial: Victims may psychologically block out the event, especially if they are minimally injured.
- Lack of support, for example

  - Victims may fear how others will judge them.
  - Family members and friends may be unsupportive and even negative.

- Lack of services: Rape crisis centers may explicitly refuse services to male victims or are highly insensitive to male victims' needs. Other agencies that offer services are rarely designed specifically for men.
- Concerns about safety: The victim or his family may have been threatened by the perpetrator.

- Concerns about privacy: The victim may resist repeating his story to health and law enforcement professionals, and/or may want to protect his family from societal judgment.
- Self-blame: The victim may blame himself for the attack because he was unable to defend himself, or he may think the assault was his fault because he became sexually aroused during the attack. Arousal (erection with or without ejaculation) is a normal physiologic response, not a sign of enjoyment.

ETIOLOGY

The etiology lies with the offender, not the victim. Like those who offend against females, most offenders who sexually abuse males are also male. Most identify themselves as heterosexual and state they have consensual sexual relationships with women. Groth and Birnbaum (1979) noted that all acts of sexual assault are acts of aggression, regardless of the gender or age of the victim or the assailant. The assault is about power and control, not sexual desire or sexual deprivation. However, there are some differences in those who assault men or boys when compared to men who assault only females. Boys are more like to be assaulted by strangers, or by authority figures such as clergy and Boy Scout leaders. Perpetrators who offend males usually choose young men and adolescents as their victims and are more likely to assault many victims. These offenders are also more likely to commit their assaults in isolated areas where help is not readily available.

ASSESSMENT

General Principles

There are no universal signs, symptoms, or forensic markers of male sexual assault victimization. Some men will experience some forms of physical injuries, some will experience some forms of psychological disturbance, and some may experience sexual dysfunction or identity questions. However, many men will not exhibit manifestations, will present to health care providers under the guise of a hidden agenda, or will present so long after the incident that connecting symptoms to sexual assault victimization may not be likely.

The *National Protocol for Sexual Assault Medical Forensic Examinations* (http://www.ncjrs.gov/pdffiles1/ovw/206554.pdf) provides detailed guidelines for criminal justice and health care practitioners in responding to the immediate needs of sexual assault victims. Specific guidelines for male victims are:

- Requests by male victims to have an advocate of a particular gender should be respected and honored if possible.
- Assure them that they are not at fault. Many male victims focus on the sexual aspect of the assault. They overlook other elements, such as coercion, power differences, and emotional abuse. Enhancing their understanding of sexual assault may help reduce their self-blame.
- Some male victims fear public disclosure of the assault and its associated stigma. Emphasize confidentiality, unless performing a forensic examination where confidentiality is limited.
- Help victims to figure out how friends and family members will react to the fact that they were sexually assaulted.
- Male victims may be less likely to seek and receive support from family members and friends, as well as from advocacy and counseling services.
- Health care providers need to be empathetic, supportive, and knowledgeable, and they need to make appropriate referrals to specialists and agencies that provide interventions for male victims of sexual assault.
- Health care providers should encourage advocacy programs and mental health providers to build their capacity to serve male sexual assault victims and increase their accessibility to this population.

History

As with female victims of sexual assault, male victims have a range of presentations. The most common response of male victims is a sense of stigma, shame, and embarrassment. Some may appear as if nothing happened, while others look as if they are on the verge of a breakdown. Some may have symptoms of acute or posttraumatic stress disorder. A number of symptoms have been reported by male sexual assault victims: headaches; decreased appetite and weight loss; sleep difficulties; depression; anxiety; somatic complaints; alcohol, drug and tobacco use; suicide attempts; hostility and aggression; nausea and vomiting; constipation and abdominal pain; and fecal incontinence. Suicidal attempts are most common among adolescent and young adult victims.

Sexual consequences include sexual anxieties, sexual dysfunction, impotence, and questioning their "true" sexuality, whether being raped makes them gay, and whether there is something about them that leads others to perceive them as gay. Men who are sexually victimized by male offenders may question their gender and gender role. This may be especially true for men who hold traditional or stereotypical views about sexuality and gender. Men who are victimized by female perpetrators may question how they could be victimized by a "weaker" female, which may also contribute to questions about gender role fulfillment.

Victimized males may question their "true" sexuality if they experienced sexual arousal during the assault. This can be very devastating and requires assurance and teaching from the health care professional. An erection (with or without ejaculation) is a common involuntary response for many men in times of intense pain, anxiety, panic, and/or fear.

Physical Assessment

Some male victims experience physical injuries; others do not. When genito-anal injuries do occur, they tend to be soft tissue injuries that are most frequently noted in the perianal and anal areas. However, general body trauma from physical assault or restraint is more common than genitor-anal trauma. Male sexual assault can be very violent if the offender uses a weapon to subdue the victim. Some victims may be too embarrassed to report that their injuries are the result of sexual assault and instead report them as having occurred from another crime such as robbery. It is therefore critical that health care providers obtain a thorough history to rule out sexual assault when males present with intentionally induced injuries.

The *National Protocol for Sexual Assault Medical Forensic Examinations* advises the following for male clients: examine the external and perineal area for injury, foreign materials, and other findings, including from the abdomen, buttocks, thighs, foreskin, urethral meatus, shaft, scrotum, perineum, glans, and testes. Document whether or not clients are circumcised.

Rectal injuries may include: anal tears; abrasions; bleeding; erythema; hematoma; discoloration with tenderness; fissures; the presence of dirt, vegetation, or hair in the anus; engorgement; and friability. The use of anoscopy for diagnosis of rectal trauma may be required in cases of forceful anal assault.

Restraint injuries may include abrasions to the throat and abdomen, bruises, broken bones, and black eyes. Common locations for injuries are head/neck/face, leg/knee/feet, and arm/hands.

Diagnostic Testing

Cultures for sexually transmitted infections may be performed post–sexual assault. The health care provider must appreciate that cultures taken in the immediate aftermath of sexual assault are not testing for infections transmitted during the assault. Many providers choose to give prophylactic medication to prevent sexually transmitted infections post-assault in lieu of cultures. That being said, if the victim/survivor presents to health care post-assault with an infection, cultures may be a necessary part of the treatment protocol.

Alcohol and illicit drugs are frequently a part of the crime of sexual assault. Alcohol and/or drugs may be given to the victim/survivor of sexual assault by the offender, but more commonly the victim/survivor consumes drugs and alcohol prior to the assault. The offender may encourage the victim to consume, but rarely administers the alcohol or drugs himself. When the victim/survivor appears to be intoxicated or drugged or both post-assault, a forensic toxicology screening is advised. Forensic toxicology screening is different from clinical toxicology screening. Clinical screening is performed via a hospital laboratory with the expectation that the results will guide clinical management. Forensic toxicology is designed to identify alcohol and/or drugs consumed and quantify the amount of these substances. Forensic toxicological screening is performed by a forensic science laboratory. The level of impairment at the time of the assault may be important to the investigative process.

INTERVENTION

Treatment of any physical injuries is of primary importance in intervention for victims of sexual assault. Documentation of injury (see chapter 3 on forensic assessment) is of forensic importance. Collection of evidence is guided via victim interview. Evidence collection after rape/sexual assault is focused on collection of semen and saliva as well as any other sources of DNA that may have transferred from the suspect to the victim (see chapter 3). If the time frame post–sexual assault is within three to five days, evidence collection is recommended. Evidence collection from the body does not vary according to whether the victim is male or female. Evidence collection from male genitalia involves swabbing of the penis and scrotum. Evidence collection from the rectal/anal area does not vary according to gender.

Prophylactic treatment for sexually transmitted diseases is recommended. Prevention for Chlamydia trachomatis and Neisseria gonorrhea should be offered. Medication to prevent the transmission of HIV should be discussed with the patient. The nature of the assault affects the clinical decision to offer HIV prophylactic medication. In a study by Pesola, Westfal, and Kuffner (1999), the victim knew the offender in one-half of the cases. The lack of information about the offender via the victim may increase the likelihood that the health care provider offers HIV prophylactic medication.

A very important intervention for male victims/survivors of sexual assault is referral to appropriate counseling. According to Masho and Anderson (2009), only 15% of males who reported sexual assault sought counseling. However, males do have long-term psychological responses to sexual assault that include depression, phobias, and psycho-physiological reactions A homosexual male may feel that he is being "punished" for his sexual orientation. Relationships may be disrupted by the assault, or by other's reactions to the assault, such as a lack of belief and support. Referral to appropriate and sensitive counseling is required for all male victims of sexual assault.

Health care providers should also refer to chapter 17 for more interventions.

PREVENTION/PATIENT TEACHING

Prevention and patient teaching follow the same guidelines as in chapter 17. However, prevention of male sexual assault first begins with helping patients understand that men can be raped. One way to accomplish this is to post brochures on male sexual assault in health care settings. Health care providers may be able to obtain these types of brochures from their local health or mental health department. If not available locally, a male sexual assault brochure can be downloaded online from the West Virginia Foundation for Rape Information and Services at http://www.fris.org/Sections/07-Publications/PDFs/Brochures/Bro-MaleSexAssault.pdf.

RESOURCES

Adult Male Sexual Assault Exam: http://www.dhss.mo.gov/ViolenceAgainstWomen/580-2893.pdf

National Organization on Male Sexual Victimization: http://www.malesurvivor.org

Rape, Abuse & Incest National Network: http://www.rainn.org/get-information/types-of-sexual-assault/male-sexual-assault

REFERENCES

Beck, A. J., & Harrison, P. M. (2007). *Bureau of Justice Statistics special report: Prison Rape Elimination Act of 2003: Sexual victimization in state and federal prisons reported by inmates, 2007* (NCJ 219414). Washington, DC: U.S. Department of Justice, Office of Justice Programs. Retrieved from http://bjs.ojp.usdoj.gov/content/pub/pdf/svsfpri07.pdf

Federal Bureau of Investigation. (2008). *Crime in the United States, 2007.* Retrieved from http://www.fbi.gov/ucr/cius2007.

Ferguson, M. T., Weiss, S. J., & Green, W. M. (2000). The utility of anoscopy and colposcopy in the evaluation of male sexual assault victims. *Annals of Emergency Medicine, 11*(36), 432–437.

Groth, N., & Birnbaum, B. (1979). *Men who rape: The psychology of the offender.* New York: Plenum.

Masho S., & Anderson L. (2009). Sexual assault in men: A population based survey in Virginia. *Violence and Victims, 24*(1), 98–100.

Mezey, G., & King, M. (1997). The effects of sexual assault in men: A survey of 22 victims. *Journal of Psychiatric Mental Health Nursing, 4*(2), 122–124.

National Centers for Victims of Crime. (2008). *Male rape.* Retrieved from http://www.ncvc.org/ncvc/main.aspx?dbName=DocumentViewer&DocumentID=32361

National Prison Rape Elimination Commission Report Executive Summary. (2009). Retrieved from http://www.ncjrs.gov/pdffiles1/226681.pdf

Pesola, G. R., Westfal, R. E., & Kuffner, C. A. (1999). Emergency department characteristics of male sexual assault. *Academic Emergency Medicine, 6*(8), 792–798.

Rape, Abuse and Incest National Network (RAINN). (n.d.). *Male sexual assault.* Retrieved from http://www.rainn.org/get-information/types-of-sexual-assault/male-sexual-assault

Tewksbury, R. (2007). Effects of sexual assaults on men: Physical, mental and sexual consequences. *International Journal of Men's Health, 6*(1), 22–35.

Tjaden, P., & Thoennes, N. (2000). *Full report of the prevalence, incidence, and consequences of violence against women: Findings from the National Violence Against Women survey* (NCJ183781). Washington, DC: National Institute of Justice, Office of Justice Programs, U.S. Department of Justice. Retrieved from http://www.ncjrs.gov/pdffiles1/nij/183781.pdf

Tjaden, P., & Thoennes, N. (2006). *Special report on the extent, nature, and consequences of rape victimization: Findings from the National Violence Against Women Survey.* Retrieved from http://www.ncjrs.gov/pdffiles1/nij/210346.pdf

Whealin, J. (2007). *Men and sexual trauma.* U.S. Department of Veteran Affairs. Retrieved from http://ncptsd.va.gov/ncmain/ncdocs/fact_shts/fs_male_sexual_assault.html

19 Elder Victims of Sexual Assault

DEFINITION

Sexual activity with an elder that is nonconsensual is sexual abuse. As with other populations this may involve rape, touching, and forced nudity. Although reported sexual abuse is 1% of all reports of elder abuse, it is disturbing to realize that this form of abuse occurs at all.

Many elderly women were raised in a time when sexual matters were not discussed in the open. Thus, becoming a victim of sexual abuse represents the worst crime possible to them. Speaking about their private sexual life in the public arena of the health care and criminal justice systems is unfathomable. They may experience profound shame in discussing the crime or in participating in the forensic medical exam and may be fearful that the information will somehow get to their families, communities, and the media. Many of these women are assaulted in their own homes during the commission of another crime such as burglary, intensifying their sense of loss of control. Embarrassment may also stem from being forced to perform oral or anal sex, concern over developing a sexually transmitted infection, and fear that their religious community will learn of the assault (see chapter 17 for more details on sexual assault).

PREVALENCE

There are no reliable estimates of the incidence or prevalence of elder sexual abuse in the community or in health care facilities. However, data from cases reported to Adult Protective Services (APS) are a source of information about elder sexual assault/abuse. In 1991, Ramsey-Klawsnik surveyed APS caseworkers in Massachusetts and identified 28 cases of women believed to have been sexually assaulted in the home, primarily by family members, including adult sons and husbands. In a similar 1998 study, Ramsey Klawsnik reported 90 suspected elder sexual assault victims, 86% of whom were female. The majority was over the age of 85, had dementia, and was frail. Most abuse occurred in the elder's domicile, and 90% of the offenders were males upon whom the victim was dependant.

Nursing homes are not immune from elder sexual abuse, as both staff and other residents have been identified as perpetrators. Teaster and colleagues (2000) reported 42 Virginia APS cases of sexual abuse in both domestic and institutional settings. They found that 75% of the identified offenders were residents in the same nursing home as their victims. Facility staff members were also identified as offenders.

ETIOLOGY

In continuing her study of APS data, Ramsey-Klawsnik (2004) identified five types of elder sexual abuse: stranger or acquaintance assault, abuse by unrelated care providers, incestuous abuse, marital or partner abuse, and resident-to-resident assault in elder care settings. She further delineated subtypes of marital and incestuous abuse. Three patterns of marital abuse seen in clinical samples are: (a) long-term domestic violence, (b) recent onset of sexual abuse within a long-term marriage, and (c) sexual victimization within a new marriage. Incestuous elder abuse involves cases perpetrated by adult children, other relatives, and quasi-relatives. Resident-to-resident sexual abuse has been substantiated in nursing homes, assisted living facilities, board and care homes, and other settings that care for elderly people.

In a study of forensic markers in 125 elder female sexual abuse cases, Burgess, Hanrahan, and Baker (2005) reported that the offender's hand was the primary mechanism of physical injury to the nongenital area of the elder's body, and the offender's hands, fingers, mouth, penis, or foreign object caused injury to the genital area. Over half of the elderly victims had at least one part of their body injured, and nearly half had signs of vaginal injury. Of the 46 cases with forensic results from a rape examination, 35% had positive evidence for the presence of sperm in the vagina, anus, or mouth.

Burgess and colleagues identified several types of offenders who commit sex crimes against elders. Opportunistic offenders show little planning or preparation. The offender is seeking immediate sexual gratification. Pervasively angry offenders use excessive force; violence is a lifestyle characteristic that is directed toward males and females alike. Sexual type offenders have a high degree of preoccupation with gratifying sexual needs. Recurrent rape fantasies, pornography, uncontrollable sexual urges, and engaging in other deviant sexual behaviors are part of this third typology.

The majority of victims are female, and these females are highly dependent. Dementia is a factor in many of these crimes. Dementia limits the ability of the victim to stop the abuse and report the crime. Victims who are highly dependent on the care giver cannot safely report the crime.

ASSESSMENT

General Principles

Elder sexual assault victims with any degree of cognitive impairment are unable to consent to sex, unable to defend themselves, and often delay in reporting a rape. Obtaining an accurate history, as much as the situation will permit, and conducting a physical examination is critical to the diagnosis and treatment of elder sexual assault.

History

Victimized elders have been noted to exhibit rape-related trauma symptoms: becoming fearful of the location of the rape (e.g., bathrooms, showers) and/or fearful of males and male caregivers if assaulted in a nursing home, experiencing flashbacks, and being easily startled (e.g., hyperarousal symptoms). They also will exhibit general symptoms of traumatic stress (e.g., fear, confusion, hypersomnia, lack of appetite, withdrawal), and an exacerbation of symptoms related to existing physical and/prior mental conditions. Elders with the presence of a preexisting cognitive deficit, such as a dementia, may have a delay in information processing and impaired communication that potentially compounds the trauma of the sexual assault and makes getting an accurate history very difficult.

Signs of emotional trauma, including observable signs such as crying, rocking, hands shaking, flushed appearance, and signs of perspiration should be noted. Elders may try to hide their feelings by being very quiet, guarded, or controlled in their demeanor. This too should be noted. Symptoms of emotional trauma include reports by the elder of what was done to her or him.

The following suggestions aid in the development of trust with the elder in order to obtain an accurate history of the sexual assault/abuse.

- Tell the elder what to expect. Talk slowly and clearly. Advise victims they will be examined and by whom for the collection of evidence if evidence is to be collected.
- Assess the victim's sensory system. Can she or he hear and see people? A quiet and well-lighted area should be used, and the health care person should face the victim and should be well in the line of vision of the elder. If there are sensory problems, learn how the elder adjusts to the deficit by asking her or him or their family or caregivers how the elder copes with sensory difficulties.
- Observe the victim's demeanor. Is she or he quiet, crying, angry, in distress? Ask how she or he is feeling and if there are any questions about what is going to happen. Allow adequate time for the elder to express emotions.

In cases of elder sexual assault/abuse, the nurse should seriously consider consultation with nursing staff members who are comfortable and familiar with the interview of elders. Many elders who are sexually victimized have physical impairments and cognitive impairments. Obtaining an accurate history is crucial to investigation. This history should be conducted in tandem with a geriatric nursing specialist.

Physical Assessment

The presence of a sexually transmitted infection (STI) is usually a hallmark of sexual abuse in a child. Children are considered an asexual population. In the cases of elder sexual assault/abuse, sexually transmitted infections may be a result of consensual sex, or the argument can be made that it was the result of a preexisting condition or it was transmitted by health care staff. However, detection and documentation of any sexually transmitted infection may be important forensic evidence as the case is investigated and ability to consent to sex determined.

In the Burgess, Hanrahan, and Baker (2005) study, almost half (45%) of the elderly victims who were examined within 72 hours had vaginal trauma, almost 20% had anal trauma, and over 10% had oral penetration. It is to be noted, however, that elderly residents in nursing homes did not necessarily have timely examinations due to delayed reporting. The time lapse between injury and examination is important to document.

Inspection of the genitalia of an elder female is a clinical challenge. Many elderly women cannot be placed into the traditional position utilized for pelvic examination. Contractures, arthritis, and many other medical conditions common to the elderly prohibit the use of this position. External genitalia can be examined in a supine position with legs supported by assistants. External genitalia must be carefully inspected utilizing a colposcope or high-intensity light source. Injury may occur at any genital location, but careful attention should be given to inspection of the posterior aspect of the entrance to the vagina and the perineum. Inspection of the vagina and cervix requires speculum inspection. If a speculum can be inserted, a small narrow speculum (not a pediatric speculum because length is required to reach the cervix) should be utilized.

Common genital injuries in elder victims of sexual assault are lacerations, abrasions, and bruises. The complicated nature of the pelvic examination of elder persons requires a very special set of nursing skills. A combined team of a forensic health care worker and a women's health nurse practitioner is needed to adequately conduct this examination.

Diagnostic Testing

See chapters 15 and 17 for suggested testing.

INTERVENTION

Elder sexual abuse cases can be reported to the criminal justice system through a local law enforcement agency in much the same route as a younger victim report. The second investigative agency, Adult Protective Services (APS), is typically the agency of first report for the mistreatment of vulnerable and older adults (Teaster, Roberto, Duke, & Kim, 2000). Across the country, laws exist requiring mandated professionals (such as those in medicine, nursing, social services, law enforcement, and aging services) to report suspected abuse of vulnerable elders to APS. Reports can also be made by nonmandated individuals such as family members and friends, as well as by victims themselves

Most sexual assaults are not witnessed. However, when the victim is infirmed via cognitive deficits, the lack of an eyewitness is a complicating issue in the investigation of these cases. The skill and challenge of investigation is to attempt to reconstruct the events surrounding the possible sexual injury. Health care providers should identify victims of elder sexual assault and consult with a team of geriatric experts to ensure an adequate history and examination is conducted.

As with all cases of assault, health and safety of the elder is the first priority. Diagnosing any injury that requires medical intervention is the first priority in cases of elder sexual assault. In a pilot study of 20 elderly women, the single most profound result of the sexual assaults against these victims was that 11 of the 20 victims died within 12 months of the assault.

The neurobiology of trauma suggests that traumatic memories cannot be totally extinguished, and sleep disturbance, mood instability, angry outbursts, and withdrawal and depression often follow. Elder victims of sexual assault/abuse require referral to an appropriate counseling service. There should be a list of counselors who have experience with elderly victims available to health care workers for purposes of referral. The impact of a sexual assault on elders is affected by the elder's age, general health status, and diminished cognitive processing. The latter explains why behavioral symptoms may be delayed and prolonged in the elder. The elder's fragility places victims at unusually high risk for severe traumatic reactions to assault.

Advocates visiting elder victims in an institution can use the technique of music therapy. The goal of this therapy is to help the victim learn to reduce the anxiety experienced after the assault. Family members need assistance when an elder is sexually assaulted/abused whether it happens when the elder is living alone, living in assisted-living facilities, or living in a nursing home.

PREVENTION/PATIENT TEACHING

Primary Prevention

Prevention programs of elder sexual abuse are aimed at public education, to help people understand what elder sexual abuse is and how it can be prevented. The programs focus on educating seniors, front-line workers, and the public about situations and behaviors indicative of sexual abuse.

Secondary Prevention

Prevention programs for elders living independently in the community, in assisted living facilities, or in nursing homes need to be part of all sexual violence community education programs. The program would include the traditional public education to teach elder safety as well as to raise awareness and to increase reporting.

The senior safety education component requires an understanding of the level of the elder's independent functioning and the social network support. In addition, there should be emphasis on a safety checklist specifically designed for seniors. It is stressed that prevention is by safety awareness and not by unreasonable fear of attack.

For seniors living alone in a neighborhood, the safety questions are as follows: Does the senior have some connection with neighbors or family? If so what is the connection and exactly who is assisting in securing the safety of the elder?

Tertiary Prevention

Seniors living independently include those living with their families and/ or partners as well as those living alone. If the senior who is raped is alert, verbal, and with minimal memory deficits, the sexual violence advocates generally follow the same protocol for support services as they do for adult victims in general. That is, they meet with the senior, assess social network support, provide crisis counseling, and work with the prosecutor's office if the case is scheduled for trial.

Living in assisted living generally implies that an elder is in a protected environment that has safety features in place. That is, staff checks on them over 24-hour shifts, and meals and cleaning services are often provided. When an elder is sexually assaulted in a perceived safe environment, such as assisted living and/or an institution, it causes additional trauma, because staff has been trusted and there is a breach in safety and security. Very often, the family feels guilty.

Interventions for elders should focus on verbal and nonverbal signs of stress. The traumatized elder needs careful observation and a good description of preassault behavior from family and staff members for a baseline to assess changes. Nursing homes are, for the residents, precisely that—a home, and the staff functions as the caregivers. The nursing home and its staff are perceived as "safe," and violations represent a betrayal of trust for the victim and the family.

RESOURCES

Elderly Victims of Sexual Abuse and Their Offenders: http://www.ncjrs.gov/pdffiles1/nij/grants/216550.pdf
Mississippi Coalition Against Sexual Assault: http://www.mscasa.org/elder_sexual_assault.php
Sexual Abuse in the Elderly: http://www.ojp.usdoj.gov/nij/topics/crime/elder-abuse/sexual-abuse.htm

REFERENCES

Burgess, A. W., Hanrahan, N. P., & Baker, T. (2005). Forensic markers in elder female sexual abuse cases. *Clinics in Geriatric Medicine, 21,* 399–412.
National Victim Assistance Academy. (1996). Chapter 18: Elderly victims of crime. Retrieved from http://www.ojp.usdoj.gov/ovc/assist/nvaa/ch18eld.htm
Ramin, S. M., Satin, A. J., Stone, I. C., & Wendel, G. D. (1992). Sexual assault in postmenopausal women. *Obstetrics & Gynecology, 80,* 860–864.
Ramsey-Klawsnik, H. (1991). Elder sexual abuse: Preliminary findings. *Journal of Elder Abuse and Neglect, 3*(3), 73–90.
Ramsey-Klawsnik, H. (1998). Dynamics of sexual assault/abuse against people with disabilities and the elderly. In *Wisconsin Coalition Against Sexual Assault. Widening the Circle: Sexual assault/abuse and people with disabilities and the elderly* (Chapter 3). Madison, WI: Author.
Ramsey-Klawsnik, H. (2003). Elder sexual abuse within the family. *Journal of Elder Abuse & Neglect, 15*(1), 43–58.
Ramsey-Klawsnik, H. (2004). Elder sexual abuse perpetrated by residents in care settings. *Victimization of the Elderly and Disabled, 6*(6), 81, 93–95.
Ramsey-Klawsnik, H., & Klawsnik, L. (2004). Interviewing victims with barriers to communication. *Victimization of the Elderly and Disabled, 7*(4), 49–50, 63–64.
Roberto, K. A., & Teaster, P. B. (2005). Sexual abuse of vulnerable young and old women. *Violence Against Women, 2*(4), 473–504.
Teaster, P. B. (2003). *A response to the abuse of vulnerable adults: The 2000 survey of state Adult Protective Services.* Washington, DC: National Center on Elder Abuse.
Teaster, P. B., Roberto, K. A., Duke, J. O., & Kim, M. (2000). Sexual abuse of older adults: Preliminary findings of cases in Virginia. *Journal of Elder Abuse and Neglect, 12*(3/4), 1–17.
U.S. Department of Justice. (2000). *Statistics on Adult Protective Services, Office of Justice Programs.* Washington, DC: Author.

20 Victims of Human Trafficking

DEFINITION

Human trafficking is modern-day slavery. The Trafficking Victims Protection Act of 2000 (TVPA) defines "Severe Forms of Trafficking in Persons" as follows:

> Sex Trafficking is the recruitment, harboring, transportation, provision, or obtaining of a person for the purpose of a commercial sex act, in which a commercial sex act is induced by force, fraud, or coercion, or in which the person forced to perform such an act is under the age of 18 years.

> Labor Trafficking is the recruitment, harboring, transportation, provision, or obtaining of a person for labor or services, through the use of force, fraud or coercion for the purpose of subjection to involuntary servitude, peonage, debt bondage or slavery.

Trafficking is different from smuggling, which is the crime of getting paid to assist another in illegally crossing a border. However, if the smuggler sells or brokers the smuggled individual into a condition of servitude, or if the smuggled individual is forced to work off the debt, the crime turns from smuggling into human trafficking. Contrary to a common assumption, human trafficking is not just a problem in other countries—cases have been reported in all 50 states, Washington, D.C., and some U.S. territories.

The reasons for coming to the United States vary, but most victims succumb to exploitation under the guise of opportunity. They may believe they are coming to the United States to be united with family, to work in a legitimate job, or to attend school. Victims may also be subject to psychological intimidation or threats of physical harm to self or family members.

PREVALENCE

According to the U.S. Department of State, approximately 600,000 to 800,000 victims annually are trafficked across international borders worldwide, and between 14,500 and 17,500 of those victims are trafficked into the United States. These estimates include women, men, and children. Victims are generally trafficked into the United States from other countries, and many of them do not speak and understand English and are therefore isolated and unable to communicate with service providers, law enforcement, and others who might be able to help them.

Victims can also be trafficked within this country. People can be moved from one portion of the country to another for the purposes of exploitative sex or labor. More than 80% of people trafficked are female, according to the U.S. Department of State, and 50% of trafficking victims are under the age of 18 years. Many American children who are victims of trafficking are runaways who have been physically and sexually abused. Due to the covert nature of the crime, accurate statistics on the prevalence of human trafficking are difficult to determine. Trafficking victims are closely guarded by their captors, and many remain "invisible" in private homes, and private businesses.

ETIOLOGY

Trafficking is exploitation that comes in many forms. Victims can be deceived into debt bondage or forced into involuntary servitude and prostitution. They may be compelled to perform sex acts for the creation of pornography. According to Kangaspunta (2003), approximately 80% of trafficking involves sexual exploitation. These victims are exploited for purposes of commercial sex, including prostitution, stripping, pornography, and live-sex shows. Victims trafficked for labor exploitation are exploited via domestic servitude, sweatshop factories, or migrant agricultural work. According to the U.S. Department of Health and Human Services, traffickers use force, fraud, and coercion to compel victims into engaging in these activities.

Force involves the use of rape, beatings, and confinement. Forceful violence is often used in the early stages of victimization for purposes of controlling the victim.

Fraud typically involves fake offers that induce people into trafficking situations. For example, women will reply to advertisements promising jobs as waitresses and maids in other countries and are then trafficked for purposes of prostitution once they arrive at their destinations.

Coercion involves threats of serious harm to, or physical restraint of any person. Traffickers subject their victims to debt-bondage, usually in the context of paying off transportation fees and housing fees. They also often threaten victims with injury or death. In international trafficking cases, traffickers usually take away the victims' travel documents and isolate them to make escape more difficult. Victims do not realize that their debts are often legally unenforceable and that it is illegal for traffickers to dictate how they have to pay off their debts. In many cases, the victims become trapped in a cycle of debt because they have to pay for all living expenses. Fines for not meeting daily service quotas or for "bad" behavior are also used by some trafficking operations to increase debt. Trafficked victims rarely see the money they are earning.

ASSESSMENT

General Principles

Health care providers are important first-line professionals in identifying victims of human trafficking. Traffickers use force and physical abuse to control their victims. Victims may come to an emergency room, an office, or a clinic displaying various medical problems that have serious health implications. Health issues seen in trafficking victims include:

- Sexually transmitted infections, HIV/AIDS, pelvic pain, rectal trauma, and urinary difficulties from working in the sex industry
- Pregnancy, resulting from rape or prostitution
- Infertility from chronic untreated sexually transmitted infections or botched or unsafe abortions
- Infections or mutilations caused by unsanitary and dangerous medical procedures performed by the trafficker's so-called doctor
- Malnourishment and serious dental problems
- Infectious diseases like tuberculosis
- Undetected or untreated diseases, such as diabetes
- Headaches
- Hearing loss
- Cardiovascular problems
- Chronic back, visual, and respiratory problems
- Bruises, scars and other signs of physical abuse and torture (sex-industry victims are often beaten in areas that won't damage their outward appearance, like their lower back)
- Substance abuse problems or addictions (either from being coerced into drug use by their traffickers or by turning to substance abuse to help cope with or mentally escape their desperate situations)
- Shock and denial
- Depression
- Symptoms of sleeping and eating disorders
- Posttraumatic stress disorder
- Phobias and panic attacks

History

Trafficking victims do not generally seek health care services, because they fear retaliation and deportation. A victim usually enters the health care system presenting with an injury or infection that requires treatment. Sometimes the traffickers move the victims to different communities on a regular basis to prevent the victim from forming social networks and identifying help resources, including health care. When victims do present to health care providers, they rarely identify themselves as victims.

According to Garza (2007), the following are factors may assist in the identification of victims of trafficking and the necessity for reporting and referral. The person is:

- Uncooperative and fearful of authority figures, even medical staff
- Not allowed to give one's own medical information to hospital staff; someone else insists upon providing this information on her or his behalf
- Not in control of one's own identification documents, including personal ID or passport
- Shows evidence of an inability to move or leave a job
- Exhibits fear, anxiety, depression, submission, tension, and/or nervousness
- Is non-English speaking
- Was recently brought to the United States from Latin America, Africa, Eastern Europe, or Asia
- Exhibits poor hygiene; is dirty, unwashed
- Has a loss of sense of time or space

If the health care provider believes he or she has encountered a victim, it is important to keep in mind these key elements before you begin communicating with a potential victim:

- Without raising suspicions, separate the possible victim from the person who is accompanying them.
- Be sensitive to cultural and language barriers, and enlist a trusted translator or interpreter if needed—do not use the person(s) who accompanied the possible victim.
- Maintain strict confidentiality to ensure the victim's safety.

Health care providers can use the following screening questions to identify trafficking victims:

- Can you leave your job or situation if you want?
- Can you come and go as you please?
- Have you been threatened if you try to leave?
- Have you been physically harmed in any way?
- What are your working or living conditions like?
- Where do you sleep and eat?
- Do you sleep in a bed, on a cot, or on the floor?

- Have you ever been deprived of food, water, sleep, or medical care?
- Do you have to ask permission to eat, sleep, or go to the bathroom?
- Are there locks on your doors and windows so you cannot get out?
- Has anyone threatened your family?
- Has your identification or documentation been taken from you?
- Is anyone forcing you to do anything that you do not want to do?

Interview questions should be culturally appropriate, and health care providers should have an understanding of the victim's community and background if they have been trafficked from another country or are part of an immigrant community here in the United States. Victims may have serious concerns about immigration and the safety of their family members, which may hinder their providing information. Health care providers should be aware of issues these people may have as survivors of abuse, neglect, and trauma. Do not make promises you cannot keep; faulty assurances will not help to heal these victims who have already been abused and betrayed.

Physical Assessment

According to Hynes and Raymond (2002), 65% of female victims of sex trafficking sustain serious physical injuries, including head injuries and broken bones. Providing sex for money is a very dangerous situation for the victim. Consumers of sex for money can further victimize the trafficked victim by inflicting physical injury upon the person. Women who have been trafficked for the purpose of sexual exploitation have a tenfold risk of contracting HIV. Female victims of sex trafficking also have a high rate of other sexually transmitted infections and tuberculosis.

Diagnostic Testing

Screen for sexually transmitted infections, as well as other infections related to lifestyle difficulties, such as tuberculosis. Diagnostic testing includes any radiological or laboratory testing needed to diagnose the medical condition with which the patient presents. Psychological testing is required to diagnose mental health disorders associated with this crime.

INTERVENTION

Interventions include treatment of medical conditions and referrals for psychological, social, and immigration issues. Identification of which agency to report to is a challenge. Any of the following hotlines are a method of reporting:

- The U.S. Department of Health and Human Services National Human Trafficking Resource Center can be reached by calling 1-888-3737-888. This toll-free, multilingual, 24-hour-a-day hotline connects victims of trafficking to available local service organizations that provide support services.
- Trafficking in Persons and Worker Exploitation Task Force: 1-888-428-7581
- National Domestic Violence Hotline: 1-800-799-SAFE
- National Sexual Assault Hotline: 1-800-656-HOPE
- National Child Abuse Hotline: 1-800-4-A-Child

Placing a call to a local law enforcement agency for assistance in creating a safe environment for a trafficked person is also an effective strategy.

PREVENTION/PATIENT TEACHING

Prevention of human trafficking is a local, state and federal initiative. Health care professionals interested in the prevention of human trafficking should find a local community prevention program.

RESOURCES

Humantrafficking.org: http://www.humantrafficking.org/updates/777
National Geographic News: U.S. Law Helps Victims of Human Trafficking: http://news.nationalgeographic.com/news/2004/07/0713_040713_tvhumantraffic.html
National Human Trafficking Resource Center: http://www.acf.hhs.gov/trafficking/hotline/index.html
Rescue & Restore: http://www.acf.hhs.gov/trafficking
U.S. Department of State: Trafficking in Persons Report 2007: http://www.state.gov/g/tip/rls/tiprpt/2007/

REFERENCES

Garza, V. (2007). Human trafficking. *On the Edge: Newsletter of the IAFN, 13*(2).
Hynes, P., & Raymond, J. (2002). Put in harm's way: The neglected health consequences of sex trafficking in the United States. In J. L. Silliman (Ed.), *Policing the national body: Sex, race and criminalization* (pp. 197–229). Cambridge, MA: South End Press.
Kangaspunta, K. (2003, December 2–4). *Mapping the inhuman trade: Preliminary findings on the human trafficking database, as presented to the United Nations division of the advancement of women.* United Nations Division for the Advancement of Women

(DAW) Consultative Meeting on Migration and Mobility and How This Movement Affects Women. Malmö, Sweden. Retrieved from http://www.un.org/womenwatch/daw/meetings/consult/CM-Dec03-CRP1.pdf

Klain, E. (1999). *Prostitution of children and child sex tourism: An analysis of domestic and international responses.* National Center for Missing & Exploited Children. Retrieved from http://www.hawaii.edu/hivandaids/Prostitution%20of%20Children%20and%20Child%20Sex%20Tourism.pdf

U.S. Health and Human Services. (n.d.). *Looking beneath the surface.* Retrieved from http://www.acf.hhs.gov/trafficking

21 Victims of Personal Injury

DEFINITION

Many people arrive in health care settings with injuries related to criminal activity. At times it is obvious to health care personnel that the person before the provider is a victim of crime. Stabbings, shootings, and homicide cases are obviously related to criminal activity. Less obvious relationships to criminal activity are victims involved in motor vehicle accidents, poisonings, fraudulent medical care, and other cases with a legal component. Many of these actions, especially motor vehicle accidents, can also be civil wrongs.

Any trauma client can become involved in the legal system. The health care provider has information related to the health of the client in front of them, not the legal aspects of the client. For example, the health care provider may not know, when caring for a person who was involved in a multivehicle crash, that the client is the victim of a drunk driver or the victim of a faulty automobile. Health care is often unaware that the client's injuries are the result of a work-related accident. Health care workers are aware of the circumstances surrounding the injury or injuries in most cases but are unaware of legal implications of client injury at the time they are providing care.

Personal injury is America's number one litigation. Most cases are auto-accident related, but other issues include product liability, slips and falls, job accidents, dog bites, and toxic exposure. Civil actions can be filed related to any client encounter. Health care providers are, in general, aware of the possibility of civil legal action related to the care they provide. All care provided must meet current standards of care. However, civil action may result from malpractice or from many other sources. Civil action can result from health care consequences of an event that occurred outside the health care arena. Common examples are chronic pain as a result of an automobile crash, posttraumatic stress disorder as a result of a crime committed, and injury as a result of institutional negligence.

Torts

A tort is a private (civil) wrong or injury for which a court provides a remedy through an action for damages. States create tort law through legislatures (statutory law) and judges (common law). Torts can even be called civil crimes. Some torts, particularly the intentional ones, such as assault (a threat of bodily harm) and battery (an offensive nonconsensual touch), have the same names as criminal crimes.

Torts fall into three general categories:

Intentional torts are those wrongs that the defendant knew or should have known would occur through his or her actions. Assault and battery are intentional torts. Sometimes called quasi-intentional torts, defamation (slander and libel), invasion of privacy, and breach of confidentiality are common causes of action, with the latter two being relevant to health care litigation.

Negligent torts occur when the defendant's actions were unreasonably unsafe, but the defendant did not intend to commit harm.

Strict liability torts do not depend either on the state of mind or on the degree of carefulness of the defendant. Instead, these pertain to the dangerousness of the activity or the existence of a statute that establishes strict liability, including workers' compensation and products liability.

The Elements of Negligence

Negligence is a type of tort, although it can also be a criminal concept. Essentially, negligence means a failure to use ordinary care through either omission or commission of an act. Thus, negligence occurs when someone (the defendant) does not exercise the care that a reasonably careful person would have used in that circumstance, or someone did something that a reasonably careful person would not do under the same circumstances.

The following are four elements of negligence that have to be proven in civil cases.

Duty: The defendant must first owe a duty to the plaintiff (injured party). Duty is a legal obligation owed by one person to another. In medically related cases, duty is often referred to as standard of care. However, a driver has a duty to stop at a red light and a company has the duty to provide a safe product.

Breach: The defendant must have breached that duty. Breach occurs when there is neglect of or failure to fulfill the duties that have been established as the responsibility of the defendant. In other words, a duty has been breached when the appropriate standard of care has not been met. Breach may also be viewed within the concept of foreseeability, which is the legal test for breach. The more foreseeable the injuries to the plaintiff, the more likely that a duty has been breached. Speeding through a red light at a busy intersection would most likely cause foreseeable injuries.

Causation: There must be a causal relationship between the defendant's breach and the plaintiff's injuries. Proximate, or legal, cause is determined by the facts that show the defendant's legal responsibility for the plaintiff's injuries. Thus, the plaintiff's attorney must establish that the plaintiff's injuries were caused by the defendant's speeding through the red light and hitting the plaintiff.

Damages: The plaintiff's injuries must be compensable through the payment of damages. Damages are monetary payments designed to compensate the plaintiff for an injury. The purpose of damages is to restore the plaintiff to the condition he or she was in prior to the injury. There are two general categories of damages: compensatory and punitive.

Compensatory damages compensate the plaintiff for losses suffered as a result of the defendant's negligent behavior. Compensatory damages can be either general and special. General damages are by their nature difficult to quantify, as in awards for pain and suffering, because different individuals experience pain so differently. Special damages are quantifiable and may include total medical bills and total lost time from work, for example.

Punitive damages punish the defendant when the judge or jury believes the defendant's actions have been especially in the wrong, showing reckless disregard or other lack of concern for consequences.

PREVALENCE AND ETIOLOGY

Injury is the leading cause of death for Americans age 1 through 44. The Centers for Disease Control and Prevention (National Committee for Injury Prevention and Control, 2009) holds statistics for the 10 leading causes of death and injury noted by age, and by nonfatal injury in people who present to a sampling of large emergency departments.

Injuries are classified by morphology (fractures, focal intracranial injury, and diffuse intracranial injury), severity (mild, moderate, and severe), and mechanism (closed vs. penetrating injury). Mechanism of injury (MOI) is the force or forces that cause injury when applied to the human body. These forces have characteristics such as size, speed, and direction. Health care providers who work in this arena should understand the mechanism of injury to provide client care and understand the legal implications related to the injury.

ASSESSMENT

History and Physical Assessment

Treat all cases as if they were trial-bound so that you always use impeccable documentation. All health care records should be legible, clear, and accurate.

Trauma warrants a complete head-to-toe assessment, and health care providers must keep in mind that some signs and symptoms may surface slowly. Documenting the health care history with as many accurate quotes from the patient as possible assists any legal process. The patient's own words, not the interpretation of the patient's words, are what are useful in both criminal and civil cases.

Motor vehicle impact occurs when a vehicle hits an object, such as another vehicle or tree. Body impact occurs when the vehicle occupant hits some structure inside the car such as the steering wheel or dashboard. Organ impact occurs when the organs impact with the supportive structures, for example, when the brain hits the skull or the lungs hit the sternum and ribs.

Frontal collisions can create injuries in the head and neck, back, brain, spine, rib and clavicle, abdomen, and arms and legs. Immediate injuries include concussions, soft tissue damage, internal injuries, fractures, dislocations, abrasions, cuts, and bruises. Internal injuries may surface as late as 48–72 hours after impact. Symptoms associated with delayed internal injury include: headache, blurred vision, dizziness, loss of taste, smell, or hearing, difficulty breathing, blood in urine or stool, and loss of motion.

Side-impact collisions can create injuries in the head and cervical spine. Spinal fractures are more common with this type of collision than with rear-end collisions. The combination of the rotation and flexion of the spine that occurs on lateral impact produces more frequent and severe cervical injuries. Other injuries include "side of impact" injuries to the chest, abdominal area, upper arm, shoulder, clavicle, pelvis, hip, and femur.

Rear-impact collision injuries usually occur as the torso and seat shoot forward. If the victim's headrest is too low, the neck will hyperextend over the top of the headrest, causing strains, torn ligaments, and more serious cervical injuries.

Rollover collision injuries are difficult to predict. If the victim was ejected, injuries usually result from the second impact. Hitting the ground can be more severe than the original impact. The distance between the victim and the vehicle can indicate how fast the car was traveling and, therefore, how much energy was absorbed by the victim. Ejected victims are more likely to be killed than those who remain in the vehicle. Health care providers should observe for evidence of secondary impact (dirt, shrubs, paint from the car, road rash). This evidence can assist in determining the degree of possible injuries.

Incursion collisions often result in the need for extraction, and when extraction is needed, victims frequently present with some type of crushing injury. The steering wheel and/or dashboard often create the entrapment, causing severe leg, pelvic, and abdominal injuries. Cervical spine injuries, as well as face and neck trauma are also common.

Restraint systems are supposed to be protective; however, they can be quite damaging in a collision when worn improperly. If worn too high or worn with the arm removed from the shoulder harness, seat belts increase their risk for the following injuries: compression injuries to abdominal organs, burst injuries to the small intestines and colon, rupture of the diaphragm from increased interabdominal pressure, and compression fractures of the lumbar spine.

Motorcycle accident injuries are similar to those seen when a victim is ejected from a vehicle. Helmets, when properly worn, help prevent head trauma but do not protect against spinal injury. The majority of motorcycle-related deaths are due to severe head trauma. Focus should be placed on head and spinal injuries, and battle signs or raccoon eyes may lead to diagnosis of basal skull fracture.

Pedestrian accidents result when a human is hit by a motor vehicle. In adults, the first impact is made by the bumper to the lower extremities. As the victim folds forward, the second impact occurs when the adult's upper legs and trunk hit the hood of the car. The third impact occurs when the victim falls off the car and hits the ground.

Penetrating injuries result when an object pierces the body. The amount of trauma depends on the amount of energy transferred into the body, and the area over which it is transferred. Penetrating injury can be low-, medium-, or high-velocity, with the difference essentially being in the amount of energy that the victim endures.

Low-velocity injuries usually involve knife attacks, falling through plate glass, or garden tool injuries. Compound fractures also fall into this category. The severity of stab wounds depends on the length of the blade, the location penetrated, and the angle of penetration.

Medium-velocity injuries usually involve handguns, arrows, long-bladed knives or swords, and objects that were used to impale with great force. The bigger the area of contact, the bigger the trauma, and the faster the object, the deeper it goes. When a medium-velocity projectile strikes bone, it may knock many bits off and push them away from the original injury site, increasing soft-tissue trauma by shrapnel effect.

High-velocity injuries usually involve a higher-caliber shotgun or rifle. The projectile strikes at such great speed that it blasts apart a channel far wider than the projectile. This process, called cavitation, forms a star-shaped exit wound if carried on to an exit point. If bone is encountered by the projectile, the bone shatters into small bits, increasing bleeding and tissue damage. The severity of firearm injury depends upon the type of weapon, caliber/size of the bullet, distance from which the weapon was fired, and tumble and yaw of the bullet as the bullet travels forward. The bullet can tumble and oscillate vertically or horizontally about its axis, resulting in a larger surface area meeting the surface of the body, and a bullet deformity (hollow-point and soft-nose bullets flatten out when they impact the victim, so the area damaged is greater).

DIAGNOSTIC TESTING AND INTERVENTION

Diagnostic testing and intervention depend on extent and type of injuries. Documentation should include narrative, diagrams, and photos.

Primary Prevention

Numerous prevention programs exist. Examples are bicycle and motorcycle helmet programs, and programs aimed at the safe use of firearms. The American Association for the Surgery of Trauma suggests the following 10 steps for the creation of an injury prevention program:

1. Gather and analyze data. Examine data related to deaths and hospitalizations. Data from your own community is the most powerful source of information. After examining the data, decide how narrowly you wish to define the target injury and the target population.
2. Select the target injury and population. Think about the severity and frequency of the injury and whether or not there is a prevention method for the injury chosen.
3. Determine intervention strategies. Consider who will provide the intervention strategies.
4. Develop an implementation plan. Be goal-specific, including objectives and a timeline.
5. Identify, select, and commit community agencies to implement the program. Forming a coalition is an effective way to engage community agencies.
6. Develop an action. Activities to accomplish the objectives are the responsibility of the coalition members. Strategies can be educational, legislative, or technological.
7. Orient and train agencies and individuals to implement the intervention plan. Orientation helps solidify roles.

8. Implement the program. Planning is important, but do not lose the initial enthusiasm of the group. Implement the plan as soon as possible.
9. Monitor and support the program. Maintain communications and monitor activities.
10. Evaluate and revise the program. Evaluate both process and outcome and use the results to revise the program.

Secondary Prevention

Programs to prevent injury can be targeted to at risk populations. Secondary programs are similar to primary prevention programs, but a specific audience is the target of the intervention.

Tertiary Prevention

Providing good health care to victims who are injured and creating good documentation of all care provided is tertiary prevention in cases of personal injury.

RESOURCES

American Association for the Surgery of Trauma: Trauma Prevention: http://www.aast. org/Library/dynamic.aspx?id=1680
American Bar Association: http://www.abanet.org
Trauma: Mechanisms of Injury: http://www.lbfdtraining.com/Pages/emt/sectionc/ mechofinjury.html

REFERENCES

American Association for the Surgery of Trauma. (2007). *You can do it: A community guide to injury prevention.* Retrieved from http://www.aast.org/Library/dynamic. aspx?id=1708
Baker, S. P., O'Neill, B., & Karpf, R. S. (1984). *The injury fact book.* Lexington, MA: Lexington Books.
Barringer, P. J., Studdent, D. M.., Kachalia, A. B., & Mello, M. M. (2008). Administrative compensation of medical injuries: A hardy perennial blooms again. *Journal of Health Politics, Policy and Law, 33*(4), 725–760.
Children's Safety Network. (1991). *A data book of child and adolescent injury.* Washington, DC: National Center for Education in Maternal and Child Health.
Hudson, K. (2009). Trauma: Mechanism of injury and appropriate nursing assessment. *Dynamic nursing education.* Retrieved from http://dynamicnursingeducation.com/ class.php?class_id=14&pid=11

National Committee for Injury Prevention and Control. (2009). *Injury prevention: Meeting the challenge.* Atlanta, GA: Program Development and Implementation Branch, Division of Injury Control, Center for Environmental Health & Injury Control, Centers for Disease Control.

Stretzler, J., Eliashof, B. A., Kline, A. E., & Goebert, D. (2000). Chronic pain disorder following physical injury. *Psychosomatic, 41*(3), 227–234.

22 Stalking

DEFINITION

Legal definitions vary by jurisdiction; however, stalking generally describes a pattern of overtly criminal and/or apparently innocent behaviors whereby an individual bestows or inflicts repeated, unwanted communications and intrusions upon another. Stalking has also been referred to as a pattern of behavior directed at a specific person that would cause a reasonable person to feel fear. It can be distinguished from other crimes in two ways: stalking involves repeated victimization, and it is partly defined by its impact on the victim. The first stalking law was passed in California in 1990. Increasing awareness has since made stalking a crime, in many cases a felony, under the law of all 50 states, the District of Columbia, the federal government, and tribal codes.

One study of a community sample of both males and females revealed two broad types of stalking. In the first type, stalking behaviors lasted for less than two weeks, usually involving one or two days of intense harassment that predominantly consisted of approaches or following. The perpetrator was usually a stranger. In the second type, stalking behaviors lasted more than two weeks, usually six months or more. Behaviors consisted of a range of unwanted communications and approaches, and the perpetrator was typically an acquaintance or ex-partner. Regardless of the time or relationship involved, stalking creates uncertainty, instills fear, and sometimes kills.

PREVALENCE

Stalking is widespread, with nearly 1 in 12 women and 1 in 45 men stalked at least once in their lifetime. Most victims know their stalkers, and most stalkers (87%) are male. Almost 60% of female victims and 30% of male victims are stalked by current or former intimate partners, with most of these cases occurring during the relationship. According to a special report on stalking by Baum, Catalano, Rand, and Rose (2009)

- Nearly three in four stalking victims knew their offender in some capacity.
- 46% of stalking victims experienced at least one unwanted contact per week.
- 11% of victims said they had been stalked for 5 years or more.
- The risk of stalking victimization was highest for divorced or separated people—34 per 1,000 individuals.
- Women were at greater risk than men for stalking victimization, but women and men were equally likely to experience harassment.
- Male (37%) and female (41%) stalking victimizations were equally likely to be reported to the police.
- About one in four stalking victims reported some form of cyberstalking, including e-mail (83%) and instant messaging (35%).
- 46% of stalking victims felt fear of not knowing what would happen next.

Stalking behaviors have been found in women and children. In a study of 190 stalkers, 40 (21%) of whom were female, researchers found that female stalkers had demographic and psychiatric profiles similar to their male counterparts but were less likely to have histories of criminality and substance abuse. The intrusiveness and duration of stalking behaviors were similar between the genders, as were the rates of associated threats and violence. Major differences were the choice of victim, underlying motivation for stalking, and the context in which the behavior emerged. Females tended to pursue victims they knew, particularly those with whom they had professional contact (therapists, physicians, legal professionals, and teachers). Almost one-half of the female stalkers were motivated by a desire to forge an intimate relationship with the victim, hopeful for a romantic or sexual relationship, friendship or even mothering alliance.

A literature review by McCann (2003) revealed that empirical literature on children and stalking is limited. However, he found that stalking behaviors, such as dating violence, spying, and leaving unwanted notes or photos were found in young populations. McCann also noted that a small study of 13 juvenile stalkers found patterns consistent with adult perpetrators.

ETIOLOGY

Stalking classifications or typologies vary. The National Center for Victims of Crime (2004) provides a typology that includes simple obsessional, love obsessional, and erotomanic stalkers. The most common type, the simple obsessional stalker, has some type of previous relationship with the victim, usually an intimate one. These cases commonly occur in the context of domestic violence; however, simple obsessional offenders may also stalk neighbors, casual acquaintances, work mates, or professional contacts. The love obsessional stalkers have no existing relationship but believe they are loved by their victims. Many of these offenders stalk celebrities and other media figures, frequently choosing what they describe as "female bombshells." Erotomanic stalkers, a grouping derived from the *Diagnostic and Statistical Manual for Mental Disorders*, 3rd edition, revised (*DSM-III-R*) for the criteria of delusional disorder erotomanic type, delusionally believe that they are loved by the victims. This group, the rarest stalking offending group, is predominately female and almost exclusively focuses their amorous aspirations on those in the entertainment industry.

Mullen (2003) provides a typology that describes five types of stalkers, based on those perpetrators who exhibit stalking behaviors for more than two weeks. This classification is based on a multiaxial approach, whereby the primary axis is a typology relating to the stalker's predominant motivation in commencing and sustaining the stalking. Mullen notes that the five types can overlap, and that in practice it is difficult to consign the vast majority of stalkers to a single type:

- Rejected stalkers are motivated by a desire for reconciliation and/ or revenge. Their stalking becomes a substitute for the lost relationship. Some derive satisfaction from inflicting pain. They often have personality disorders and are among the most persistent and intrusive stalkers.

- Intimacy seekers identify the object of their affection as their true love. Some imagine that the person they are stalking reciprocates such feelings. Many "celebrity-stalkers" fall into this category. Their sought-after partner's indifference may enrage them. Many intimacy seekers have serious mental illnesses such as delusional disorders and need psychiatric intervention.

- Incompetent suitors are those whose stalking is sustained by hopefulness. Their stalking of a particular person usually lasts only a short time. However, these perpetrators, who are often intellectually limited and socially impaired and unable or unwilling to appreciate the negative responses to their approaches, may then pursue others. Incompetent suitors are probably the most common type of stalker in the community.

- Resentful stalkers often are aggrieved workers who feel humiliated or treated unfairly. They may carry out a vendetta against a specific person or choose someone at random as representative of those they believe harmed them. Resentful stalkers are primarily motivated by the desire to frighten and distress their victims, and the majority are suspicious, oversensitive personalities with a tendency to be obsessive and to ruminate.

- Predatory stalkers stalk someone as preparation for a physical or sexual assault and take pleasure in causing sadistic pain. Many have paraphilias, particularly sexual sadism, and prior convictions for sexual offenses. The very process of stalking may provide satisfaction, because it gives the stalker a sense of power and control. This may be heightened by the stalker leaving the victims subtle hints that they are being observed (silent phone calls, entering their homes to move the furniture), causing unease and confusion in the victim. Victims are frequently the object of ridicule when they share their fears and suspicions about being followed or their home being entered.

ASSESSMENT

Offender Behavior

Spitzberg (2003) categorized stalking behaviors into the following forms: hyperintimacy (the difference between an occasional phone call and dozens per day), surveillance and pursuit (driving by the victim's residence, checking up on the victim's whereabouts, waiting at places the victim frequents), invasion (violating the victim's privacy), intimidation and harassment (attempts to harangue), proxy pursuit (gaining the willing or unwitting assistance of others in the stalking process), coercion (threats), and violence.

Stalking is not a one-time event, but a pattern of conduct that may involve criminal activities and/or seemingly nonthreatening acts. According to the National Centers for Victims of Crime (2004), stalking often includes:

- Assaulting the victim
- Violating protective orders
- Sexually assaulting the victim
- Vandalizing the victim's property
- Burglarizing the victim's home or otherwise stealing from the victim
- Threatening the victim
- Killing the victim's pet

Other common stalking behaviors include:

- Sending unwanted cards or gifts
- Leaving phone and/or e-mail messages
- Voyeurism
- Identity theft
- Disclosing to the victim personal information the offender has uncovered about said victim
- Disseminating personal information about the victim
- Following the victim
- Visiting the victim at the victim's workplace; workplace violence
- Waiting outside the victim's home
- Sending the victim photographs taken of the victim without consent
- Monitoring the victim's computer usage
- Using technology to gather images of or information about the victim
- Violating protective orders.

Stalking is often a feature of domestic violence, and, like domestic violence, it is often not taken sufficiently seriously, because it involves acts that health care and law enforcement professionals may perceive as everyday courtship. However, when gestures are part of a course of conduct that instills fear in the victim, they are being used to terrorize.

Victim Reactions

Victim impact is critical in stalking cases, not only for health care intervention, but also for potential evidence, since the legal definition of stalking includes its effect on the victim. Many victims feel constantly hypervigilant, vulnerable, out of control, and anxious. Stalking can rob them of their energy, leaving them with a loss of trust, long-term emotional distress, and significant disruption in everyday living. Symptoms may worsen with each new incident and may be compounded by the victims' concerns about the effects on their children and other secondary victims. Victims may experience:

- Anxiety, fear, and/or depression
- Posttraumatic stress disorder
- Altered thought or perceptual processes (lowered self-esteem, confusion, irrational beliefs)
- Impaired physical health (eating disorders, sleep disorders, digestive distress)
- Financial changes (job loss, investing in home security)
- Altered normal routines to avoid detection by the offender
- Changing phone numbers, e-mail addresses, driver's license, social security number
- Relocating (temporary or permanent)
- Changing identity, uprooting themselves and their immediate families, while leaving behind friends and other relatives.

Some victims may experience resilience through stronger relationships with family and friends and therefore a heightened sense of personal safety. However, these positive aspects are unlikely to outweigh the detriments caused by the victimization.

INTERVENTIONS

Health care professionals need to be knowledgeable of this crime, its behaviors, and the impact it has on victims. To better assist victims:

- Ascertain why a victim believes he or she is being stalked—assess for stalking behaviors.
- Do not challenge or belittle the victim's concerns.
- Assess for and intervene with physiologic and psychological consequences, such as eating and sleep disorders, posttraumatic stress disorder, anxiety, and depression.
- Refer victims for counseling.
- Enable the victim to access victims' resource services, both local resources and Web-based resources. Local victim groups can also assist victims in coping with the legal process if the case comes to trial.
- Encourage the victim to report her or his concerns to the proper authorities (usually local or state police).
- Encourage the victim to obtain a protective/restraining order. These orders are not "bulletproof"; therefore, victims must also take other measures to protect their safety:

  - Obtain an unlisted telephone number, caller ID, voice mail, and cellular phone.
  - Install and utilize quality deadbolt locks, solid core doors, and security systems.
  - Install adequate outdoor lighting; trim bushes and shrubs to avoid hiding places.
  - Notify family, friends, and trusted neighbors of stalking. Provide them with a photo and the vehicle information of the stalker, if possible.
  - Create a contingency plan should going to or staying home not be possible; keep a suitcase packed with necessary supplies.
  - Stay alert and be aware of surroundings.
  - Vary routes of travel to and from work.
  - Park in secure and well-lit areas. Ask a trusted person for an escort to the car.
  - Do not dismiss threats. Report them immediately to the authorities.

- Encourage the victim to collect evidence of stalking:

  - Document all incidents.

    - Keep a stalking journal or log (the Stalking Resource Center has a Stalking Incident and Behavior Log that can be downloaded from its Web site: http://www.ncvc.org/src). Since this information can possibly be used as evidence or inadvertently shared with the stalker at a future time, encourage the victim to not include any information that they do not want the offender to see.

- ◆ Take photographs.
- ◆ Obtain affidavits from witnesses.
- ◆ Videotape the stalker in action, if possible.
- ◆ Keep phone answering machine messages.
- ◆ Keep a list of potential witnesses.

- ■ Carefully preserve all evidence:

  - ◆ Letters, notes, e-mails
  - ◆ Gifts
  - ◆ Damaged property

Given the incidence of stalking against health care professionals, providers should assist health care facilities in developing workplace violence policies that address stalking and its management. Forensic professionals prove invaluable in implementing these policies by working with the risk management department to create safety measures to minimize stalking incidents and to intervene should one occur.

RESOURCES

Antistalking Laws: http://www.ncvc.org/src/main.aspx?dbID=DB_Register204
Cornell University's Antistalking Site: http://www.humec.cornell.edu/stalking
Penn State Resources for Stalking Victims: http://www.sa.psu.edu/cws/sr.shtml
Stalking Help.org (University of Texas): http://homepage.psy.utexas.edu/homepage/Group/BussLAB/stalkinghelp.org
Stalking Resource Center National Center for Victims of Crime: http://www.ncvc.org/src

REFERENCES

American Psychiatric Association. (1987). *Diagnostic and statistical manual of mental disorders* (3rd ed., revised). Washington, DC: Author.

Baum, K., Catalano, S., Rand, M., & Rose, K. (2009). *Stalking victimization in the United States.* National Institute of Justice Bureau of Justice Statistics Special Report (NCJ 224527). Retrieved from http://bjs.ojp.usdoj.gov/content/pub/pdf/svus.pdf

Crime Victims Services, Office of the Attorney General of Texas. (n.d.). *Information on stalking.* Retrieved from http://www.oag.state.tx.us/victims/stalking.shtml#safety

McCann, J. (2003). Stalking and obsessional forms of harassment in children and adolescents. *Psychiatric Annals, 33*(10), 637–640.

Mullen, P. (2003). Multiple classifications of stalkers and stalking behavior available to clinicians. *Psychiatric Annals, 33*(10), 650–658.

Mullen, P., Pathe, M., & Purcell, R. (2001). The management of stalkers. *Advances in Psychiatric Treatment, 7,* 335–342.

National Center for Victims of Crime. (2004). Stalking (Problem-Oriented Guides for Police Problem-Specific Guides Series, No. 22). U.S. Department of Justice, Office of Community Oriented Policing Services (COPS). Retrieved from http://www.cops.usdoj.gov/files/RIC/Publications/e12032163.pdf

National Center for Victims of Crime, Stalking Resource Center. (n.d.). *Stalking fact sheet.* Retrieved from http://www.ncvc.org/src/main.aspx?dbID=DB_Online_National111

Pathe, M., & Mullen, P. E. (1997). The impact of stalkers on their victims. *British Journal of Psychiatry, 170,* 12–17.

Purcell, R., Pathe, M., & Mullen. P. (2001). A study of women who stalk. *The American Journal of Psychiatry, 12,* 2056–2060.

Purcell, R., Pathe, M., & Mullen. P. (2002). The prevalence and nature of stalking in the Australian Community. *Australian New Zealand Journal, 36*(1), 114–120.

Spitzberg, B. (2003). Reclaiming control in stalking cases. *Journal of Psychosocial Nursing & Mental Health Services, 41,* 38–47.

Zona, M. A., Palarea, R. E., & Lane, J. (1998). Psychiatric diagnosis and offender-victim typology of stalking. In J. R. Meloy (Ed.), *The psychology of stalking: Clinical and forensic perspectives* (pp. 70–84). San Diego, CA: Academic Press.

23 Victim Services

Young (2001) notes that while the majority of victims and survivors cope quite well with a little assistance at the time of the crisis, some require additional counseling support for several reasons. These reasons can be organized into four categories, including:

1. Victims who are involved with the criminal justice system often need continuing counseling during the criminal justice process. Postarraignment activities and pretrial issues become a source of annoyance and concern, and the trial itself may trigger stress reactions. After the trial is over, victims may again be placed in trauma by the verdict, the sentence, or the way the sentence is administered.
2. In cases where there is no arrest, victims may need continuing support over the years because of the perceived failure of the criminal justice system.
3. There may be events that occur during victims' lives that trigger additional crisis reactions. These may occur on a continuing basis or years after the crime. The anniversary date of the crime may distress some victims, who may need to talk to a counselor only once each year. Others may find that they are doing okay until another crisis arises or another event such as a marriage, a divorce, the

birth of a child, or the death of a loved one causes them to relive the original crime.

4. Some victims may just take longer to cope with their victimization and to reconstruct a new life.

A multitude of services exists for victims of violence. Health care providers need to be aware of the agencies that exist in their area and also the services that they provide in order to refer victims to the correct resources. The Office for Victims of Crime (n.d.) Victims Assistance Training Program describes four types of service agencies: community-based, faith-based, criminal-justice-based, and reservation-based. Victims may need assistance from one or more of these types of agencies.

COMMUNITY-BASED SERVICES

Community-based organizations (CBOs) are usually created by communities to meet the general needs of community members. These agencies offer a variety of services within a particular focus, such as victims of domestic violence, people with HIV/AIDS, the homeless, and other underserved populations. CBOs offer comprehensive services for their clients, tailor their services to meet the needs of their client populations, and help their clients to navigate through larger service organizations, including criminal justice and public assistance.

CBOs can help a crime victim recover after a crime has occurred by helping them with safety planning, financial planning, and referrals for mental health support. Types of CBOs include: emergency shelters, crisis centers, hospital emergency rooms, homeless shelters, community counseling centers, group support meetings, rape crisis centers, and day care centers. These organizations can provide a number of services to victims:

Crisis intervention and/or supportive counseling

Emergency shelter

Support groups for victims or family members of victims

Assistance with completing or locating victim compensation claims and insurance forms

Referrals for longer-term rehabilitation or hospital treatment

Community education on victimization issues or crime prevention

Immediate assistance with practical needs such as food, clothing, or shelter

Advocacy with other systems (such as the criminal justice system or child protective services)

FAITH-BASED SERVICES

Many victims turn to their religious leaders or community for help. Victims may experience various spiritual reactions, including: questioning of faith and questioning of God; self-blame; anger at God and/or the faith community; realization of vulnerability and mortality; redefinition of moral values; searching for meaning and hope; concern about vengeance, justice, forgiveness; spiritual awakening and strengthening; and reliance on faith/faith community/faith practice.

Faith-based organizations (FBOs) are nonprofit organizations that are religious in nature or have faith as the core value. These organizations deliver traditional social and community services. Examples include the Metropolitan Council on Jewish Poverty, Catholic Charities, and the Salvation Army. Besides counseling and education, FBOs provide meeting space, food, clothing, and emergency supplies.

CRIMINAL JUSTICE–BASED SERVICES

The U.S. criminal justice system is actually made up of many systems. The federal criminal justice system deals with the violation of U.S. criminal law; the U.S. military justice system deals with the violation of the Uniform Code of Military Justice; and tribal-based criminal justice deals with violation of tribal codes within specific tribes' criminal code. Criminal justice systems are also based on violation of each state's criminal law. These systems have services that work with victims.

Criminal justice system providers usually provide services to victims of violent crimes; however, they also help victims of financial and property crimes. These systems also have different rules in different situations, which may include these varieties of situations:

- A victim's entitlement to services depends on the seriousness of the crime.

- Basic rights are afforded only to victims of felonies.

- Victims of any violent crime, felony, or misdemeanor may enjoy such rights.

- Rights have been extended to include victims of juvenile offenders, although these rights may be greatly reduced in comparison to cases involving adult offenders.

- Victims of financial and property crimes, including identity theft, may be covered by victim rights laws and even crime victim compensation.

- A victim may include a business or nonprofit agency.

All crime victims have certain rights from the time when the crime is reported, through the investigation, to the court proceedings and sentencing. Criminal justice agencies have multiple opportunities and some legal obligation to provide crime victims with assistance and services, and these services should be available at every stage of the criminal justice system. In addition to the direct victims of applicable crimes, victims' rights may also be exercised by a family member of a homicide victim; the parent, guardian, or other relative of a minor, or a disabled or incompetent victim; or a victim's legal representative or another person designated by the victim.

A victim's right to be informed is crucial, because without notice of their rights and the services available, victims cannot assert those rights, and without notice of court proceedings, victims may miss the opportunity to exercise the rights they have been afforded. The federal government and most states give victims and/or their families the right to be notified of the status of an investigation or arrest and of scheduled criminal proceedings and the outcomes of those proceedings. In addition, victims may also have the right to be informed of various rights, including the rights to: attend a proceeding and/or submit a victim impact statement, seek restitution for losses, sue the offender for monetary damages in the civil justice system, have a court order that they be protected from the offender and/or the offender's family and associates, and collect witness fees for their testimony.

Victims may have the right to attend and address the court. They usually have the right to make an oral or written statement at sentencing or parole hearings, stating the impact that the crime has had on their lives. Overall, victims may be heard at or during: bail or pretrial release hearings of the offender, entry of plea agreements, posttrial relief or release hearings, probation hearings, change of security status hearings, and commutation or pardon hearings.

Victims have the right to reasonable protection from intimidation and harassment by the offender or the offender's family or associates. This protection may, under certain circumstances, be extended to a victim's family members. Examples of this protection include: safety planning consultation; police escorts to and from court; assistance with restraining orders; secure waiting areas separate from those of the accused and his or her family, witnesses, and friends during court proceedings; closed courtrooms to those who are not parties to a case; assistance in helping a victim to change their name and social security number; assistance in entering local, state, or federal short- and long-term protection programs; residence relocation; denial of bail or imposition of specific conditions of bail release for offenders found to present a danger to the community or to protect the safety of victims and/or witnesses; and/or emergency shelter.

In general, criminal justice–based services provide some or all of the following services:

Orientation to the criminal justice system and process

Assistance to victims and witnesses who must testify

Crisis intervention

Information about individual case status and outcome

Assistance with compensation and restitution, including referrals for civil remedies

Facilitating property return

Information and referral to community services

Education and training for the public, justice system personnel, and other local service providers about the needs and rights of victims

Witness coordination and postdisposition services

RESERVATION-BASED SERVICES

As of July 1, 2002, 4.3 million people in the United States recognized themselves as American Indians/Alaska Natives (AI/AN), and 72% of people from this group reported that they are members in a tribal nation. AI/AN people hold dual citizenship in the United States and in the federally recognized tribe in which they are enrolled. To promote effective relationships with Native American victims of crime, it is important to learn more about the core values inherent to many tribal people. AI/AN people honor their ancestral history, seek reclamation of their tribal identity, and desire to provide a prosperous future for their children.

American Indians experienced a per capita rate of violence twice that of the U.S. resident population. Tribal nations have authority over crimes committed on their own land, with some limitations. According to the amendments to the Indian Civil Rights Act, tribes have the right to govern their own tribally enrolled citizen members living on the Tribal nation's land base, and they have jurisdiction over other Tribal nation members who are living on their land base but are on the roll of another federally recognized tribe. Today more non-Indians live on reservations than do Indians, and tribes do not have authority or jurisdiction over non-Indians who perpetrate crimes on reservation or Indian trust land. The tribe also does not have authority over the crime unless they have in place tribal code that specifically addresses the crime.

REFERENCES

Office for Victims of Crime. (n.d.). *Victim's assistance training: Systems.* Retrieved from http://www.ovcttac.gov/VATOnline_Course/HOME/index.cfm

U.S. Department of Interior, Indian Affairs. (2009). *Victim services.* Retrieved from http://www.bia.gov/WhoWeAre/BIA/OJS/VictimServices/index.htm

Young, M. (2001). Supportive counseling and advocacy. In M. A. Young (Ed.), *Victim assistance: Frontiers and fundamentals.* National Organization for Victim Assistance. Retrieved from http://www.trynova.org/publications

Adults and Older Adults as Offenders

24 Substance Abuse and Offending

DEFINITION

Substance abuse has been associated with numerous crimes, including drug possession and trafficking, driving under the influence, domestic violence, and sexual assault. The U.S. Office of National Drug Control Policy describes four types of substance-related offenses:

- Drug-defined offenses are violations of laws prohibiting or regulating the possession, use, distribution, or manufacture of illegal drugs. Examples of these crimes include: drug possession or use; marijuana cultivation; methamphetamine production; and cocaine, heroin, or marijuana sales.
- Drug-related offenses are those offenses to which a drug's pharmacologic effects contribute; offenses motivated by the user's need for money to support continued use; and offenses connected to drug distribution itself. Examples of these offenses include: violent behavior resulting from drug effects, stealing to get money to buy drugs, and violence against rival drug dealers.
- Drug-using lifestyle offenses result from a lifestyle in which the likelihood and frequency of involvement in illegal activity are increased because drug users may not participate in the legitimate economy

and are exposed to situations that encourage crime. Examples of these offenses include: a life orientation with an emphasis on short-term goals supported by illegal activities, opportunities to offend resulting from contacts with offenders and illegal markets, and criminal skills learned from other offenders.

■ Alcohol-usage offenses result from the inappropriate usage of alcohol. Examples of these offenses include: underage drinking, driving while intoxicated/driving under the influence, and public drunkenness.

Substance abuse is the excessive use of a substance that persists despite negative consequences, which include being arrested for driving under the influence, poor work performance, and marital problems. Substance dependence indicates the presence of problems such as tolerance (increased amounts of substance are needed to produce a desired effect), withdrawal (physiologic symptoms develop when substance use is discontinued abruptly), and giving up pleasurable or important activities because of substances. In substance dependence, the substance dominates the user's life.

PREVALENCE

According to the Bureau of Justice Statistics, in 2004 17% of state inmates and 18% of federal inmates claimed to have committed their current offense to obtain money for drugs. These numbers represent a slight increase for federal prisoners (16% in 1997) and a slight decrease for state prisoners (19% in 1997). In 2002 about 25% of convicted property and drug offenders in local jails had committed their crimes to get money for drugs, compared to 5% of violent and public order offenders. According to the National Crime Victimization Survey (NCVS), there were 5.2 million violent victimizations of residents age 12 or older in 2007, and approximately 26% of the victims reported that the offender was using drugs or alcohol.

According to the World Psychiatric Association, substance abuse seems to be a major determinant of violence. This is true whether or not it occurs in the context of a concurrent mental illness. Persons with substance abuse disorders are major contributors to community violence and may account for as much as one-third of self-reported violent acts, and 7 out of every 10 crimes of violence among mentally disordered offenders.

The Office of National Drug Control Policy (2000/2006) notes that the drug/crime relationship is difficult to quantify because: (a) Crimes usually result from a variety of factors (personal, situational, cultural, and economic); even when drugs are a cause, they are likely to be only one factor among many. (b) The meaning of "drug-related" varies from study to study; some studies interpret the mere presence of drugs as having causal relevance, whereas other studies interpret the relationship more narrowly. (c) Offender self-reports of drug use may be exaggerated or minimized.

Regarding driving under the influence, the 2005 National Survey on Drug Use and Health noted that an estimated 30.7 million persons aged 21 or older (16.6% of adult drivers) reported driving under the influence of alcohol or illegal drugs during the past year. Of these, 1.2 million (0.6% of adult drivers) were arrested for driving under the influence of alcohol or illicit drugs during the past year.

ETIOLOGY

The etiology of substance abuse remains unknown; however, evidence indicates that it is likely multifactorial. Biopsychosocial influences related to substance abuse include:

- Biological: genetic predisposition, biologic vulnerability, inborn metabolism differences, neurotransmitter reward, and reinforcement
- Psychological: immature ego defenses, psychopathology, mood disorders, unresolved conflicts from the past, self-concept disturbance
- Social: accessibility and availability, family influences, peer influence, conditioning and learned behavior, cultural factors, social maladaption, and deviance

Domestic Violence (Intimate Partner Violence)

A batterer's violent behavior can interfere with treatment for substance abuse, and substance abuse can interfere with interventions aimed at changing the violent behavior. Substances can hinder a person's capacity to make a safe and sane choice against violence by impairing the ability to accurately perceive and process information about another's behavior toward him or her. Intoxication seems to increase the chance that a batterer may misinterpret his or her partner's demeanor, remarks, or actions, because it dulls the batterer's cognitive regulators. Abstinence does not alter battering behavior; however, substance abuse negatively affects a batterer's capacity to change and increases the chance that violence will occur.

Driving Under the Influence (DUI)/Driving While Intoxicated (DWI)

Alcohol is a depressant that is quickly absorbed and remains in the body for an extended period of time. It has a significant effect on driving skills.

- Concentration: Attention to driving may decrease and/or drowsiness may occur.
- Comprehension: Alcohol hinders the ability to make rational decisions.
- Vision: Eye muscles function more slowly; eye movement and perception are altered and may result in blurred vision; night vision and color perception are also impaired.
- Tracking: The ability to judge the car's position on the road, the location of other vehicles, the center line, road signs, and other objects can be adversely affected.
- Reaction time: Slow reflexes can decrease the ability to react quickly to situations.
- Coordination: Driving mechanics can be affected by decreased eye/hand/foot coordination.

The legal limit for drinking is the alcohol level above which an individual is subject to legal penalties, such as arrest for DUI. Measured using either a blood alcohol test or a breathalyzer, legal limits are usually defined by state law and may vary based on individual characteristics such as age and occupation. All states have adopted 0.08% (80 mg/dL) as the legal limit for operating a motor vehicle for drivers aged 21 years or older. However, drivers under age 21 years are not allowed to operate a motor vehicle with any level of alcohol in their system. Legal limits do not define a level below which it is safe to operate a vehicle or engage in other activities, since impairment due to alcohol use begins to occur at levels well below the legal limit.

ASSESSMENT

General Principles

Health care professionals can play a critical role in early identification of substance abuse problems to prevent clients from becoming offenders, as well as in assisting those offenders with substance abuse disorders in the reentry process. More Americans abuse alcohol than illicit drugs; thus, primary care providers will encounter substantially more clients with alcohol problems than with drug problems—although many who abuse one substance abuse others. Most people who consume alcoholic beverages do not experience problems related to their use, but primary care providers can expect that 15% to 20% of their male patients and 5% to 10% of their female patients will be at risk for or already are experiencing related medical, legal, and/or psychosocial problems.

History and Physical Assessment

Clients do not typically present with complaints of substance abuse problems; however, they can present with "red flags." Red flag manifestations can be detected through physical examination or by screening during consultation for atypical progress of medical problems. None of the red flags is pathognomonic for alcohol or drug problems, but the presence of even one should raise suspicion, as should a history of relationship difficulties, poorly explained trauma, or convictions for driving while intoxicated (DWI).

Red flag signs and symptoms include:

- Frequent absences from school or work
- History of frequent trauma or accidental injuries
- Depression or anxiety
- Labile hypertension
- Gastrointestinal symptoms (e.g., epigastric distress, diarrhea, or weight changes)
- Sexual dysfunction
- Sleep disorders
- Mild tremor
- Odor of alcohol on breath
- Enlarged, tender liver
- Nasal irritation (suggestive of cocaine snorting)
- Conjunctival irritation (suggestive of exposure to marijuana smoke)
- Labile blood pressure, tachycardia (suggestive of alcohol withdrawal)
- Heavy aftershave/cologne/mouthwash usage (to mask the odor of alcohol)
- Odor of marijuana on clothing
- Signs of chronic obstructive pulmonary disease, hepatitis B or C, HIV infection

Screening

Screening for Substance Problems in Health Care Settings

Screening can vary from one simple question to extensive assessment using a standardized questionnaire. The level of screening usually depends on the client's characteristics, the presence of other medical or psychiatric problems, the health care provider's skills, and the amount of time available. A number of screening methods are available (please be advised that these are screening tools and not diagnostic measures), including:

1. The single-screening question, recommended by the National Institute of Alcohol Abuse and Alcoholism (NIAAA), accurately identifies unhealthy alcohol use in primary-care patients. The recommended question is, "How many times in the past year have you had X or more drinks in a day?" (X stands for 5 for men and 4 for women). A positive response to this single-question screen was defined as more than one.

2. The NIAAA also has guidelines on screening and brief intervention for primary care and mental health practitioners in their *Helping Patients Who Drink Too Much: A Clinician's Guide* (see resource section). It includes the Alcohol Use Disorders Identification (AUDIT) screening tool, both in English and Spanish, as a self-report option.

3. The American Society of Addiction Medicine has developed standards for a positive screen based on the number of drinks ingested per week. A positive screen is considered consumption of more than 14 drinks per week or more than 4 drinks per occasion for men, and more than 7 drinks per week or more than 3 drinks per occasion for women.

4. The CAGE questionnaire is useful in primary care because it is short, simple, and easy to remember. It has also been proven effective for detecting a range of alcohol problems.

   C: Have you ever felt you should *cut down* on your drinking?

   A: Have people *annoyed* or *angered* you by criticizing your drinking?

   G: Have you ever felt bad or *guilty* about your drinking?

   E: Have you ever had an *eye opener* (drink) first thing in the morning to steady your nerves or to get rid of a hangover?

When using the CAGE, two positive responses are considered a positive test and indicate further assessment is warranted.

5. The Michigan Alcohol Screening Test (MAST) is a self-scoring screening tool that uses 22 yes/no questions. It can be found at: http://www.ncadd-sfv.org/symptoms/mast_test.html

6. The Drug Abuse Screening Test (DAST) is a self-report scale that parallels the MAST. It comes in 10-, 20-, and 28-question versions. All versions are easy to use and all have been found to yield satisfactory measures of reliability and validity for use as clinical or research tools. The 10-item version can be found at: http://www.drugabuse.gov/diagnosis-treatment/DAST10.html.

7. The Conjoint Screening Test involves only two questions: "In the past year, have you ever drunk or used drugs more than you meant to?" and "Have you felt you wanted or needed to cut down on your drinking or drug use in the past year?" When studied in primary care, at least one positive response detected current substance-use disorders with nearly 80% sensitivity and specificity.

Screening for Substance Problems in the Criminal Justice Setting

Most states mandate screening and assessment of DUI offenders to evaluate the extent of their alcohol use problems and their need for treatment. Sentencing guidelines also recommend that all DUI offenders be screened for alcohol use problems and recidivism risk. However, existing screening programs differ in their evaluations. Some programs conduct a simple screening, while others combine screening with assessment, referral guidelines, and specific treatment recommendations. Screening for substance disorders in the criminal justice setting creates unique challenges. Effectiveness may be limited due to the use of instruments, such as the MAST, that were developed in populations other than criminal justice populations and that were not designed specifically for use in court-mandated screening. These instruments also rely on the offenders' self-report, making it more difficult to truly gauge alcohol consumption.

INTERVENTION

If problem drinking is diagnosed, even brief health care provider advice can be helpful. The NIAAA Guide, *Helping Patients Who Drink Too*

Much: A Clinician's Guide and Related Professional Support (link in resource section), provides guidelines for brief interventions. Clients with alcohol dependency or other substance disorders warrant referral to an addiction specialist or treatment center.

PREVENTION/PATIENT TEACHING

Primary Prevention

For most adults, moderate alcohol use (up to two drinks per day for men and one drink per day for women and older people) causes few if any problems. (One drink equals one 12-ounce bottle of beer or wine cooler, one 5-ounce glass of wine, or 1.5 ounces of 80-proof distilled spirits.) However, certain people should not drink at all:

■ People younger than age 21
■ Women who are pregnant or trying to become pregnant
■ People who plan to drive or engage in other activities that require alertness and skill (such as driving a boat, or using heavy machinery)
■ People taking certain over-the-counter or prescription medications
■ People with medical conditions that can be made worse by drinking
■ Recovering alcoholics

Clients should be taught the following:

■ If you do choose to drink, have a designated driver before drinking.
■ Drink slowly, and alternate alcoholic beverages with nonalcoholic ones. The body can efficiently metabolize only one drink in an hour.
■ Do not drink on an empty stomach. Eat foods with a high fat content, such as meats or cheeses, because these foods are metabolized at a slower rate.
■ Choose drinks that are heavily diluted with juices, cream, or nonalcoholic mixers to help slow the metabolic rate. Avoid carbonated mixers and alcoholic beverages such as champagne, sparkling wine, or wine coolers; these increase alcohol absorption.
■ Avoid drinking games, which can be deadly.

- Avoid alcohol if you are taking any medication, including aspirin.
- Do not be pressured into consuming more alcohol than is safe.

Tertiary Prevention

Several treatment options are available to address offenders' needs and situations in the correctional system. Therapeutic communities (TCs) are intensive, long-term, self-help, highly structured, residential treatment modalities for chronic, hardcore drug users. Pharmacological maintenance programs involve the long-term administration of a medication that either replaces the illicit drug or blocks its actions. Inmates can participate in outpatient drug treatment, which includes a range of protocols, from highly professional psychotherapies to informal peer discussions. Counseling services include individual, group, or family counseling, peer group support, vocational therapy, and cognitive therapy. Aftercare, an important tool in relapse prevention, usually consists of 12-step meetings, group and/or individual counseling, recovery training, self-help and relapse-prevention strategies, and/or vocational counseling. Offenders who need more intensive rehabilitative services during the transition or aftercare phase may be referred to residential treatment. Finally, multimodality programs provide a combination of services, including inpatient treatment, medical care, vocational training, family therapy, TCs, methadone maintenance, group psychotherapy, individual psychotherapy, drug education, and stress-coping techniques.

RESOURCES

American Society of Addiction Medicine: http://www.asam.org

Assessing Alcohol Problems: A Guide for Clinicians and Researchers, 2nd Edition: http://pubs.niaaa.nih.gov/publications/Assesing%20Alcohol/index.htm

Centers for Disease Control and Prevention Alcohol and Public Health: http://www.cdc.gov/alcohol/index.htm

Helping Patients Who Drink Too Much: A Clinician's Guide and Related Professional Support Resources: http://www.niaaa.nih.gov/Publications/EducationTrainingMaterials/guide.htm

National Institute on Drug Abuse: http://www.nida.nih.gov

REFERENCES

Center for Substance Abuse Treatment. (2005). *Substance abuse treatment for adults in the criminal justice system.* Treatment Improvement Protocol (TIP) Series 44.

DHHS Publication No. (SMA) 05-4056. Rockville, MD: Substance Abuse and Mental Health Services Administration.

Ewing, J. A. (1984). Detecting alcoholism: The CAGE questionnaire. *JAMA: Journal of the American Medical Association, 252*(14), 1905–1907.

Mersey, D. (2003). Recognition of alcohol and substance abuse. *American Family Physician, 67*(7), 1529–1532.

National Institute of Alcohol Abuse and Alcoholism (NIAAA). (2005). Screening for alcohol use and alcohol related problems. *Alcohol Alert, 65*. Retrieved from http://pubs.niaaa.nih.gov/publications/aa65/AA65.htm

National Institute on Alcohol Abuse and Alcoholism (NIAAA). (2007). FAQs for the general public. Retrieved from http://www.niaaa.nih.gov/FAQs/General-English/default.htm#safe_level.

National Survey on Drug Use and Health. (2005). Retrieved from http://www.oas.samhsa.gov/nhsda.htm

Office of National Drug Control Policy. (2000/2006). *Drug related crime.* Retrieved from http://www.whitehousedrugpolicy.gov/publications/factsht/crime/index.html

Palmera, R., Younga, S., Hopferb, C., Corleya, R., Stallings, M., Crowleyb, T., et al. (2009). Developmental epidemiology of drug use and abuse in adolescence and young adulthood: Evidence of generalized risk. *Drug and Alcohol Dependence, 102*, 78–87.

Substance Abuse and Mental Health Services Administration (SAMHSA). (2005). *National Survey on Drug Use and Health.* Retrieved from http://www.oas.samhsa.gov/2k5/DUIarrests/DUIarrests.htm

U.S. Department of Justice Bureau of Justice Statistics. (2009). *Drug and crime facts.* Retrieved from http://www.ojp.usdoj.gov/bjs/dcf/contents.htm

West Virginia University School of Medicine. (n.d.). *Driving and alcohol.* Retrieved from http://www.hsc.wvu.edu/som/cmed/alcohol/driving.htm

Yudko, E., Lozhkina, O., & Fouts, A. (2007). A comprehensive review of the psychometric properties of the Drug Abuse Screening Test. *Journal of Substance Abuse Treatment, 32*(2), 189–198.

Offenders With Mental Illness and Cognitive Impairment

DEFINITION

From a health care perspective, psychiatric and cognitive disorders usually refer to diagnostic labels as per the *Diagnostic and Statistical Manual of Mental Disorders,* 4th edition, text revision (*DSM-IV-TR*). However, the legal world uses terms such as "mental disorder" (usually for psychiatric illnesses) or "mental defect" (usually for mental retardation).

Competency refers to the "here-and-now" ability of an offender to function, such as competency to stand trial or to plead guilty, as well as competency to waive Miranda warnings; competency to confess; competency to waive trial by jury; competency to waive counsel; competency to testify; competency to be sentenced; and competency to be executed. Criminal responsibility, as in the insanity defense, refers to the offender's mental state at the time of the offense (MSO).

Competency to Proceed

Competency denotes the person's capacity to function knowingly and meaningfully in a legal proceeding, understanding the legal proceedings, communicating with attorneys, appreciating one's role in the proceedings, and making legally relevant decisions. Competency to stand trial

(CST), also termed "fitness," serves three legal purposes: (a) being fit to stand trial safeguards the accuracy of the criminal adjudication and thereby guarantees a fair trial; (b) fitness preserves the dignity and integrity of the legal process and ensures that the defendant knows why he or she will be punished if found guilty; and (c) trying incompetent defendants violates their constitutional rights, including the 14th Amendment right to due process. This is known as the Dusky standard for competency to stand trial, set by the U.S. Supreme Court in *Dusky v. U.S.* in 1960. All states now have competency statutes that are either exact or modified versions of the original Dusky standard. The standard is whether a defendant has adequate present ability to consult with his attorney with a reasonable degree of rational understanding of the proceedings against him. It is not sufficient that the defendant be oriented to time, place, and some events. Defendants may be in need of brief competency assessments while awaiting trial if they exhibit bizarre behavior.

Requests for evaluations may also come from the defendant's defense attorney or the court. Assessments involve a mental status exam (MSE), clinical interview, and psychological tests. Tests utilized in competency to proceed evaluations include the Competency Screening Test (CST), and the Competency Assessment Instrument (CAI). Competency to proceed determines the defendant's capacity in the present, and the defendant's competency must be determined each time he or she goes to court. A previous determination of incompetence does not preclude a subsequent finding of competency in a later, unrelated case. If a defendant is found competent, the prosecution proceeds with its case. If a defendant is found incompetent, either the trial is postponed until competency is regained, or the charges are dismissed, usually without prejudice. The offender may be committed or given an alternative to commitment, if found incompetent.

Criminal Responsibility

The law recognizes that the responsibility for committing a crime depends on two factors: *actus reus* (evidence that the accused engaged in the act) and *mens rea* (evidence that the accused had the required mental state to have intended to commit the act or have foreseen its consequences). Intent is critical in homicide cases, because it helps separate different degrees of killing, from negligence for manslaughter to premeditation for first-degree murder. Sanity is a legal, not clinical, term related to a plea of "not guilty by reason of insanity" (NGRI). Sanity evaluations may be entered into evidence at a criminal trial to help a judge or jury determine whether a defendant is criminally responsible for an alleged offense. The definition of legal sanity varies from one jurisdiction to another but usually denotes the defendant's ability to tell right from wrong regarding the offense.

Most jurisdictions also view insanity, automatism (somnambulism, hypnotic states, fugues, epilepsy, and metabolic disorders), and diminished capacity (impaired mental state short of insanity), as separate defenses. A defense of diminished capacity is typically used to aid in determining the degree of the offense or the punishment.

Currently all insanity standards require that the defendant had a mental disease or defect at the time of the offense. However, the terms "mental disease" and "mental defect" do not equate with particular disorders listed in the *DSM-IV-TR*. Courts typically rule that serious psychotic and mood disorders qualify as a mental disease, and mental retardation qualifies as a mental defect. However, the courts do not usually qualify personality disorders, paraphilias, and voluntary intoxication as a disease or defect. Forensic mental health specialists typically review all pertinent medical and legal records and perform a mental status exam (MSE), interview, and psychological testing of the offender. An instrument that may be used in this assessment is the Rogers Criminal Responsibility Assessment Scales (R-CRAS).

PREVALENCE

Persons with mental illness are more likely to be a victim of a crime than commit one; however, at midyear 2005 more than half of all prison and jail inmates had a mental health problem, including 705,600 inmates in state prisons (56% of state prisoners), 78,800 in federal prisons (45% of federal prisoners), and 479,900 in local jails (64% of jail inmates). Female inmates had much higher rates of mental health problems than male inmates, and the prevalence of mental health problems varied by racial or ethnic group.

White inmates were more likely to have a mental illness than Blacks and Latinos. The rate of mental health problems also varied by the age of inmates, with inmates ages 24 or younger having the highest rate of mental health problems and those ages 55 or older having the lowest rate. Prisoners with mental illnesses also had higher rates of homelessness, violent crime, histories of being in foster care or institutions, substance abuse, histories of sexual abuse, and higher rates of family members with substance abuse and incarceration.

Prisoners with mental illness also had lower rates of employment, and one-third of them used drugs at the time of their offense. Offenders with a triple diagnosis—substance abuse, mental illness, and developmental disability, are a small subgroup of criminal offenders with complex needs. Offenders with dual diagnosis are at high risk for a range of other problems in functioning, including homelessness, lack of employment, physical health problems, and interpersonal conflicts.

Individuals with developmental disabilities constitute a small, but growing percentage of offenders within the criminal justice system. Persons with intellectual disabilities comprise 2% to 3% of the general population, but they represent 4% to 10% of the prison population, with an even greater number in jails. Some people with intellectual disabilities commit crimes because of their unique personal experiences, environmental influences, and individual differences. Offenses range from property crimes, including theft and robbery, to physical and sexual assault.

ETIOLOGY

While a variety of disorders present in the offender population, some are more common than others. It is important to note that symptoms, more than diagnostic labels, are more likely to correlate with offending behaviors and that comorbid substance abuse increases the chances for offending.

Antisocial personality disorder is a pervasive pattern of disregard for the rights of others, which includes characteristics such as: failure to conform to social norms and observe lawful behaviors; deceitfulness, repeated lying, use of aliases, or conning others; impulsivity or failure to develop long-term plans; irritability and aggressiveness; disregard for the safety of others; consistent irresponsibility; and lack of remorse and indifference to harming, mistreating, or stealing from another.

Psychopathy is not in the *DSM-IV-TR*, but it should be differentiated from antisocial personality disorder. Characteristics include being: hot-headed, manipulative, exploitative, irresponsible, self-centered, shallow, and unable to bond. Affected persons may lack empathy or anxiety, lack remorse, or may exhibit: shallow emotions, serial relationships, lying, glibness, low frustration tolerance, parasitic lifestyle, and persistent violation of norms.

Narcissistic personality disorder is characterized by a pattern of grandiosity and an excessive need for admiration. People with a narcissistic personality disorder tend to have manifestations that include: an exaggerated sense of being special, such that they limit their associations only to others deemed worthy; exploitation of others to advance their own ambitions; lack of empathy; belief that others envy them; preoccupation with fantasies of unlimited power and success; belief that they deserve ideal love; a sense of entitlement; and arrogant behaviors. Lack of empathy coupled with exploitation can lead to abuse, as well as financial crimes.

Persons with borderline personality disorder have a pervasive pattern of unstable relationships, poor self-image, and affects with marked impulsivity. Manifestations include: frantic efforts to avoid real or perceived abandonment, unstable and intense interpersonal relationships, identity disturbance, poor impulse control, volatile affect, black-and-white thinking, chronic feelings of emptiness, inappropriate anger and handling of anger, and self-mutilation and/or recurrent suicidal behavior. Inappropriate anger and impulsivity can lead to fights and other types of violence.

People with histrionic personality disorder show excessive mood instability and are often unpredictable and theatrical. They desperately seek attention and may believe that a relationship is a lot more than it actually is, thus making them candidates for becoming stalkers (they refuse to accept the reality of the relationship).

Schizophrenia is a group of mental disorders characterized by major disturbances in thought, perception, emotion, and behavior. Thinking is illogical and often accompanied by delusional beliefs. Distorted perceptions may take the form of hallucinations, and emotions are flat or inappropriate. Paranoid schizophrenia is a common concern in criminal justice as it describes those who hear voices that command them to kill, stalk, or destroy property. As many as 5% of prison inmates may have schizophrenia.

Also known as manic-depressive disorder, bipolar disorder is a cyclic disturbance usually characterized by periods of mania and depression. Mania is manifested by an elevated, expansive, or irritable mood, beyond what would be considered normal or typical. Individuals may appear to have an inflated sense of self-worth or grandiosity, and their thoughts or speech may be very rapid and difficult to follow. Judgment is usually poor, and they may behave recklessly in many areas, including driving. Mania often co-occurs with substance abuse, making diagnosis difficult. Bipolar disorder is thought to affect up to 6% of the prison population.

Cognitive impairment problems vary among offenders and include mental retardation (MR), learning disorders, and organic brain syndrome. The latter may be due to problems such as traumatic brain injury syndrome (TBI) or Wernicke-Korsakoff syndrome. Persons with TBI can have general and executive cognitive impairments that may result in antisocial behaviors, and persons with MR and learning disorders may have associated factors that combine to result in offending behaviors. Research has focused on global cognitive impairment, learning disability, or mental retardation, and thus the impact of even minor cognitive impairments has generally not been recognized or explored.

ASSESSMENT

General Principles

Most clients with psychotic disorders are not violent, but clients with acute psychosis who are paranoid and having command auditory hallucinations, or who have a history of being violent, being a victim of violence, or abusing alcohol or drugs are at high risk for violent behavior.

History and Physical Assessment

While screening tools exist for specific disorders, such as depression, nothing is available for general screening at this time. Therefore, health care providers should utilize the clinical interview and mental status exam to assess for signs of mental illness.

INTERVENTION

Persons with significant mental illness warrant referral to the appropriate mental health specialist. Offenders with mental illness warrant appropriate treatment to assist them in the reentry process and to minimize recidivism. Some offenders enter the mental health system through mental health courts. Mental health courts require collaboration from practitioners in both the criminal justice and mental health fields. These courts generally deal with nonviolent offenders who have been diagnosed with a mental illness or comorbid mental health and substance abuse disorders.

PREVENTION/PATIENT TEACHING

Primary Prevention

Minimize risk factors for mental illness:

- Access to drugs and alcohol
- Displacement
- Isolation and alienation
- Lack of education, transport, housing
- Peer rejection
- Poor social circumstances
- Poor nutrition
- Poverty
- Work stress
- Unemployment

Promote protective factors for mental illness:

- Empowerment
- Positive interpersonal interactions
- Social participation
- Social services
- Social support and community networks

Secondary Prevention

Mental health courts are one of many initiatives launched in the past two decades to address the large numbers of people with mental illnesses involved in the criminal justice system. Mental health courts are specialized court dockets for certain defendants with mental illnesses. These courts substitute a problem-solving model for traditional criminal court processing. Participants are identified through mental health assessments and voluntarily participate in a judicially supervised treatment plan developed jointly by a team of court staff and mental health professionals. Offenders are rewarded with incentives for adherence to the treatment plan or other court conditions and are sanctioned for nonadherence. Mental health courts vary widely in factors such as target population, charge accepted (for example, misdemeanor versus felony), plea arrangement, intensity of supervision, program duration, and type of treatment available.

Without adequate treatment while incarcerated or linkage to community services upon release, many offenders with mental illnesses cycle repeatedly through the justice system.

RESOURCES

American Psychiatric Association: http://www.psych.org
American Psychological Association: http://www.apa.org
Effective Prison Mental Health Services: http://www.nicic.org/pubs/2004/018604.pdf
Substance Abuse and Mental Health Services Administration (SAMHSA): http://mental health.samhsa.gov/

REFERENCES

Abrams, A. A. (2002). Assessing competency in criminal proceedings. In B. V. Dorsten (Ed.), *Forensic psychology: From classroom to courtroom* (pp 105–142). New York: Kluwer Academic/Plenum Publishers.

American Psychiatric Association. (2000). *Diagnostic and statistical manual of mental disorders* (4th ed., text revision). Washington, DC: Author.

Council of State Governments Justice Center Criminal Justice/Mental Health Consensus Project New York, New York for the Bureau of Justice Assistance Office of Justice Programs U.S. Department of Justice. (2008). *Mental health courts: A primer for policymakers and practitioners.* Retrieved from http://www.ojp.usdoj.gov/BJA/pdf/MHC_Primer.pdf

Fethouse, A. (2003). Competency to stand trial. *Behavioral Sciences and the Law, 21,* 281–283.

Ireland, C. (2008). Cognitive impairment and sex offending: Management during therapy and factors in offending. *The British Journal of Forensic Practice, 10*(2), 18–25.

Jame, D., & Glaze, R. (2006). *Mental health problems of prison and jail inmates.* Bureau of Justice Statistics Special Report (NCJ 213600). Retrieved from http://www.ojp.usdoj.gov/bjs/pub/pdf/mhppji.pdf

West, S., & Noffsinger, S. (2006). How to assess a defendant's mental state at the time of the offense. *Journal of Family Practice, 5*(8). Retrieved from http://www.jfponline.com/Pages.asp?AID=4312

World Health Organization (WHO). (2004). *Prevention of mental disorders, effective interventions and policy options.* Retrieved from http://www.who.int/mental_health/evidence/en/prevention_of_mental_disorders_sr.pdf

26 | Violence Risk Assessment

DEFINITION

Risk assessment is a broad concept that encompasses multiple meanings that depend on context. In public health, risk assessment is the process of quantifying the probability of a harmful effect to individuals or populations. Thus, risk assessment requires determination of quantitative and/or qualitative values of risk related to a situation and a recognized threat. This chapter explores factors related to formal risk assessment, as well as those that can assist health care providers in the clinical arena.

Violence risk assessment also encompasses multiple meanings, as it can relate to a number of types of violence, such as intimate partner violence, workplace violence, sexual violence, or violence risk in general, and can be either clinical or forensic in nature. Clinicians assess the risk for harm that individuals pose to themselves and others, the need for involuntary treatment, readiness for discharge, and the potential for violent recidivism, while the courts and department of corrections assess risk for pretrial release, sentencing, and parole. Lately, employers and school officials have been asked to estimate the nature and degree of risk a particular individual may pose to others.

While health care professionals cannot predict which clients will succumb to heart attacks or strokes, they are expected to screen for those at risk and do something to try to prevent these events from happening. The same is true for violence. No professional can predict which clients will become violent. However, like physiologic illnesses, violence has risk factors, and thus health care providers can determine risk, or at least screen for those at risk and refer them for more accurate assessment.

PREVALENCE

The U.S. Department of Justice Bureau of Statistics reported that the violent crime rate decreased 1.4% from 2006 to 2007 and 17.7% from 1998 to 2007. The rate of family violence fell between 1993 and 2002 from an estimated 5.4 victims to 2.1 victims per 1,000 U.S. residents age 12 or older. The FBI reported that violent crimes in all population groups declined: murder by 4.4%, aggravated assault by 4.1%, forcible rape by 3.3%, and robbery by 2.2%. They also reported increases in some areas:

- Murder and nonnegligent manslaughter increased in midsized cities with populations of 50,000 to 99,999 (3.3%), as well as in smaller cities of populations under 10,000 (9.8%).
- Increases were noted in the northeast. Forcible rapes were up slightly (0.6%), as were burglaries (2.7%) and larceny-theft (2.9%) during the same 6-month period in 2007. Property crimes rose in the northeast by 1.7%.
- Cities with populations of one million or more recorded a 3.4% jump in forcible rapes.
- The South demonstrated an increase in burglaries (0.6%) and larceny-thefts (0.5%).

ETIOLOGY

Mental illness is not a sufficient cause of violence. Instead, major determinants of violence continue to be sociodemographic and economic factors. The literature is rich in etiology of specific forms of violence, particularly youth violence. This section examines general etiological factors.

Risk and Mental Illness

According to the National Crime Victimization Survey for 1993 to 1999, the annual rate of nonfatal, job-related, violent crime was 12.6 per 1,000 workers in all occupations. The rate increases to 16.2 per 1,000 for physicians, and 21.9 per 1,000 for nurses. For psychiatrists and mental health professionals, the rate was 68.2 per 1,000. However, clinical experiences with violence are not representative of the behaviors of the majority of mentally ill individuals. The MacArthur Violence Risk Assessment Study (Monahan et al., 2001) stands out as the most sophisticated attempt to date to disentangle the complex interrelationships related to mental illness and violence.

The researchers collected extensive follow-up data on a large cohort of subjects ($N = 1,136$) and used multiple measures of violence, including patient self-report. In this study, the prevalence of violence among those with a major mental disorder who did not abuse substances was indistinguishable from their nonsubstance-abusing neighborhood controls. A concurrent substance-abuse disorder doubled the risk of violence. Subjects with schizophrenia had the lowest occurrence of violence over the course of the year (14.8%), compared to those with a bipolar disorder (22.0%) or major depression (28.5%). Delusions were not associated with violence, including "threat-control override" delusions that cause an individual to think that someone is out to harm them or that someone can control their thoughts.

- Neuropsychiatric disorders

  - Traumatic brain injury
  - Cerebral vascular accidents
  - Huntington's disease
  - Dementia

- Medical and neurological conditions and dementia may precipitate aggression in patients who are not normally violent.
- Medical disorders

  - Delirium
  - Metabolic disorders
  - Encephalitis

- Axis I psychiatric disorders

  - Schizophrenia
  - Mania
  - Process usually occurs from delusions of hallucinations related to medication noncompliance or failure

- Axis II cluster B personality disorders
  - Antisocial
  - Borderline
  - Narcissistic
  - Histrionic
- Other psychiatric disorders

  - Mental retardation
  - Pervasive developmental disorders
  - Impulse-control disorders
  - Attention deficit hyperactivity disorder (ADHD)
  - Oppositional defiant disorder (ODD)
  - Conduct disorder (CD)
  - Tourette syndrome
  - Posttraumatic stress disorder (PTSD)

Risk and Substance Abuse

The majority of people who drink alcohol do not become violent; however, overwhelming evidence implicates alcohol in the expression of violence. According to Stuart (2003), substance abuse appears to be a major factor in violence, which is true whether it occurs in the context of a concurrent mental illness or not. Persons with substance disorders are major contributors to community violence, possibly accounting for as much as a third of self-reported violent acts, and 7 out of every 10 crimes of violence among mentally disordered offenders.

Research evidence indicates that drug users are more likely than nonusers to commit crimes, arrestees frequently were under the influence of a drug at the time they committed their offense, and drugs including alcohol, cocaine, PCP, and amphetamines generate violence. Other issues related to substance abuse and violence are:

- Problems related to violence:

  - Drug-seeking behavior
  - Violence under the influence
  - Withdrawal leading to aggression due to drug-seeking behavior, paranoia, or extreme anxiety

Other problem substances can include: caffeine; water (intoxication); antihistamines; inhalants; anabolic steroids, which can lead to road rage. Problems with anabolic steroids include the following:

- Many users report feeling good about themselves while on anabolic steroids.
- Users may experience extreme mood swings, including manic-like symptoms leading to violence.
- Depression is often seen when drugs are stopped and may contribute to dependence on anabolic steroids.
- Users may suffer from paranoid jealousy, extreme irritability, delusions, and impaired judgment stemming from feelings of invincibility.

Risk and Psychopathy

Characteristics of psychopathy include lack of a conscience or sense of guilt, lack of empathy, egocentricity, pathological lying, repeated violations of social norms, disregard for the law, shallow emotions, and a history of victimizing others. Not all psychopaths are violent. However, psychopaths are more likely to commit violence, use weapons, and be aggressive in prison than other criminals and are more likely to commit other crimes when released from prison. They are more likely to choose sadistic techniques and are motivated more by gain than arousal.

ASSESSMENT

There are three basic approaches to risk assessment:

1. Clinical assessment relies on personal judgment and experience. The logic behind this approach to assessment is that the clinician has a basis of experience, expertise, and perhaps even natural insight that allows for an impressionistic interpretation of the client's risk. This has been shown to be fairly unreliable.
2. Actuarial assessments are based upon risk factors that have been researched and demonstrated to be statistically significant in the prediction of reoffense or dangerousness. They identify specific criteria used and assign weight to each based on significance. Actuarial assessment does not consider case-specific information.
3. Structured clinical assessments allow clinicians to consider a number of variables that will have some application to the assessment of risk in the case under consideration.

Assessment tools include the following.

The Historical, Clinical, and Risk Management 20-item checklist (HCR-20) consists of 10 historical items (such as previous violence and young age at first violence), 5 clinical items (such as lack of insight and negative attitude), and 5 risk management items (such as lack of personal support and noncompliance with remediation efforts) shown to predict violence. Information on the HCR-20 can be found at http://www3.par inc.com/products/product.aspx?Productid=HCR-20.

The Violence Risk Appraisal Guide (VRAG) gives the probability (from zero to 100%) that an offender will commit a new violent offense within a specified period of community access and shows how one offender's risk compares to others. The VRAG is for men who have committed serious, violent, or sexual offenses. The VRAG may be found at http://www.tennes see.gov/mental/policy/forms/MHDDvrag.pdf.

The Psychopathy Checklist—Revised (PCL-R) is a 20-item scale that measures the degree to which an individual displays the prototypical characteristics of a psychopath. The scale consists of two factors, one representing an antisocial and irresponsible lifestyle and the other representing an affective and interpersonal style. Information on the PCL-R may be found at http://www.hare.org/scales/pclr.html.

REFERENCES

Durose, M., Harlow, C., Langan, P., Motivans, M., Rantala, R., & Smith, E. (2005). *Family violence statistics including statistics on strangers and acquaintances* (NCJ 207846). U.S. Department of Justice Office of Justice Programs Bureau of Justice Statistics.

Federal Bureau of Investigation (FBI). (2009). *Crime in the United States Preliminary Semiannual Uniform Crime Report January to June 2008.* Retrieved from http://www.fbi.gov/ucr/2009prelimsem/index.html

Friedman, R. (2006). Violence and mental illness—How strong is the link? *New England Journal of Medicine, 355*(20), 2064–2066.

Lamber, L. (2007). New tools aid violence risk assessment. *The Journal of the American Medical Association, JAMA, 298*, 499–501.

Link, B. G., Stueve, A., & Phelan, J. (1997). Psychotic symptoms and violent behaviors: Probing the components of "threat/control-override" symptoms. *Social Psychiatry & Psychiatric Epidemiology, 33*(Suppl. 1), S55–S60.

Monahan, J., Steadman, S., Silver, E., Appelbaum, P., Robbins, P., Mulvey, E., et al. (2001). *Risk assessment: The MacArthur Study of Mental Disorder and Violence.* Oxford: Oxford University Press.

Stuart, H. (2003). Violence and mental illness: An overview. *World Psychiatry, 2*(2), 121–124.

Woods, P., & Lasiuk, G. (2008). Risk prediction: A review of the literature. *Journal of Forensic Nursing, 4*, 1–11.

27 Long-Term Offenders

DEFINITION

A new offender is someone arrested and convicted of a crime for the first time. First arrest and conviction may not mean that this is the first crime the offender committed. It simply means this is the first crime for which an offender was arrested and convicted.

The long-term offender is the person who has been arrested and convicted on several occasions. Recidivism refers to a person's relapse into criminal behavior, often after receiving sanctions or undergoing intervention for a previous crime. Recidivism is the termed used to describe offenders who reoffend; however this term is also used for rearrest, reconviction, and resentencing. There is no one accepted definition of recidivism, even though it is one of the most fundamental concepts in criminal justice. Much of criminal justice research is focused on this topic.

Desistance is continuous abstinence from offending as former criminals reintegrate into productive society. Some professionals believe that people must choose not to engage in crime at all, while others say desistance can be gradual, defined as a switch from serious felonies to misdemeanors. A more specific definition is that desistance is a process in which criminal activity decreases, and reintegration into the community increases, over time. The mere absence of criminal activity during an observed period of time, which would qualify as a showing no recidivism, is not the same as desistance. The hallmark of desistance is an eventual permanent abstention from criminal behavior.

PREVALENCE

The Bureau of Justice Statistics published a study in 2002 on the recidivism rates of 272,111 prisoners released in 1994, a number that represented two-thirds of the U.S. prison population at that time. The prisoners were followed for a three-year period following their release, and four measures of recidivism were used to assess them: rearrest, reconviction, resentence to prison, and return to prison with or without a new sentence. Results showed that 67.5% of the prisoners were rearrested for a new crime within that three-year period after release. Of this number, 46.9% were reconvicted in state or federal court after a new crime; 25.4% were resentenced in state or federal court after a new crime; and 51.8% were back in prison, 25.4% for a new sentence and 26.4% for a technical parole violation.

Released prisoners with the highest rearrest rates were those convicted of motor vehicle theft (78.8%), stolen property (77.4%), larceny (74.6%), burglary (74%), robbery (70.2%), and illegal weapons (70.2%). Lowest rates were for those convicted of driving under the influence (51.5%), rape (46%), other sexual assault (41.4%), and homicide (40.7%). The study also showed that men were more likely to recidivate than women, blacks more than whites, and younger prisoners more often than older ones. Prior criminal history was also significant for recidivism; 70% of the discharged prisoners had five or more prior arrests, and those with longer records were more likely to recidivate than those with shorter ones.

RECIDIVISM

Recidivism is relapse back into criminal activity. It is usually, but not always, measured by a person's return to prison for a new offense. Recidivism rates reflect the degree to which released inmates have been rehabilitated and the role correctional programs play in reintegrating prisoners into society. High rates of recidivism result in huge costs in terms of public safety, as well as tax dollars spent to arrest, prosecute, and incarcerate reoffenders. High rates of recidivism also lead to devastating social costs to the communities and families of offenders, as well as to the offenders themselves.

There is no "average" prisoner or parolee; they are a heterogeneous group. However, parolees with short criminal records seem to have higher rates of postrelease desistance than those with long criminal histories. That is, releasees paroled from their first prison sentence are more likely to desist than those who have served one or more previous sentences. Individuals incarcerated for violent offenses are more likely to desist from crime when released than those convicted of drug and property crimes, regardless of the parolee's sex, age, race, or the specific type of offense committed. The likelihood of recidivism is highest a few months, weeks, or even days after the offender is released. Deaths of releasees are also very common within the first weeks after release, more than 12 times the average for the general population. Thus the initial period after release is the riskiest time for both the public and former inmates.

All professionals need to stop believing that "nothing works" to decrease repeat offending, and they also need to realize that not every intervention will work with every individual. Some programs work for some releasees. The key is matching the program to the individual. Cognitive-behavioral therapy programs seem to have positive effects on the greatest number of releasees. Substance abuse treatment, especially when combined with frequent drug testing, also work for some people, and employment training and mentoring programs also show promise. Certain other factors help prevent former inmates from reoffending. These include a stable marriage and a job that the releasee wants to keep.

INTERVENTION

According to the National Institutes of Justice, prisoner reentry, the transition from life as an inmate to life in the community, has profound implications for public safety. Reentry programs aim to increase public safety and reduce offender recidivism. A key way to accomplish this is to institutionalize the cross-agency and community teamwork needed to make reentry succeed. Reentry efforts must begin in the prison and be actively carried into the community after release. Services that are individualized to prisoners' needs help them reintegrate into society. Examples of reentry services include housing, education, employment aid, peer mentoring, case management, health services, family reunification, and heightened surveillance. Many prisoners must be taught how to interact with the community in the first place—that is, they were not functioning productively in the community before their incarceration.

Many responsibilities for reentry have fallen upon the community. Some communities have relied upon faith-based organizations, even though very little research has been conducted to assess offender outcomes after receipt of services by faith-based providers. However, a growing number of correctional administrators and community reentry experts have found that faith-based organizations can provide much-needed services to offenders through volunteers. These services are important because they may prepare prisoners to more easily use the community services that will aid in their transition after release. Faith-based organizations often help prisoners' families and provide assistance that reflects the values of the community where the offender will live upon release. Because they are part of the community, faith-based volunteers can offer invaluable knowledge and assistance to offenders who are trying to manage transportation, housing, employment assistance, and health issues.

Health care providers may choose to collaborate with faith-based organizations in providing a health care connection for offenders released to the community. Offenders in the community have multiple health care needs, including psychological needs. There is a great need for nursing to become involved with the physical and psychological treatment of offenders, both in jail and prison and postrelease.

Reentry programs are under close scrutiny by the criminal justice community. Questions about the effectiveness of sanctions and interventions are numerous. Health care is part of the process in seeking answers to questions such as: How can static risk factors such as unalterable events in the past be addressed for long-term offenders? How can antisocial attitudes and ineffective problem-solving skills be addressed in offenders? What are the reentry programs that are most effective for released offenders? What are successful strategies for monitoring offenders who reenter the community? What are the outcomes of jail and prison programs?

REFERENCES

Bhati, A. (2006). *Studying the effects of incarceration on offending trajectories: An information-theoretic approach.* Retrieved from http://www.ncjrs.gov/pdffiles1/nij/grants/216639.pdf

Burrowes, N. (2009). Needs, a time to contemplate change? A framework for assessing readiness to change with offenders. *Aggression and Violent Behavior, 14*(1), 39–49.

Cullen, F. (2009). Nothing works: Deconstructing Farabee's rethinking rehabilitation. *Victims and Offenders, 4*(2), 101–123.

Department of Justice Bureau of Statistics. (2004). *Recidivism rates of prisoners released in 1994.* Retrieved from http://www.ojp.usdoj.gov/bjs/abstract/rpr94.htm

Douglas, K., Guy, L., & Hart S. (2009). Psychosis as a risk factor for violence to others. *Psychology Bulletin, 135*(3), 679–706.

National Institutes of Justice. (2007). *Reentry.* Retrieved from http://www.ojp.usdoj.gov/nij/topics/corrections/reentry/welcome.htm

Rosenfeld, R., Petersilia, J., & Visher, C. (2008). The first days after release can make a difference (NCJ 222983). Retrieved from http://nij.ncjrs.gov/publications/Pub_Search.asp?category=99&searchtype=basic&location=top&PSID=40

Zanis, D. (2009). Predictors of drug treatment: Completion among parole violators. *Journal of Psychoactive Drugs, 4*(2), 173–180.

28 Offenders in Correctional Facilities

DEFINITIONS

Jails are usually run by sheriffs and/or county/local governments. These facilities are designed to hold individuals awaiting trial or a serving short sentences (usually one or two years or less). Jails operate work-release programs, boot camps, and other specialized services and try to address educational needs, substance abuse needs, and vocational needs while managing inmate behavior.

Prisons are operated by state correctional departments and the Federal Bureau of Prisons (BOP). These facilities are designed to hold individuals convicted of crimes and sentenced to longer terms. State prison systems operate halfway houses, work-release centers, and community restitution centers—all considered medium or minimum custody. Inmates assigned to such facilities are usually reaching the end of their sentences.

Prisoners are entitled to health care as determined in the 1976 Supreme Court *Estelle v. Gamble* decision, in which the Court held that deprivation of health care constituted cruel and unusual punishment and thus a violation of the Eighth Amendment to the U.S. Constitution. This interpretation created a de facto right to health care for all persons in custody. Prisoners also have a right to privacy, and health care providers have a duty to protect the confidentiality of all medical information. However, this can be especially challenging in correctional facilities, because of the tension that exists between maintaining optimal security and safety and maintaining confidentiality of inmate medical information (custody versus caring).

Patients in custody are ingenious in creating weapons out of medical devices and materials, including shanks (homemade knives) and garrotes using the metal, plastic, and other material in everyday medical equipment. Therefore, most facilities that care for patients in custody have a policy to never give prisoners anything that could be used as weapons (scissors, syringes, scalpels). Prisoners must never be left alone in a clinic or emergency area, and all braces or splints must have the metal and plastic parts removed and plaster substituted. Correctional officers must stay with prisoners at all times, and the health care provider must be educated in this unique aspect of correctional health. Prisoners make weapons for fighting, escape attempts, or protection from other prisoners. Prisoners can also be very clever in planning escape attempts and should not be informed of specific dates arranged for their follow-up appointments.

PREVALENCE

A report by Pew's Public Safety Performance Project (The Pew Center on the States, 2008) details that, for the first time in history, more than one in every 100 adults in America are in jail or prison.

A report by the Bureau of Justice Statistics (Maruschak, 2010) showed:

- Approximately 44% of state inmates and 39% of federal inmates reported a current medical problem other than a cold or virus.
- Arthritis (state 15%; federal 12%) and hypertension (state 14%; federal 13%) were the two most commonly reported medical problems.
- Among inmates with medical problems, 70% of state and 76% of federal inmates reported seeing a medical professional because of the problem.
- 36% of state inmates and 24% of federal inmates reported having an impairment.
- Learning disability was the most commonly reported impairment among state and federal inmates (23% and 13%, respectively).
- 16% of state inmates and 8% of federal inmates reported having multiple impairments.

■ Among both state and federal inmates, females were more than 1.5 times more likely to report two or more current medical problems than male inmates.

HEALTH PROBLEMS OF INMATES

According to the National Commission on Correctional Health Care (NCCHC, http://www.ncchc.org) prisoners are usually from high-risk groups and have poor health histories, increasing their susceptibility to disease. But prisoner health problems are not contained within correctional facilities. Prisoner health problems are public health problems.

Traumatic Brain Injury

A traumatic brain injury (TBI) results from a blow or jolt to the head or a penetrating head injury that disrupts the normal function of the brain. Many prisoners live with TBI-related problems that complicate their management and treatment during incarceration. Prisoners who have had head injuries may also experience mental health problems such as severe depression, anxiety, substance use disorders, difficulty controlling anger, or suicidal ideation and/or attempts. TBI can cause supervision and treatment issues:

■ Attention deficits can make it difficult for the prisoner to focus on a required task or respond to directions given by a correctional officer. These behaviors can be misinterpreted, leading to an impression of deliberate defiance.
■ Memory deficits can make it difficult to understand or remember rules and directions, which can lead to disciplinary actions.
■ Uncontrolled anger might can lead to an incident with another prisoner or correctional officer and to further injury for the person and others.
■ Slowed verbal and physical responses may be interpreted by correctional officers as uncooperative behavior.
■ Uninhibited or impulsive behavior, including unacceptable sexual behavior, may provoke other prisoners or result in disciplinary action by jail or prison staff.

The Commission on Safety and Abuse in America's Prisons (http://www.prisoncommission.org) recommends increased health screenings, evaluations, and treatment for inmates. Other suggestions include:

- Routine screening of inmates to identify a history of TBI, checking for the following symptoms:
    - Headaches or neck pain that do not go away
    - Problems with memory, concentration, or decision making
    - Slowness in thinking, speaking, moving, or reading
    - Getting lost or easily confused
    - Feeling tired all of the time
    - Lack of motivation
    - Mood changes
    - Changes in sleep patterns
    - Light-headedness, dizziness, or loss of balance
    - Nausea
    - Increased sensitivity to lights, sounds, or distractions
- Blurred vision or eyes that tire easily
- Loss of sense of smell or taste
- Tinnitus
- Assessing inmates with TBI for possible alcohol and/or substance abuse and appropriate treatment for these co-occurring conditions.
- Additional evaluations to identify and treat specific TBI-related problems; special attention should be given to impulsive behavior, including violence, sexual behavior, and suicide risk.

Infectious Disease

Infectious diseases common in the incarcerated population include human immunodeficiency virus (HIV), tuberculosis, hepatitis, sexually transmitted diseases, meningitis, and soft tissue infections including abscesses, cellulitis, and fasciitis. The overcrowding of many jails and close inmate proximity creates an ideal environment for the spread of infectious diseases. Detection and early treatment of infectious diseases is critical, not only for the prisoners, but also for the public and correctional staff. Correctional officers have reported injuries from human bites, needles, and other sharp instruments, as well as skin and mucous membrane exposures to blood and body fluids, all of which can result in the transmission of infectious diseases.

The prevalence of HIV varies widely among the correctional systems; however, 21,980 state and federal prison inmates were known to be infected with HIV or to have confirmed AIDS (1.7% of the total custody population). The prevalence of HIV in U.S. prisons is related to intravenous drug use and prostitution. Some correctional HIV testing policies are determined by state or federal statutes. Clinical guidelines for medical management of HIV infection and other issues surrounding HIV infection may be found online (http://aidsinfo.nih.gov/guidelines/Guideline Detail.aspx?MenuItem=Guidelines&Search=Off&GuidelineID=7&Cla ssID=1).

Tuberculosis (TB) outbreaks have been documented in prisons. Control can be difficult in correctional and detention facilities in which persons are housed in close proximity for varying periods. At least three factors contribute to the high rate of TB in correctional and detention facilities: (1) The population is high-risk (users of illicit substances, persons of low socioeconomic status, and persons with human immunodeficiency virus [HIV] infection). These persons often have not received standard public health interventions or appropriate medical care before incarceration. (2) The physical structure of the facilities contributes to disease transmission, as facilities often provide close living quarters, might have inadequate ventilation, and can be overcrowded. (3) Movement of inmates into and out of facilities, coupled with existing TB-related risk factors of the inmates, combine to make correctional and detention facilities a high-risk environment for the transmission of *M. tuberculosis* and make implementation of TB-control measures particularly difficult. Despite control measures, outbreaks of TB continue to occur in these settings. Effective TB prevention and control measures include early identification of prisoners with TB disease through entry and periodic follow-up screening, successful treatment of TB disease and latent TB infection, appropriate use of airborne precautions, comprehensive discharge planning, and thorough and efficient contact investigation. These measures should be instituted in close collaboration with local or state health department TB control programs. Continuing education of prisoners and correctional facility staff is necessary to maximize cooperation and participation.

Prostitution and drugs are some of the most common reasons for arrest in women, and female inmates are at risk for sexually transmitted disease, including hepatitis and syphilis, complicated pregnancies, and possibly poor fetal outcome. Several studies have emphasized the need for rapid screening, detection, and treatment of syphilis and pregnancy to improve outcomes.

Prisoners are also at risk for other respiratory-borne diseases, including pneumococcal disease and meningococcal meningitis. The latter has led to the idea of requiring men sentenced for one month or more to receive the quadrivalent meningococcal vaccine. Outbreaks in prison of other infectious disease such as varicella and tetanus have occurred because the population may be underimmunized. Because of the high prevalence of infectious disease and the at-risk population in the detention system, complete documentation and updating of vaccination status (including diphtheria, tetanus, measles, rubella, and meningococcus) is highly recommended.

Outbreaks of methicillin-resistant staphylococcus aureus (MRSA) have occurred among prisoners and correctional staff. Physical contact among and between inmates and correctional officers is routine. Inmates share towels, linens, or other personal items potentially contaminated by wound drainage; they lance their own boils or other inmates' boils with fingernails or tweezers; they use unsafe tattoo practices; and they undergo physical searches. All these and more can cause MRSA transmission in a prison environment. Poor inmate hygiene, including limited access to showering and soap, and overcrowding can make the spread of MRSA more likely. The Federal Bureau of Prisons Clinical Practice Guidelines for the Management of Methicillin-Resistant Staphylococcus aureus (MRSA) Infections may be found online (http://www.bop.gov/news/PDFs/mrsa.pdf).

Foreign Body Ingestions

Metal objects, razor blades, needles, and plastic are ingested by prisoners with a history of psychiatric illness, sometimes with suicidal intent or in a desire to conceal contraband. Many of these prisoners have a history of multiple ingestions. Prisoners are also brought to emergency departments because of court orders for body cavity searches for drugs or weapons. Health care providers should realize that the vagina, rectum, and gastrointestinal tract may be considered safe hiding spots for keys, drugs, or other prison contraband, but body cavity searches require a court order unless the patient consents to examination.

Assessment includes radiographs, but many ingestions are not radiopaque. Therefore, a negative radiograph does not rule out a foreign body. Management consists of a surgical consultation, although treatment in many cases is usually conservative, with the prisoner observed with serial examinations as the foreign object is followed radiologically as it passes through the gastrointestinal tract. A high-fiber diet and serial stool examinations for blood or the object are also required. If the foreign body is lodged in the esophagus or cricopharyngeal area, it is usually removal under anesthesia. Perforation is rare; however, if clinical evidence of pain, obstruction, bleeding, or peritonitis develops, a laparotomy is recommended. Prevention of recurrent ingestions is critical, and discharge instructions should include limiting prisoner access to objects that can be swallowed.

Reproductive Problems

A history of both substance abuse and commercial sex work places incarcerated women at an elevated risk for reproductive health problems, including high-risk pregnancies and increased rates of HIV and other sexually transmitted diseases (STDs). Pregnancies among female prisoners are usually unplanned and high-risk and have poor outcomes, for several reasons: (a) many of these women lack or fail to access/attend prenatal care; (b) drug abuse leads to preterm deliveries, spontaneous abortions, low–birth weight infants, and preeclampsia; (c) high rates of psychiatric illness can result in fetal exposure to teratogenic medications; (d) prenatal alcohol use may cause fetal alcohol syndrome; and (e) many of these women have poor nutrition and STDs.

Upon release from prison, women have many competing needs for food, shelter, and safety, which often result in neglect of reproductive health care. Incarceration creates an opportunity to provide reproductive health services to a large population of high-risk women who might not otherwise seek health services.

Other health problems include arthritis and heart disease, due to the aging of the prison population (heart disease can also be due to cocaine use).

PREVENTION/PATIENT TEACHING

Primary Prevention

The risk of infectious disease transmission can be reduced by encouraging the following:

- Practice good hand hygiene.
- Provide inmates access to showers and soap to maintain hygiene.

- Discourage sharing of personal items.
- Encourage inmates with symptoms of infections to report to the health care staff.
- Use contact precautions for wound care.
- Clean wounds and cover them with a clean, dry bandage.
- House individuals with draining wounds separately from other inmates, to the extent possible.
- Wear gloves when handling dirty laundry.
- Clean and disinfect contaminated surfaces and equipment, including handcuffs, shackles, pagers, and cell phones. (Contaminated surfaces should be cleaned and then disinfected using an EPA-registered cleaner or a bleach solution [1/4 cup bleach to 1 gallon of water or 1 tablespoon bleach per quart of water].)
- Clean sinks, showers, and toilets on a regular basis.
- Disinfect shared athletic equipment on a regular basis.
- Follow the facility's infection control policy.

Secondary Prevention

Project START is an individual-level, multisession intervention for offenders who are being released from a correctional facility and returning to the community. It is based on the conceptual framework of Incremental Risk Reduction, and focuses on increasing offenders' awareness of their HIV, STI, and hepatitis risk behaviors after release and providing them with tools and resources to reduce their risk.

Tertiary Prevention

As with other populations, prisoners should receive early intervention of medical problems to prevent potential complications.

RESOURCES

Federal Bureau of Prisons Clinical Practice Guidelines: http://www.bop.gov/news/medresources.jsp
National Commission of Correctional Health Care: http://www.ncchc.org
Project START: http://www.effectiveinterventions.org/go/interventions/project-start

REFERENCES

Centers for Disease Control and Prevention. (2009). Correctional health educational materials. Retrieved from http://www.cdc.gov/correctionalhealth/health-ed.html

Clarke, J., Hebert, M., Rosengard, C., Rose, J., DSilva, K., & Stein, M. (2006). Reproductive health care and family planning needs among incarcerated women. *American Journal of Public Health, 96*(5), 834–839.

Maruschak, L. (2010). *Medical problems of prisoners.* Bureau of Justice Statistics. Retrieved from http://www.ojp.usdoj.gov/bjs/pub/pdf/mpp.pdf

The Pew Center on the States. (2008). *One in 100: Behind bars in America 2008.* Retrieved from http://www.pewcenteronthestates.org/uploadedFiles/8015PCTS_Prison08_FINAL_2-1-1_FORWEB.pdf

29 Offenders in the Community

DEFINITION

Parole is the release of a convicted offender prior to his or her maximum release date. A person convicted of a crime may serve his or her entire sentence or may be released from jail or prison after a shorter interval on parole. Parolees include adults conditionally released to community supervision whether by parole board decision or by mandatory conditional release after serving a prison term. They can be returned to jail or prison for rule violations or other offenses. Thus, monitoring is required for people on parole, and the type and frequency of monitoring is determined by the criminal justice system on a case-by-case basis.

Probation is a sentence given rather than jail time or prison time, usually because a judge decides that a person convicted of a crime may return to the community rather than serve time. Probation for adult offenders in lieu of incarceration involves supervision within the community. Probation, like parole, requires varying degrees of monitoring in the community, and the type and frequency of monitoring are usually determined by a judge. Probation and parole officers serve to monitor people in the community on probation or parole. These officers follow specific guidelines handed down by the criminal justice system.

PREVALENCE

According to the Department of Justice (2008), at the end of 2007, over 5.1 million adult men and women were supervised in the community, either on probation or parole. More than 8 in 10 were on probation (4,293,163), while less than 2 in 10 were on parole (826,097). Approximately 1 in every 45 adults in the United States was supervised in the community, either on probation or parole, at the end of 2007. The total community supervision population grew by 104,100 offenders during 2007. The parole population (up 3.3%) increased at a faster pace than the probation population (up 1.8%) during the year; however, probation accounted for three-quarters (77,800) of the growth in the number of offenders under community supervision. At the end of 2007:

> 51% of offenders on probation had been convicted for committing a misdemeanor; 47% for a felony, and 3% for other infractions. The most common type of offense for which offenders were on probation was a drug offense (27%). 95% of offenders on parole had been sentenced to a period of incarceration of one year or more. The most common type of offense for which offenders were on parole was a drug offense (37%). Women account for 23% of the nation's probationers and 12% of the nation's parolees. 55% of adults on probation were white, 29% were black, and 13% were Hispanic. 41% of parolees where white, 38% were black, and 19% were Hispanic.
>
> Entries to probation supervision (2.4 million) exceeded exits from supervision (2.3 million) during 2007. Entries to parole supervision (554,500) also exceeded exits from parole (529,200) during 2007.

According to the Bureau of Prisons at least 95% of all state-incarcerated prisoners will be released from prison at some point; nearly 80% will be released to parole supervision (see http://www.bop.gov/).

ETIOLOGY

Probation and parole serve to decrease the prison and jail populations and to return offenders to the community as soon as safely possible. Confinement to a jail or prison is a serious violation of personal freedom and is not taken lightly by the judiciary. If it is at all possible to decrease the amount of time served in confinement, especially for nonviolent offenders, the judicial system will do so. Safety of the community is the largest judicial concern related to probation and parole. Judges do not release offenders into the community who apparently threaten the safety of the community.

ASSESSMENT

General Principles

When a person is released from jail and returns to the community, the individual is referred to a community health center for follow-up care, as well as a parole center to monitor the released offender's activities. Inside the jail, health care is a right. In the community health care is a privilege. The responsibility for health care after release falls to the individual. An untold number of people who are released from jail do not follow through on health-related issues. They stop taking their psychiatric medications. They stop treating their heart disease or diabetes or hypertension. They stop taking their antibiotics for sexually transmitted diseases. They return to their communities with their illnesses, including their substance abuse tendencies, and they often commit another crime or crimes that return them to jail.

First and foremost is the issue of poverty as it applies to health-related concerns. The number one correlate to incarceration is poverty. Therefore, release from incarceration translates into returning to a poverty living situation and all the health-related aspects that are related to poverty. In addition, people who have been incarcerated for a long period of time have lost what means of income they had acquired before incarceration and often have lost personal and family connections they established prior to incarceration. If the person released had job skills when they were incarcerated, those skills may now be antique. Living arrangements are lost during incarceration due to lack of rent payments or mortgage payments. No current address, no current job, lack of friends and family, and health care concerns impede the offender reintegrating into the community.

A felony conviction can haunt an offender for life. State laws vary, but convicted felons may: have difficulty finding a job and/or receiving government clearance for security jobs; be unable to enter some foreign countries; be disqualified from serving as jurors; forfeit their right to vote, be a candidate for public office, or hold public office; be unable to qualify for federal assistance including loans, grants, and work study; be disallowed to possess firearms; and may be disallowed from obtaining licensure in certain professions. They may also be denied becoming a foster or adoptive parent, especially those branded as sex offenders.

History and Physical Assessment

Offenders reentering the community have multiple barriers to overcome. The ability of health care providers to elicit an unbiased health-related history is important. People who have committed crimes and are reintroduced to the community have served their time or been placed on probation and deserve to be treated with respect and support in the same manner as any other client.

Conditions of probation and parole must be strictly followed. An offender reintroduced to a community must specifically meet the requirements of probation and parole, including drug screening, attending school or work, and maintaining curfews. Any arrest for any violation—small or large—usually means reincarceration or incarceration for the first time. For the person returning to the community, health care can become less of priority than meeting the conditions of probation or parole and finding a place to live and a place to work. An increased understanding of these pressures will assist nurses in helping the person on probation or parole maneuver the health care system and receive the best health care possible.

Offenders leave incarceration experiencing nutritional inadequacy, possible undiagnosed infection, undertreated infections, stress-related illnesses, effects of drug and alcohol misuse, and various mental health issues. Kidney and liver disease are frequently diagnosed in prisons and jails related to drug use. Stress-related illnesses such as irritable bowel, headaches, nausea, and muscular aches have an increased rate of occurrence in incarcerated populations

Mental Illness

Mental health issues are prevalent in incarcerated individuals. While incarcerated individuals with mental health diagnoses are treated by mental health care workers, finding a mental health care provider in the community is a difficult process for many offenders. The most common form of treatment in jails and prisons for mental health issues is medication. While it van be beneficial, cognitive therapy is not a common treatment modality in correctional facilities. Continuing psychiatric medications upon return to the community requires that the offender establish a connection with mental health services in the community. For many offenders, this connection is not made, and stabilizing medications are discontinued. For people released back into poverty with less personal and social support than they had prior to their incarceration, treatment is likely to discontinue. This is particularly true of individuals who are diagnosed as paranoid.

People with diagnosed mental health issues may reoffend related to a lack of psychiatric treatment. Thus, maintaining a mental health treatment regime in the community is vital to keeping people with a mental health diagnosis out of jails and prisons. Incarceration provides a predictable rhythm of life. For people with mental health issues, such stability, even though it comes at the high price of no freedom, can decrease mental health symptoms. Returning to the community and all the stresses that are associated with living in the community can exacerbate mental health symptoms.

Substance Abuse

Substance abuse is often connected to criminal activity. People who have been incarcerated for drug-related crimes often return to communities where drug trade and drug use are common. Those who used and or sold drugs prior to their incarceration frequently return to the drug-related activity such as committing fraud, stealing, and resisting arrest, when released, as they are also returning to people and situations and circumstances that encourage returning to such activity. If the selling of drugs is related to the reason for incarceration, returning to this method of obtaining income is likely. Returning to drug sales is also affected by the fact that after leaving incarceration the chances of obtaining a job that pays an adequate living decreases due to the person's criminal record and the lack of job skills.

Violence

Imprisonment means lack of all freedoms and also means residing in very close living arrangements. Living in such a close environment with a variety of people increases the likelihood of violence. Fighting, verbal and physical, is common in correctional facilities. Incompatibility of people incarcerated together is a factor in the violence, as is opposing gang members incarcerated together. People returning to the community after incarceration have endured not only close living arrangements but also violence of all types and of varying durations. The result of living with violence while incarcerated creates physical injuries and posttraumatic stress disorder of varying degrees, requiring assessment.

Infection

Close living arrangements can cause infections among inmates. Tuberculosis is also diagnosed more often in prisons and jails than it is in the general population, and probationers may still be on medication. Skin abnormalities are common and may be undetected prior to release into the community. Common infections and parasitic conditions seen in prisons and jails include scabies, lice, and fungal infections. Minimal outdoor activity, lack of sunshine, and close living arrangements contribute to these infections.

Males and females are incarcerated in separate areas or separate buildings. This division creates an environment in which same-sex relationships occur. People who are not sexually attracted to the same gender in the community may form same-sex relationships while incarcerated. These same-sex relationships do not usually survive after release from prison or jail, but the sexually transmitted infections from such relationships may and do survive after reentry into the community.

Nutrition

Nutrition is adequate in prisons and jails in the sense of caloric consumption per day. In fact, in most jails or prisons an overconsumption of calories per day is likely and common. In both jails and prisons but more often in jails, the consumption of starches and sugars over protein is a nutritional issue. The taste of the food is not agreeable to many incarcerated people. If in addition to meals, a commissary is available for inmates, this commissary often provides food sources of empty calories and more starch and sugar. The commissaries sell what most people call junk food. This junk food is consumed by inmates in addition to or in place of meals. Money for the commissary comes from financial support from the outside (friends and family) and from prison and jail jobs such as cleaning and cooking.

Women's Health

Women who are incarcerated require additional health care. Prenatal care is provided in correctional facilities. While it may not be provided during probation or parole, obtaining adequate prenatal care is usually a condition of parole for pregnant offenders. Parenting is another issue (also an issue for male offenders). Depending upon the facility, women may be able to keep their children with them up to age 18 months to encourage bonding. Some of these women may be single mothers; some may have been incarcerated for crimes committed with and by male offenders. When released from jail or prison, reconnecting to the community without their co-offending male partner can be difficult. Thus, assessment of living arrangements and parenting skills is essential, as is knowing about the health and well-being of the children. Women who were incarcerated for many years may have lost all legal rights to their children. Their children may be living with family members, in foster care, or with an adoptive family. Lack of legal rights to the children makes reuniting with them difficult or impossible.

INTERVENTION

When readmitted to the community, offenders require health care intervention. These interventions should include:

Continuation of mental health and/or substance abuse treatment

Careful screening and treatment for STIs including HIV

Careful screening and treatment of respiratory infections including TB

Treatment of skin diseases

Screening and treatment of kidney and liver disease

Screening for nutritional deficiencies

Nutritional counseling and possible supplementation

Referrals to social work for assistance with family reunions

Prenatal care (as pertinent)

Parenting classes (as pertinent)

PREVENTION/PATIENT TEACHING

Primary Prevention

Primary prevention should target problems related to criminal offending, including mental illness, substance abuse, and poverty.

Secondary Prevention

Assisting communities who have increased rates of incarceration via innovative social work, health care, and public health initiatives is an example of secondary prevention.

Assisting children of incarcerated parents via innovative programs is another example of secondary prevention.

Tertiary Prevention

Programs aimed at preventing recidivism are examples of tertiary prevention. These include:

- Faith based initiatives designed to assist offenders in successfully completing requirements for probation or parole.
- Adequate mental health screening and treatment. Offenders who receive adequate mental health care while incarcerated and after they return to the community are less likely to reoffend.
- Assisting probation/parole officers with their increasing workloads and paper work, which decreases the risk of people on probation and parole becoming incarcerated.
- Assisting anyone who has been arrested with obtaining medical benefits.
- Tracking outcomes of offenders in the community. Health care could assist in the evaluation of probation and parole initiatives by tracking the health outcomes of people on probation and parole.
- Assisting offenders who return to the community to achieve and maintain good physical and mental. Health care professionals have an important role in assisting people on parole and probation to be as healthy as possible. Being of sound mind, body, and spirit will increase the probability that the offender will keep the conditions of his or her parole or probation and decrease the chances of reoffending. Continued treatment after release will lead to a more successful return to the community and a decreased probability of spread of infections including HIV, hepatitis C, and tuberculosis.

RESOURCES

American Probation and Parole Association: http://www.appa-net.org/eweb
National Institute of Justice: Successful Job Placement of Ex-Offenders: http://www.ncjrs.gov/pdffiles/168102.pdf

REFERENCES

Astbury B. (2008). Problems of implementing offender programs in the community. *Journal of Offender Rehabilitation, 46*(3/4), 31–47.

How will pleading guilty to a felony affect your life? (2007). Criminal Info Network. Retrieved from http://www.criminalinfonetwork.com/pleading-guilty.htm

Minnesota Department of Corrections. (2001). *Safe homes, safe communities.* Retrieved from http://www.doc.state.mn.us/publications/documents/housing.pdf

Reinhart, C. (2003). *Consequences of a felony conviction.* State of Connecticut General Assembly. Retrieved from http://www.cga.ct.gov/2003/olrdata/jud/rpt/2003-R-0333.htm

U.S. Department of Justice Bureau of Statistics. (2007). *Probation and parole.* Retrieved from http://www.ojp.usdoj.gov/bjs/pandp.htm

U.S. Department of Justice, National Institute of Justice. (2008). *Corrections today and tomorrow: A compilation of correction related articles.* Retrieved from http://nij.ncjrs.org/publications/pub_search.asp?Submit=Submit&author=&category=99&dateend=&datestart=&keyword=&title=&topic=32????

30 Perpetrators of Intimate Partner Violence

DEFINITION

The most common definition of perpetrators of intimate partner violence (IPV) is persons who commit acts of violence against current or former intimate partners. These persons used to be called batterers. The legal definition of IPV varies from state to state. IPV, as defined by many intervention providers, is physical, sexual, and psychological abuse that may include physical violence, intimidation, threats, emotional abuse, isolation, sexual abuse, manipulation, the using of children, and economic coercion.

Abusers come from all social, economic, ethnic, professional, educational, and religious groups. Most have no criminal record and are rarely violent with anyone except their partner. To people outside their household, abusers appear to be good providers, loving parents, and law-abiding citizens. In actuality, they are Jekyll and Hyde personalities, which often helps conceal abusive behavior and frequently makes it difficult for victims to be believed at disclosure.

Health care providers may believe that intimate partner violence is perpetrated by men only. This is related to the fact that nursing sees the effects of physical violence more often than any other form of violence. Men are most often the perpetrators of physical violence, and men are more likely to use a weapon in an act of physical violence. However, women do commit acts of physical violence, and when the broader definition of violence is utilized, both men and women are perpetrators of IPV.

PREVALENCE

According to the U.S. Department of Justice Bureau of Justice Statistics (2007), nonfatal intimate partner violence is most frequently committed against victims by individuals of the opposite gender. From 2001 to 2005, about 96% of females experiencing nonfatal intimate partner violence were victimized by a male and about 3% reported that the offender was another female. Approximately 82% of males experiencing nonfatal intimate partner violence were victimized by a female and about 16% of males reported that the offender was another male.

Nearly 11% of murder victims have been killed by an intimate, with female murder victims substantially more likely than male murder victims to have been killed by an intimate. The U.S. Department of Justice Bureau of Justice Statistics (2007) further notes that:

Approximately one-third of female murder victims were killed by an intimate.

Approximately 3% of male murder victims were killed by an intimate.

Of all female murder victims, the proportion killed by an intimate has been increasing.

Of male murder victims, the proportion killed by an intimate has been decreasing.

ETIOLOGY

The etiology of IPV has not been well established, but several theories exist. Social and cultural theories attribute domestic violence to social structure and cultural values. Feminist theories of IPV are based on women's social and cultural experiences. Family-based theories blame violent behaviors on the structure of the family and family interactions rather than on an individual within a family. Individual-based theories attribute IPV to psychological problems such as personality disorders, the offender's childhood experiences, or biological disposition.

Regardless of the theory, IPV usually involves a need to control the victim. Abusers may want to control their partner because of low self-esteem, extreme jealousy, difficulties in regulating anger and other strong emotions, or when they feel inferior to the other partner in education, financial achievement, or socioeconomic background. Men with very traditional gender-role beliefs may think they have the right to control women because they believe women are not equal to men. Domination then takes the form of emotional, physical, or sexual abuse. The violent behavior often results from an interaction of situational and individual factors, and thus, abusers may learn violent behavior from their family, their community, and other cultural influences. Some may have witnessed frequent violence or may have been victims themselves.

Alcohol consumption, especially at hazardous levels, is a major contributor to IPV, and the links between the two are manifold:

- Alcohol use directly affects cognitive and physical function. It reduces self-control and leaves individuals less capable of negotiating a nonviolent resolution to conflicts within relationships.
- Excessive drinking can exacerbate financial difficulties, child-care problems, infidelity, or other family stressors, creating marital tension and conflict, and increasing the risk of violence between partners.
- Beliefs that alcohol causes aggression can fuel excuses for violent behavior.
- Experiencing violence can lead to alcohol consumption as a method of coping or self-medicating.
- Children who witness violence or threats of violence between parents are more likely to display harmful drinking patterns later in life.

Perpetrators of IPV use a variety of tactics to control their victims. These include:

- Dominance: Perpetrators make decisions for their partners and the family, telling them what to do, and expecting them to obey without question. The perpetrator may treat his partner like a servant, a child, or even as his possession.

- Humiliation: Perpetrators use insults, name-calling, and other humiliating gestures to make their partners feel bad about themselves and feel powerless.
- Isolation: Perpetrators cut their partners off from the outside world, keeping them from seeing family or friends, or even preventing them from going to work or school.
- Threats: Perpetrators use threats to keep their partners from leaving or to scare them into dropping charges. They may threaten to hurt or kill the partner, the children, other family members, or pets. Some threaten to commit suicide, file false charges against the partner, or report the partner to child services.
- Intimidation: Perpetrators use a variety of intimidation tactics designed to scare their partners into submission, such as making threatening looks or gestures, destroying property, hurting the pets, or putting weapons on display. The clear message is that there will be violent consequences if the partner does not obey.
- Denial and blame: Perpetrators make excuses for the inexcusable and blame their abusive and violent behavior on a bad childhood, a bad day, and even their partner.

Female Perpetrators of IPV

Research on female batterers is limited. However, studies suggest that they tend to be young (age 18–34), highly anxious, emotional, worrisome, prone to substance abuse, tough-minded, uncaring, insensitive to others, antisocial, and have a history of family violence. Women can use the same battering methods as men, but they tend to:

Withhold approval, appreciation, or affection as punishment

Take away car keys or money

Regularly threaten to leave or to make the partner leave

Punish or deprive the children when angry at the partner

Threaten to kidnap the children if the partner leaves

Harass the partner about affairs the batterer imagines the partner is having

Manipulate with lies and contradictions

Harass the partner on the job

Threaten suicide

Drive unsafely

Drug the partner

Create a sense of impending punishment

Same-Sex Perpetrators of IPV

Power and control issues underlie same-sex IPV, just as they do any other form of IPV. However, the offender may use additional methods to control the partner:

Outing or threatening to out their partner

Telling the partner that no one will believe him or her because the police are homophobic

Telling the partner he will not be believed because homosexuals do not rape their partners

Telling the partner he or she deserves it because of being homosexual

Telling the partner he or she is not a real homosexual

Convincing the partner the abuse is normal behavior

For male couples, telling the partner that violence is an expression of masculinity

ASSESSMENT

General Principles

The most frequent method for the detection of IPV is history given by the victim/partner. Usually physical violence is what is reported to a health care professional. Most commonly a female reports that a male physically abuses her. Health care providers may also observe behavior in a patient's home or in a health care setting that alerts them to a possible IPV situation. Law enforcement may be called by the victim, family, friends, or community. Health care providers may have the opportunity to meet the offender or the victim or both after law enforcement involvement.

History

The history is most frequently derived from the victim and validated via the investigation of the offender. However, IPV offenders may provide a history of violence if asked. When a health history is obtained, asking about violence in the home may lead to an offender revealing that he or she abuses his or her partner or former partner in some way.

The following behaviors, if identified by the health care provider via history and/or observation, may indicate a client is an IPV perpetrator. None of these behaviors specifically identify a perpetrator of IPV, but a combination of these behaviors may raise the health care provider's level of suspicion:

Demonstrating extreme jealousy or possessiveness

Switching from charm to anger without warning

Blaming others for his or her own negative actions

Withdrawing love, money, or approval as punishment

Undermining the partner's feelings and accomplishments

Isolating the partner from friends and family

Exhibiting problems with drugs or alcohol.

Psychological assessment should include:

Previous episodes of violence

Duration of the violent relationship

Most recent incident of violent behavior in current or recent relationship

Worst incident of violent behavior in current or recent relationship

Violence in past relationships, including child abuse and neglect

Violent behavior in family of origin

Current work or employment situation, finances, social network or support system

Number of children

Current relationship status

Any relevant treatment history, including previous counseling for domestic violence, medical conditions, medication, hospitalizations, head injuries, psychiatric history, and chemical and alcohol use

Past records, including police reports, civil or criminal court cases, arrest records, injunctions for protection orders, and probation records, may link the abuser's history to the presenting concern. Past records can identify meaningful data that the abuser may have been unwilling to disclose, especially since self-report information from batterers is often unreliable.

Physical Assessment

The offender may be injured during a physical violence episode. The victim may resist the abuse, or the victim may purposefully injure the offender with a weapon. Children, friends, or family members may intervene in a violent encounter and injure the offender. The offender may also be injured by law enforcement. Diagnosis, treatment, and documentation of injury for the offender is appropriate in any of these circumstances (see chapter 3 on forensic assessment).

Diagnostic Testing

The Abusive Relationships Inventory (ARI) was developed to assess the attitudes and beliefs of men who have been abusive toward their partners. It measures the batterer's tendency to rationalize abusive behaviors and to project blame onto the partner. The questions related to rationalization measure excuses that batterers use to justify their abusive behavior toward others. Another group of questions relate to attribution of blame and sexual stereotyping and measures the tendency to project blame onto the spouse and the tendency to stereotype women. These two measures were found to be correlated and are considered to essentially be a single factor. The ARI was found to be internally consistent in a study of 195 male offenders in federal penitentiaries. However, further research is necessary to establish the ARI's reliability over time, its ability to discriminate batterers from nonbatterers, and its relationship to other constructs related to domestic violence, such as hostility and aggression. This tool can be found at http://www.csc-scc.gc.ca/text/pblct/forum/e051/e051d-eng.shtml.

INTERVENTION

Health care providers should first ascertain the safety of the victims, including the partner, children, other adults in the household, and pets. In states with mandatory reporting, law enforcement is notified. Health care providers should also tend to any physical injuries.

Therapy for IPV perpetrators is offered in most jurisdictions throughout the United States. Therapy is often stipulated by the court at sentencing as a condition of probation for those who are arrested and convicted of assault or other IPV-related crimes. Therapy as a sentence may also be combined with punishment. The offender may serve a sentence and attend therapy during and after release. Therapy for IPV perpetrators usually incorporates multiple phases:

- Intake: Initial contact, usually referred by the criminal justice system.
- Assessment: Perpetrator agrees with terms of the program and is assessed for dangerousness, extent of abuse, substance abuse, mental illness, illiteracy, or other obstacles to treatment.
- Victim Contact: Partner may be notified about the offender's status in the program and any imminent danger, and may be referred to victim services.
- Orientation: An initial phase of group intervention.
- Group Treatment: Structured discussions about relationships, anger-management skills, or group psychotherapy.
- Leaving the Program: Offenders may complete the program, be terminated for noncompliance, or be asked to restart the program.
- Follow-up: May consist of informal self-help groups of program graduates or less frequent group meetings.

The curriculum for IPV offenders is dependent upon the institution or community agency responsible for delivering it. Programs construct curricula based upon individual theory, family theory, or social/cultural theory, or some combination of all three theories. Success rates vary with the type of program and the skill set of the providers. Barriers to successful therapy are denial of the abuse by the offender, minimizing the abuse by the offender, and blaming the victim for the offender's behavior.

Intervention program also categorize offenders in treatment based upon risk. The following is a categorization used by treatment programs:

Low-risk offenders must not have caused any physical injury and must not have committed any previous violent offenses against the victim. This group of offenders is likely to be offered deferred prosecution wherein they are allowed to enter a guilty plea with the understanding that they complete an accredited program and do not reoffend.

Medium-risk offenders have committed criminal acts in the past. Probation officers typically recommend that medium-risk offenders be sentenced to probation with a condition of program completion.

High-risk offenders include any offender with a significant history of IPV and/or a history of past violent behavior. This group may not be appropriate for participation in IPV programs. A high-risk offender may be entered into a program but also be sentenced to other programs simultaneously, such as addictions programs and anger management programs.

PREVENTION/PATIENT TEACHING

Primary Prevention

Primary prevention for IPV requires national, state, and local initiatives. Cross-discipline education is needed as well as education in all school systems, both public and private. In order for initiatives designed to prevent IPV to be successful there needs to be a national plan based on improved data collection from many resources, including health care. State-wide initiatives require cooperation from all agencies that encounter victims and offenders of interpersonal violence: people directly affected both directly and indirectly by the problem, working together to design prevention strategies. Stronger communities with coordinated responses to signs and symptoms of interpersonal violence can help prevent much of the physical, psychological, social, and economic impact of IPV.

Secondary Prevention

Secondary prevention includes early intervention programs for people who demonstrate excessive controlling behavior. Programs designed to prevent cruelty to animals and programs designed to prevent child abuse also serve to decrease IPV.

Tertiary Prevention

Programs designed for early assessment of dangerousness of the offender help ensure the safety of the victim. Lethality assessment screening tools are designed to initiate interventions prior to homicide by perpetrators of IPV. Treatment of IPV offenders is tertiary prevention. Successful treatment of IPV offenders increases the safety of the family. Future safety of the victims, including children and pets, is the ultimate goal of tertiary prevention.

RESOURCES

Intimate Partner Violence (IPV) Guidelines for Medical Providers: http://endabuse.org/userfiles/file/Maternal_Health/Intimate_Partner_Violence_Intervention.pdf
National Center for Victims of Crime: Perpetrators of Domestic Violence: http://www.ncvc.org/ncvc/main.aspx?dbName=DocumentViewer&DocumentID=32347#5
WHO: Intervening with Perpetrator of IPV: A global perspective: http://www.who.int/violence_injury_prevention/publications/violence/intervening/en/index.html
Who Is a Perpetrator of Domestic Violence: http://www.enotalone.com/article/10004.html

REFERENCES

Campbell, J. (1995). *Assessing dangerousness: Violence by sexual offenders, batterers, and child abusers.* Thousand Oaks, CA: Sage.
Campbell, J. C. (2007). Prediction of homicide of and by battered women. In J. C. Campbell (Ed.), *Assessing dangerousness: Violence by sexual offenders, batterers, and child abusers* (pp. 96–113). Thousand Oaks, CA: Sage.
Day, A., Chang, D., O'Leary, P., & Carson, E. (2009). Programs for men who perpetrate domestic violence: An examination of effectiveness of intervention programs. *Journal of Family Violence, 24*(3), 203–212.
Dixon, C., & Peterman, L. (2001). Assessment and evaluation of men who batter women. *Journal of Rehabilitation, 67*(4), 38–42.
Goldsmith, T. (2006). What causes domestic violence? *PsychCentral.* Retrieved from http://psychcentral.com/lib/2006/what-causes-domestic-violence
Guterman, N. (2004). Advancing prevention research in child abuse, youth violence and domestic violence. *Journal of Interpersonal Violence, 19*(3), 299–321.

Hamberger, L. (2009). Treatment approaches for men who batter their partners. In *Intimate Partner Violence* (pp. 459–471). New York: Oxford University Press.

Healey, K., Smith, C., & O'Sullivan, C. (1998). Batterer intervention program approaches. *U.S. Department of Justice* (NCJ 168638). Retrieved from http://www.ncjrs.gov/pdffiles/168638.pdf

Mauricio, A., & Lopez, F. (2009). A latent classification of male batterers. *Violence and Victims, 24*(4), 419–438.

Sabol, W., Coulton, J., & Korbin, J. (2004). Building community capacity for violence prevention. *Journal of Interpsersonal Violence, 12*(3), 322–340.

Smith, M., Davies, P., & Segal, J. (2009). Domestic violence and abuse. *HelpGuide.org*. Retrieved from http://www.helpguide.org/mental/domestic_violence_abuse_types_signs_causes_effects.htm

U.S. Department of Justice Bureau of Statistics. (2007). Intimate partner violence in the U.S. Retrieved from http://www.ojp.usdoj.gov/bjs/intimate/ipv.htm

World Health Organization. (2006). *Intimate partner violence and alcohol.* Retrieved from http://www.who.int/violence_injury_prevention/violence/world_report/fact sheets/ft_intimate.pdf

31 | Abusive Parents

DEFINITION

Federal law provides states with a minimum set of acts or behaviors that define child abuse and neglect. The Federal Child Abuse Prevention and Treatment Act (CAPTA) (42 U.S.C.A. §5106g), as amended by the Keeping Children and Families Safe Act of 2003, defines child abuse and neglect as, at minimum:

- Any recent act or failure to act on the part of a parent or caretaker which results in death, serious physical or emotional harm, sexual abuse or exploitation; or
- An act or failure to act which presents an imminent risk of serious harm.

This definition of child abuse and neglect refers specifically to parents and other caregivers. A "child" under this definition generally means a person who is under the age of 18 or who is not an emancipated minor (except in the case of sexual abuse, in which the age is specified by the child protection law of the state in which the child resides).

CAPTA provides definitions for sexual abuse and the special cases related to withholding or failing to provide medically indicated treatment;

however, it does not provide specific definitions for other types of maltreatment such as physical abuse, neglect, or emotional abuse. Federal legislation sets minimum standards, but each state is responsible for providing its own definition of maltreatment within civil and criminal contexts. Individual state statutes may be found at http://www.childwelfare.gov/systemwide/laws_policies/state.

PREVALENCE

Data are collected from the National Child Abuse and Neglect Data System (NCANDS) and reported in the U.S. Department of Health and Human Services, Administration on Children, Youth and Families (2009). Its document, *Child Maltreatment 2007,* shows:

- During federal fiscal year (FFY) 2007, there were approximately 859,000 perpetrators. Nearly 79.9% of perpetrators were parents of the victim, and 61.1% of perpetrators were found to have neglected children.
- A little more than half (56.5%) of the perpetrators were women, 42.4% were men, and 1.1% were of unknown sex.
- Women were younger than men. The median age was 30 years for women and 33 years for men. 45.0% of the female perpetrators were younger than 30 years of age, compared with 34.5% of the men. These proportions have remained consistent for the past few years.
- 48.5% of perpetrators were White; 19.0% were African American; 19.8% were Hispanic. These proportions also have remained consistent for the past few years.
- 79.9% of perpetrators were parents. Other relatives accounted for an additional 6.6%. Unmarried partners of parents accounted for 4.5%. Of the parents who were perpetrators, 87.7% were biological parents. 4.2% were step-parents, and 0.6% were adoptive parents.
- 61.1% of all perpetrators were found to have neglected children. 12.7% of all perpetrators were associated with more than one type of maltreatment. 10.3% of perpetrators physically abused children, and 7.1% sexually abused children.
- Neglect represented both the most frequent form of maltreatment and the greatest number of perpetrators. Physical abuse ranked second.

■ 7.2% of all perpetrators were associated with sexually abusing a child. The percentage of perpetrators of sexual abuse was highest among friends or neighbors (57.7%), other relatives (32.0%), and child day-care providers (23.9%).

Statistics for child abuse fatalities reveal that, in 2007, one or both parents were responsible for 69.9% of child abuse or neglect fatalities; 27.1% of these fatalities were perpetrated by the mother acting alone. Child fatalities with unknown perpetrators accounted for 16.4% of the total.

ETIOLOGY

The exact etiology of child abuse is unclear. However, parents who abuse children tend to have factors that include: abuse or harsh and inconsistent discipline as children; social isolation; low frustration tolerance; marital/relationship issues; financial problems; health problems; legal difficulties; substance abuse; and/or psychopathology.

ASSESSMENT

General Principles

Patterns common to abusive parents, according to the Office of Juvenile Justice and Delinquency Prevention (Bavolek, 2000), include the following.

Inappropriate parental expectations for the child: Many abusive parents have unrealistic expectations for their children's developmental skill level. They may expect and demand that their infants and children behave in a manner that is developmentally inappropriate for their ages. Inappropriate expectations stem from their own inadequate perceptions of self and from a lack of knowledge about the capabilities and needs of children at each developmental stage.

Lack of empathy toward children's needs: Abusive parents have an inability to be empathically aware of their children's needs and to respond to those needs in an appropriate fashion. Abusive parents often ignore their children because they do not want to spoil them, resulting in the child's basic needs being left unattended. They place a high premium on the child's "being good, acting right," and learning to be obedient. However, they seldom clarify that which constitutes good and right behavior. At the extreme are those parents who are violent, cruel, and physically or psychologically abusive under the guise of teaching, helping, and controlling.

Parental valuing of physical punishment: Abusive parents often believe children should not be allowed to "get away with anything." They believe that their children must periodically be shown that the parent is the authority figure and made to respect that authority so they will not become disobedient. Abusive parents consider physical punishment a proper disciplinary measure and strongly defend their right to use physical force. Physical attacks by abusive parents are often not haphazard, uncontrolled, impulsive discharges of aggression toward their children. Instead, abusive parents use physical punishment as a behavior designed to punish and correct specific bad conduct or perceived inadequacies. Much of what abusive parents find wrong with their children reflects the behaviors for which they were criticized and punished as children.

Parental role reversal: In this role reversal, the parent behaves as a helpless, needy child who looks to his or her own children as though they were adults who could provide parental care and comfort. Potential abusers both seek and shun intimate relationships. These parents attempt to manipulate and structure the family interactions in an effort to meet their own needs. They perceive their children as being inadequate and, in their frustration, beat, chastise, belittle, or ignore the children.

Parents who kill their children: Children may die as the result of abuse, but there are also times when the parent intentionally kills his or her child. There is no single profile of a perpetrator of fatal child abuse, although certain characteristics exist. The perpetrator is often a young adult in his or her mid-20s, without a high school diploma, living at or below the poverty level, depressed, and who may have difficulty coping with stressful situations. The perpetrator often has experienced violence firsthand. Most physical abuse fatalities are caused by fathers and other male caregivers, while deaths from neglect are most often caused by the mother. While this chapter focuses on abusive parents, it is critical for health care providers to realize that at least one study showed that being a biologically unrelated caregiver is the strongest predictor of fatal child maltreatment.

Postpartum (puerperal) psychosis is a relatively rare disorder that affects approximately 1 to 2 per 1000 women and occurs within 1 to 4 weeks from delivery. Data suggest that postpartum psychosis is a presentation of bipolar disorder that coincides with tremendous hormonal shifts after delivery. Results of one study suggested that the immediate time period following childbirth entailed a substantially increased risk of psychotic illness of the first-time mother. This also held true for mothers without any previous psychiatric hospitalization, who account for almost half of the psychosis cases during the first 90 days postpartum. Among women without any previous psychiatric hospitalization, greater maternal age and lower infant birth weight are correlated with an increased risk of psychoses during the postpartum period, while maternal diabetes and high birth weight of the infant appear to be protective. Presentation is often dramatic, with rapid onset of symptoms as early as the first 48 to 72 hours after delivery. Manifestations resemble those of a rapidly evolving manic (or mixed) episode; the earliest signs are restlessness, irritability, and insomnia. Women may exhibit a rapidly shifting depressed or elated mood, disorientation or confusion, erratic or disorganized behavior, delusional beliefs that often center on the infant, and auditory hallucinations that instruct the mother to harm herself or her infant. The risk for infanticide, as well as suicide, is significant.

History, Physical Assessment, and Diagnostic Testing

The literature focuses on identification of child abuse via the presentation of the child, and thus there is no specific assessment for parents for possible abuse. However, health care providers, particularly those who work in primary care and emergency services, should be alert for risk factors when performing psychosocial assessments, particularly: criminality, inappropriate expectations of the child, psychopathology, substance abuse, and inappropriate expectations about child development.

Health care providers caring for pregnant and puerperal women should maintain a high index of suspicion for postpartum mood disorders and should ask all mothers about their postpartum adjustments. Useful tools to screen for depression and mania/hypomania include the Edinburgh Postnatal Depression Scale (EPDS; http://www.fresno.ucsf.edu/pediatrics/downloads/edinburghscale.pdf) and the Mood Disorder Questionnaire (MDQ; http://www.dbsalliance.org/pdfs/MDQ.pdf). The EPDS is a self-rating instrument that uncovers the presence of persistent low mood, anhedonia, guilt, anxiety, and thoughts of self-harm, while the MDQ assesses past and current symptoms of high, hyper, or irritable mood; excess energy; racing thoughts; pressured speech; and symptoms that are linked with mania/hypomania. The initial evaluation requires a thorough history, physical examination with complete neurological assessment, and laboratory investigations to exclude an organic cause for acute psychosis, which include cerebral vascular accident, systemic lupus erythematosus, metabolic and nutritional disorders, neurological infections, substance abuse, and medication effects. Diagnostic tests may include: complete blood count (CBC), electrolytes, blood urea nitrogen (BUN), creatinine, glucose, vitamin B12, folate, thyroid function tests, calcium, urinalysis and urine culture in the patient with fever, and a urine drug screen. The client may warrant a head CT or MRI scan to rule out the presence of a stroke related to ischemia (vascular occlusion) or hemorrhage (uncontrolled hypertension, ruptured arteriovenous malformation, or aneurysm). Clients who report confusion, threats to harm self or others, difficulty caring for their children, or poor self-care warrant immediate psychiatric referral.

INTERVENTION

All states mandate health care providers to report suspected child abuse, and some states have laws that void all confidential privileges. Failure to report suspected child abuse can result in criminal and/or civil liability. Abusive parents should be referred to appropriate child protective and mental health services.

Lack of treatment for postpartum psychosis increases the risk for mortality. These patients respond best to pharmacotherapy with atypical antipsychotic drugs; however, if the health care provider suspects the presence of comorbid depression, the addition of an antidepressant medication is highly recommended. Another option for treatment is the use of antidepressants and a mood stabilizer, such as lithium, valproic acid, and carbamazepine, in combination with antipsychotics. Mothers taking lithium and antipsychotics should be advised to not breast-feed due to the risks of toxicity to the infant. If medication treatment fails or in cases where rapid stabilization is required, electroconvulsive therapy (ECT) is a possible course of treatment. ECT also has the benefit of avoiding infant exposure to medications excreted in breast milk.

PREVENTION/PATIENT TEACHING

Primary Prevention

Primary prevention methods seek to raise the awareness of the general public, service providers, and decision makers about the scope and problems associated with child maltreatment. Health care provider approaches might include: parent education programs and support groups that focus on child development, age-appropriate expectations, and the roles and responsibilities of parenting; family support and strengthening programs that enhance the ability of families to access existing services; and resources to support positive interactions among family members.

Secondary Prevention

Activities with a high-risk focus can be offered to populations that have one or more risk factors associated with child maltreatment, such as poverty, parental substance abuse, young parental age, parental mental health concerns, and parental or child disabilities. Programs may target services for communities or neighborhoods that have a high incidence of any or all of these risk factors. Health care providers can participate in secondary prevention through: parent education programs in high schools that focus on teen parents, or substance abuse treatment programs for mothers and families with young children; helping parents deal with their everyday stresses and meet the challenges and responsibilities of parenting; referral to home visiting programs that provide support and assistance to expecting and new mothers in their homes; referral to respite care for families that have children with special needs; and providing information on family resource centers that offer information and referral services to families living in low-income neighborhoods.

Women with bipolar disorder and a personal or family history of postpartum psychosis (PP) are at substantial risk for PP. They and their families should be taught how to recognize symptoms: mood swings, confusion, strange beliefs, and hallucinations, especially in the first 2 to 4 weeks post-delivery, and to contact their physician immediately if these symptoms arise. Prior to delivery, encourage at-risk clients to consult with a psychiatrist to help them consider treatment options or treatment prophylaxis at delivery to avoid illness.

Tertiary Prevention

Tertiary prevention focuses on families where maltreatment has already occurred and aims to reduce the negative consequences of the maltreatment and to prevent its recurrence. Health care providers can: refer parents to intensive family preservation services with trained mental health counselors that are available to families 24 hours per day for a short period of time (approximately 6 to 8 weeks); refer to parent mentor programs with stable, nonabusive families who act as role models and who provide support to families in crisis; develop or refer to parent support groups that help parents transform negative practices and beliefs into positive parenting behaviors and attitudes; and refer to mental health services for children and families affected by maltreatment to improve family communication and functioning.

RESOURCES

Child Welfare Information Gateway: http://www.childwelfare.gov/
Federal Child Abuse Prevention and Treatment Act: http://www.acf.hhs.gov/programs/cb/laws_policies/cblaws/capta/index.htm
Nurse Family Partnership: http://www.nursefamilypartnership.org/index.cfm?fuseaction=home

REFERENCES

Baker, J., Mancuso, M., Montenegro, M., & Lyons, B. (2002). Treating postpartum depression. *Physician Assistant, 26*(10), 37–44.

Bavolek, S. (2000). *The nurturing parenting programs.* Office of Juvenile Justice & Delinquency Prevention Juvenile Justice Bulletin (NCJ172848). Retrieved from http://www.ncjrs.gov/html/ojjdp/2000_11_1/contents.html

Child Welfare Information Gateway. Fact sheets. Retrieved from http://www.childwelfare.gov/pubs/factsheets/fatality.cfm#perps

Massachusetts General Hospital Postpartum Psychiatric Disorders. Retrieved from http://www.womensmentalhealth.org/specialty-clinics/postpartum-psychiatric-disorders

Sit, D., Rothschild, A., & Wisner, K. (2006). A review of postpartum psychosis. *Journal of Women's Health, 15*(4), 352–368.

U.S. Department of Health and Human Services, Administration on Children, Youth and Families. (2009). *Child maltreatment 2007.* Washington, DC: U.S. Government Printing Office. Retrieved from http://www.acf.hhs.gov/programs/cb/pubs/cm07/cm07.pdf

Valdimarsdóttir, U., Hultman, C., Harlow, H., Cnattingius, S., & Sparén, P. (2009). Psychotic illness in first-time mothers with no previous psychiatric hospitalizations: A population-based study. *PLoS Medicine, 10*(6), 27. Retrieved from http://www.plosmedicine.org/article/info:doi/10.1371/journal.pmed.1000013

Yampolskaya, S., Greenbaum, P., & Berson, I. (2009). Profiles of child maltreatment perpetrators and risk for fatal assault: A latent class analysis. *Journal of Family Violence, 24,* 337–348.

32 | Perpetrators of Elder Abuse

DEFINITION

The term elder is usually used to refer to persons over the age of 65. The legal definition of abuse includes the element of intentionality. It is required by law that the person who committed the abusive act(s) be aware that the behavior or lack of behavior is abusive. This definition excludes behavior that is accidental. The law also describes an abuser as a person who has responsibility or "duty" to protect and does so in an abusive manner. In other words, the general public is not responsible (legally) for the abuse of an elder, but the person or people responsible for the elder who are legally bound to care for the elder is responsible.

ETIOLOGY

Ramsey-Klawsnick (2000) developed a typology for people who abuse elders. In this typology she describes five types of offenders.

Overwhelmed: Overwhelmed offenders are well-intentioned. They become caregivers expecting to provide adequate care and are qualified or fit care providers in personality, intelligence, caregiving skills, and motivation. However, when the amount of care exceeds that which they can comfortably provide, they lash out verbally or physically. Alternatively, or additionally, the quality of their care can degrade to the point of neglect, which is the most common form of abuse for this type of offender. This offender has difficulty asking for help or assistance and difficulty setting limits. The offender's own needs for sleep and food may not be met. The elder may have issues such as being impatient, being critical, and being uncooperative. The offender does not have enough help and often not enough finances. These offenders are ashamed and remorseful and may hide the maltreatment. Once identified, they will accept interventions. In long-term care facilities these offenders are overwhelmed workers who have been working too many hours with too little support and poor training.

Impaired: These offenders are well intentioned but have their own problems with age, fragility, and/or mental illness, disability, or substance abuse. They do not recognize the inappropriateness of their behavior and do not hide their maltreatment. The abuse can be chronic or episodic. Neglect is the most frequent form of abuse, but restraints may be used improperly and drugs given inappropriately. Impaired offenders often mismanage, but rarely steal, financial resources. In long-term care facilities, the impaired offenders are unqualified when they are hired, and they are inadequately trained.

Narcissistic: These offenders are involved in the care for reasons of personal gain and are concerned only with their own needs. They have no empathy and are self-centered. Narcissistic offenders use other people and other people's assets and will use the elder's income or valuables. The most common forms of abuse by this type of offender are neglect and financial exploitation. Their goal may be inheriting an elderly person's home, receiving Social Security or pension checks, or exploiting other valuables. Narcissists can be socially sophisticated, presenting themselves well in order to gain a position of trust over vulnerable elders. Once they gain that position, they begin to maltreat those in their care. Their maltreatment tends to be chronic and often escalates in severity over time. Victims typically feel used and neglected by their offenders but do not necessarily fear them. Narcissists can be attracted to paid or volunteer service in long-term care facilities for the elderly in order to gain the opportunity to exploit them.

Domineering (bullying): These offenders chronically abuse and feel justified in doing so. The domineering abuser blames the victim for the maltreatment and says the victim deserves it. The offender has power and authority over the victim and is very demanding. Domineering offenders can be extremely harmful to older people, particularly those unable to meet their own needs.

Their maltreatment tends to be chronic, multifaceted, and ongoing, characterized by frequent explosions of temper. Their victims are fearful and may take extreme measures to appease and placate them. The abuse may include serious psychological and physical mistreatment, sometimes life-threatening. Some domineering offenders also engage in sexual abuse and/or exert coercive control over victims and their financial and material resources. Neglect often occurs when this type of person is responsible for meeting the needs of dependent elders. These people are very difficult to live with, work with, or deal with; they are dangerous in positions of authority, including as teachers, police officers, or supervisors, and may work in long-term care facilities. When confronted with evidence of maltreatment, these offenders may lash out in anger toward those questioning them, or they may attempt to charm and manipulate those who confront them into perceiving the victim as a disturbed and unreliable source of information.

Sadistic: Humiliating, terrifying, and harming others is important to this type of offender. These offenders take pleasure in their victims' fear, and victims' pleas to avoid abuse bring the offenders feelings of excitement and control. Sadists typically exhibit sociopathic personalities, lacking guilt, shame, or remorse for their behavior, and they perpetrate severe, chronic, multifaceted abuse. Victim red flags for sadistic abuse include human bite marks, scars from inflicted burns, evidence that a victim has been tied or restrained, signs of physical assault to genitals and other sensitive areas, and observations of offenders' behavior designed to humiliate victims. Sadistic offenders often deprive victims of basic necessities to exert control, and some torture, murder, or mutilate.

Victims experience terror and will take extreme measures to avoid continuing abuse. However, extensive psychological abuse is used to control victims, including threats to harm the victim's loved ones and pets, which prevents many victims from seeking and accepting assistance. When confronted about their abuse, some sadists create a positive impression of themselves by using their intelligence or charm to manipulate; others may intimidate, threaten, and attempt to control professionals who are trying to stop the abuse.

Families Who Abuse Elders

Most cases of elder abuse occur within families. The perpetrator can be a spouse, domestic partner, child, or grandchild. A red flag for identification of families in which an elder is being abused is: *Family members who abuse elders are usually financially dependent upon the elder.* When adult children or grandchildren are the perpetrators of abuse, the offender is usually both emotionally and financially dependent on the victim. The family member, in this context, is dependent upon the elder for finances and often a place to live. Family abusers of elders often have mental health issues and/or are drug and alcohol dependent. The family member may or may not have been abused by the elder in the past. There are no statistics on how often this is the case, but former abuse by the person who is now an elder can be a factor. Victims in the circumstances in which their own children abuse them often feel guilty and fear that if they report the abuse, they will be moved to a facility and the child will go to jail or a psychiatric institution.

Elders who are abused by spouses or partners are in one of the following three situations: (1) The offender and victim are involved in a long-term relationship that has an early onset of intimate partner violence (IPV), and the couple has grown old in this context. (2) The offender and victim are in a short-term relationship with early onset of abuse. This situation most often occurs after a divorce or death of a spouse or partner. (3) The victim and offender are involved in a long-term relationship, but the abuse began recently. The abuse, in these cases, may be related to a mental or physical illness.

Caregivers Who Abuse Elders

Caregiver abusers work with elders but typically do not like the job. However, they enjoy having power over the vulnerable elders. This position of power allows the caregiver to abuse an elder or elders. They use punishment and domination against people they have power over. Overall, they are not reliable employees and deficiencies are noted in other areas of their work. They, like family members who abuse elders, often have mental health issues and/or are drug dependent. The abusing care giver may or may not have a past criminal record.

Resident-on-Resident Abuse

According to Rosen, Pillemer, and Lachs (2008), resident-to-resident aggression (RRA) between long-term care residents includes negative and aggressive physical, sexual, or verbal interactions that can have a high potential to cause physical or psychological distress in the victim. The most common reason for police to be called to a long-term care facility is for intervention in a simple assault. The calls to police about simple assault are about one resident assaulting another resident, not a caregiver assaulting a resident. Rosen, Pillemer, and Lachs (2008) also note that in interviews conducted in long-term care facilities, screaming and yelling is the number one offense reported.

ASSESSMENT

General Principles

There is not one single description of offenders who abuse elders. Offenders come from all socioeconomic backgrounds, races, religions, and occupations. The offenders are often motivated to protect themselves from the consequences of their abusive behavior. They will, therefore, minimize their abuse or deny that it is occurring.

Issues of power and control might be missed in cases of elder abuse, because people who intervene may assume that the cause of the abuse is caregiver stress. As with other offenders who abuse people, the underlying mechanism is most commonly power and control. People who abuse elders purposefully inflict pain and suffering that causes the victim untold emotional and physical harm.

History and Physical Assessment

Health care providers should interview the victim and the suspect separately. Health care providers must use good listening skills when interviewing both the victim and the suspect. Keeping an open mind assists the health care provider in interviewing suspects. Allowing the suspect to talk may encourage the suspect to reveal the abuse. Family members may verbally portray a sense of entitlement related to the elder. Either caregivers or family members who abuse elders may display their mental health issues during an interview.

Physical examination of both victim and offender is needed to determine mental capacity and any underlying physical (organic) conditions that may affect abusive behavior. Physical exam of the suspect is usually not necessary upon detection of elder abuse. The victims of elder abuse typically do not injure the offender.

Being aware of the signs and symptoms of drug and alcohol abuse will assist in detecting this issue in offenders. Health care professionals working within a system that deals with elders should become familiar with the overall signs and symptoms of mental health issues.

Caregiver abuse may be revealed via victims giving a history of abuse or displaying behavior indicative of abuse. Behaviors such as withdrawal, rapidly declining health, or fear may indicate elder abuse. Security cameras may reveal elder abuse. Review of strategically placed security cameras may validate suspicions of abuse of an elder or elders.

Diagnostic Testing

Psychiatric and psychological evaluation is required for both victims and offenders. Few diagnostic screening tools exist related to elder abuse offenders, and these are not readily available to clinicians. However, the *Nursing Home Abuse Prevention Profile & Checklist* is a comprehensive but user-friendly tool designed to unearth risk factors to vulnerable nursing home residents and to inspire and catalyze action. The Nursing Home Abuse Risk Prevention Profile—Part One describes three groups of risk factors: Resident risks, social risks of relationships, and facility administration. Part Two of the Profile presents a self-evaluation checklist with instructions that can serve as the foundation for creating a safer environment. Part Three discusses ideas for team action and prevention. The *Nursing Home Abuse Prevention Profile & Checklist* is available at http://mnvac.pbworks.com/f/NursingHomeRisk.pdf.

INTERVENTION

Once elder abuse is suspected, it should be reported to adult protective services per state statute and agency protocol. Mandatory reporting of elder abuse varies by state. For your state law, refer to http://www.rainn.org/public-policy/legal-resources/mandatory-reporting-database.

Too often health care professionals explain elder abuse on the basis of caregiver stress. Caregiver stress implies that the abuse is caused by the difficulty of caring for the elder. The abuser often minimizes and attempts to justify his or her behavior to the health care provider. The abuser may blame the victim for being dependent and the stress of the dependency for causing the abuse. When health care professionals allow the victim to be blamed, they are shifting the responsibility from the offender to the victim. Believing that the victim is difficult and therefore creating overwhelming stress also means that the health care professional is believing the offender's justifications for the abuse. In truth many people experience stress, but few use it as an excuse to hurt others. Many people who offend against elders believe that that they are entitled to abuse the elder and know that the victims they dominate are unlikely to report their abuse.

Focusing on abuser justifications does not protect the victim. Focusing on treating the offender does not keep the victim safe. Health care professionals who fail to call law enforcement are not intervening in order to protect the victim. Suspected elder abuse should be reported and thoroughly investigated. A complete and though investigation by trained professionals should follow every allegation of elder abuse. After the investigation, appropriate interventions specific to the offender and the victim can be carefully crafted.

Intervention in cases of elder abuse requires a team approach. Both the victim and the perpetrator require intervention. The offender may be referred to appropriate resources for assistance with mental health issues and/or addiction issues. The law enforcement community makes decisions regarding prosecution. Offenders who truly are in the category of overwhelmed or impaired are generally not prosecuted. Rather they are offered supportive interventions.

PREVENTION/PATIENT TEACHING

Primary Prevention

Providers of nursing care for the vulnerable elderly should be carefully selected. Health care professionals can and should recommend hiring people who are committed to caring for the elderly, do not have mental health issues, have no criminal background, and do not have drug- and alcohol-related problems. Health care professionals are very effective screeners for mental health and substance abuse issues and should have the ability to accept or reject candidates for employment with and among elders. Potential employees should also have criminal background checks.

Those who will work with the elderly should receive adequate training and education. Careful management and assessment of vulnerable elders will allow for effective care plans for vulnerable elders. Careful attention to the living situation of vulnerable elders by nursing would help prevent elder abuse.

Secondary Prevention

Ongoing training and careful supervision of the care of vulnerable elders allows for early detection and intervention. Paying very close attention to changes in behavior and patterns of injury in vulnerable elders and scheduling regular interviews of people who are working with vulnerable elders promote early detection of elder abuse.

If a caretaker reveals that he or she is very stressed by caring for the elder, careful listening skills will enhance the consideration of possible elder abuse. If the caregiver shows disdain for the population he or she is working with, listening carefully and encouraging conversation will encourage the worker to speak about how she or he cares for the elder(s).

Health care professionals working in outpatient settings should carefully track visits by and to elders. If the family stops bringing the elder in for visits, follow up on whether or not the elder has changed health care facilities or is not being seen for heath care visits at all. Health care professionals can give families and caregivers information about how to care appropriately for elders, but follow-up is needed as to whether or not the caregiver or family follow the nursing instructions.

Tertiary Prevention

Tertiary care involves identification and treatment of abusers, and disallowing them to continue to care for elders or other vulnerable populations.

RESOURCES

Characteristics of Fraud Perpetrators: http://www.da18.org/SeniorFraudCharOfFraud Perp.html

National Institute of Justice: Perpetrators of Elder Abuse: http://www.ojp.usdoj.gov/nij/ topics/crime/elder-abuse/perpetrators.htm

REFERENCES

Brandle, B., & Raymond, J. (2009). Dynamics of abuse in later life. *Family and Intimate Partner Violence Quarterly, 2*(1), 91–95.

Cledscoe, W. (2007). Criminal offender residing in long term care facilities. *Journal of Forensic Science, 3*(1), 142–146.

Fisher, J., & Dyer, C. (2005). The hidden menace of elder abuse: Physicians can help patients surmount IPV. *Postgraduate Medicine, 113*(4), 21–24.

Just, M. (2007). Issues in caregiving: Elder abuse and substance abuse. *Journal of Human Behavior in the Social Environment, 14*(1–2), 117–137.

Kaye, L. (2003). Intervention with abused older males. *Journal of Elder Abuse and Neglect, 19*(1–2), 153–172.

Lelsey, M., Kupstas, P., & Cooper, A. (2009). Domestic violence in the second half of life. *Journal of Elder Abuse and Neglect, 21*(2), 141–155.

O'Connor, D., Hall, M., & Donnelly, M. (2009). Assessing capacity within the context of abuse and neglect. *Journal of Elder Abuse and Neglect, 21*(2), 156–169.

Ramset-Klawsnik, H. (1993). Recognizing and responding to elder maltreatment. *Journal of Long Term Home Care, 12*(3), 12–20.

Ramsey-Klawsnik, H. (2000). Elder-abuse offender: A typology. *Generations, 24*(2), 17–22.

Rosen, T., Pillemer, K., & Lachs, M. (2008). Resident-to-resident aggression in long-term care facilities: An understudied problem. *Aggression and Violent Behavior, 13*(2), 77–87.

Stanford, M., Houston, R., & Baldridge, R. (2008). Comparison of impulsive and premeditated perpetrators of interpersonal violence. *Behavioral Sciences and the Law, 26*(6), 709–722.

U.S. Prevention Task Force. (2004). Screening women and elderly adults for family and IPV: A review of the evidence for the U.S. Prevention Services Task Force. *Annals of Internal Medicine, 149*(5), 387–396.

33 Adult Perpetrators of Sexual Violence

DEFINITION

While most health care providers will not assess sex offenders for treatment or forensic purposes, it is still important that they understand sexual offending and the basic elements related to treatment and forensic assessment. Convicted sex offenders get sick and require health care just like the rest of the population. Hospital and other health care risk managers should develop a uniform policy about how to handle sex offenders, and they, or a designee, can notify the staff of a client's sex offender status if that client has been convicted and registered, thus making this public information.

The term "sex offender" is a generic term for a very heterogeneous population. Contrary to popular belief, research has consistently shown that there is no such thing as a "sex offender profile." People of all ages commit sex offenses, including children and older adults, and while male offenders are far more common, females also commit sex offenses.

Offense Pathways

Several different pathways to offending have been noted. There is even a pathways model that suggests five pathways: a multiple dysfunctional mechanisms pathway; an intimacy deficits pathway; an emotional dysregulation pathway; deviant sexual scripts; and an antisocial cognitions pathway (Ward & Seigert, 2002). The latter two are discussed here since sexual deviance and criminality are the two major risk factors for recidivism.

Sexually Deviant Pathway

Offenders who follow a sexually deviant pathway to sexual offending typically show signs of one or more paraphilias. According to the *Diagnostic and Statistical Manual of Mental Disorders*, 4th edition, text revision (*DSM-IV-TR*), paraphilias are disorders characterized by recurrent, intense sexually arousing fantasies, sexual urges, or behaviors that generally involve: nonhuman objects, the suffering or humiliation of oneself or one's partner, or children or other nonconsenting persons, over a period of at least 6 months. The *DSM-IV-TR* lists eight paraphilias identified by previous classifications: exhibitionism (exposure of one's genitals), fetishism (use of nonliving objects), frotteurism (touching and rubbing against a nonconsenting person), pedophilia (focus on prepubertal children), sexual masochism (receiving humiliation or suffering), sexual sadism (inflicting humiliation or suffering), transvestic fetishism (cross-dressing), and voyeurism (peeping), as well as paraphilia not otherwise specified (NOS). Paraphilia NOS includes other paraphilias less frequently encountered, such as hebephilia (focus on postpubertal children), urophilia (urine), necrophilia (corpses), zoophilia (animals), and telephone scatophilia (obscene phone calls). There is also a paraphilia NOS nonconsent.

Paraphilias are most typically present in white males, ages 15 to 25. These disorders are said to be rare in persons over 50; however, information on paraphilias in older persons is limited. Most persons who have one paraphilia are likely to possess at least two or three more. Most paraphilic fantasies begin in adolescence, although sadistic fantasies may begin in childhood, and more than 50% of all paraphilias have their onset before age 18. Persons with paraphilias selectively view, read, purchase, or photograph depictions of their preferred stimulus, and they may select a career or hobby that gives them contact with their desired stimulus (pedophiles may work with children [scouting, teaching, clergy]; sexual sadists may drive ambulances). Paraphilias more commonly noted in sex crimes are:

- Pedophilia: *DSM-IV-TR* criteria include: (a) fantasies, sexual urges, or behaviors that involve sexual activity with a prepubescent child or children; (b) the person has acted on these urges or the urges/fantasies cause personal difficulty or marked distress; and (c) the person is at least 16 years old and at least 5 years older than the victim(s). Pedophiles may be attracted to females (usually 8- to 10-year-olds), males (slightly older), or both; they may limit their victimization to incest, and they may or may not be exclusively attracted to children. Sexual activities range from undressing the child and looking to fondling to penetration, and these activities are rationalized as "having educational value" for the child, "giving the child sexual pleasure," and "performed because the child was sexually provocative." Prior to sexual behavior, pedophiles may "groom" their victims using behaviors such as: gift giving; acting as the child's buddy; physical contact with wrestling, pats on the buttocks, or tickling; "accidentally" walking in on the child when the child is using the bathroom; "accidentally" exposing one's genitals; providing drugs or alcohol; and exposing the child to adult and child pornography. Pedophilia is egosyntonic in nature; thus, many individuals with this disorder may not be distressed by it. Therefore, it is important to realize that experiencing distress over fantasies, urges, or behaviors is not necessary for a diagnosis of pedophilia. Persons who have a pedophilic arousal pattern and act on their urges or fantasies qualify for a diagnosis of pedophilia.

- Voyeurism: *DSM-IV-TR* criteria include: (a) recurrent, intense, sexually arousing fantasies, urges, or behaviors involving the act of observing an unsuspecting person who is naked, disrobing, or engaging in sexual activity; and (b) the urges or fantasies cause marked distress or interpersonal difficulty, or the person has acted on the urges or fantasies. Masturbation and orgasm may occur during the voyeuristic activity or afterward as a response to the memory of what the voyeur witnessed. Voyeurs often fantasize about having a sexual experience with their victim (which rarely occurs), and some experience their voyeuristic behaviors as their only form of sexual activity. Some voyeurs limit their acts to looking—peeping in windows or at pools and public rest areas, while others use technology.

- Exhibitionism: *DSM-IV-TR* criteria include: (a) recurrent, intense sexually arousing fantasies, urges, or behaviors involving the exposure of one's genitals to unsuspecting strangers; and (b) the urges or fantasies cause marked distress or interpersonal difficulty, or the person has acted on the urges or fantasies. Exhibitionists expose themselves to strangers, sometimes masturbating during the exposure, usually to surprise, frighten, or shock the victim. Some fantasize that the victim becomes sexually aroused, but generally, there is no attempt at further sexual activity. Exhibitionists typically have a target victim population and location as part of their offending cycle. They may target specific ages, hair colorings, or body size, and may prefer locations such as mall parking lots, public parks, or playgrounds, with easy escape routes. Many use a car and drive about town hunting for potential victims, and some others drive around with their genitals exposed.

■ Frotteurism (frottage): *DSM-IV-TR* criteria include: (a) recurrent, intense sexually arousing fantasies, urges, or behaviors involving the touching or rubbing against nonconsenting persons; and (b) the urges or fantasies cause marked distress or interpersonal difficulty, or the person has acted on the urges or fantasies. Like exhibitionists, frotteurs choose places with easy escape routes or those where they can go undetected—busy sidewalks, elevators, or subways, for example. Frotteurs may rub their genitals on their victim's buttocks, or fondle the victim's breasts or genitals with their hands, usually while fantasizing a caring relationship with the victim. Victims are nonconsenting, unknown to the frotteur, and may be unaware of the violation.

■ Sexual sadism: *DSM-IV-TR* criteria include: (a) recurrent, intense sexually arousing fantasies, urges, or behaviors involving real (not simulated) acts in which the psychological or physical suffering of the victim is sexually exciting; and (b) the urges or fantasies cause marked distress or interpersonal difficulty, or the person has acted on the urges or fantasies against a nonconsenting person. The sadists of concern here are those who perpetrate acts on nonconsenting victims. They derive sexual excitement from the suffering of the victim (not the infliction of pain). Named after Marquis de Sade, an eighteenth-century French writer and officer who committed violent acts against women, sadism includes: using restraints, spanking, whipping, beating, burning, shocking, cutting, strangling, torturing, mutilating, or killing. Sadistic rape tends to be aggressive and eroticized with ritualistic acts and language that is degrading, commanding, or alternately threatening and reassuring. The rapist's mood is typically intensely excited and depersonalized. Victim choice is predetermined from special features or symbolic representation. Sadistic offending patterns include careful planning of the offense, taking the victim to a predetermined location, detached affect during the offense, intentional torture, and sexual dysfunction during the offense. Characteristics associated with sadism include a history of childhood physical abuse, cross-dressing, peeping, and obscene phone calls or flashing, and perpetrators may have a history that includes marriage, solid reputation, education past high school, and an incestuous relationship with a son or daughter.

Antisocial Pathway

Offenders who follow a generally antisocial pathway to sexual offending have a pervasive pattern of disregard for, and violation of, the rights of others. These individuals' behaviors fall into patterns that include: failing to conform to social norms with respect to lawful behavior, impulsivity, frequent deceit and manipulation for personal gain, irritability, aggression, recklessness, irresponsibility, and high risk-taking behaviors.

Offenders with an antisocial personality disorder exhibit a pervasive pattern of disregard for and violation of the rights of others, beginning in childhood or early adolescence and continuing into adulthood. *DSM-IV-TR* criteria for this disorder are: (a) a pervasive pattern of disregard for and violation of the rights of others occurring since age 15, as indicated by three or more of the following: failure to conform to social norms with respect for lawful behaviors, deceitfulness, impulsivity or failure to plan ahead, irritability or aggressiveness, reckless disregard for the safety of self or others, consistent irresponsibility, and lack of remorse; (b) being at least 18 years of age; (c) evidence of a conduct disorder before age 15; and (d) the occurrence of the antisocial behavior is not exclusively during the course of a manic episode or schizophrenia. Offenders may also present with personality disorder not otherwise specified (NOS) with antisocial traits, and characteristics of one or more other personality disorders.

Self-Regulation Model Pathway

Ward and Hudson (1998) proposed a self-regulation model specific to sexual offenders. Self-regulation refers to the internal and external processes that allow a person to engage in goal-directed actions over time and across contexts. It includes the selection of goals, planning, monitoring, evaluation, and modification of behavior to achieve approach or avoidance goals. Approach (acquisition) goals relate to the successful achievement of a certain state or situation, while avoidance (inhibitory) goals relate to a reduction of a particular state or situation.

There are three general self-regulation styles related to offending: (1) Under-regulation is a passive route to attempting to avoid offending. It involves a failure to control behavior and can be associated with either positive or negative emotions. (2) Misregulation involves engaging in some effort to avoid offending, but the effort is misplaced, such as using drugs or alcohol to control deviant fantasies. This style is typically associated with negative emotional states. (3) Effective regulation describes the offender whose goal is to commit the sexual offense. The problem here is the choice of goals, not dysfunctional self-regulation; thus, these offenders would experience positive emotions.

Four pathways to offending are based on these goals and self-regulation styles:

1. Avoidant-passive is characterized by under-regulation and a desire to avoid offending, but the offender lacks the coping skills to prevent it.
2. Avoidant-active involves misregulation. The offender attempts to control deviant thoughts and fantasies but uses counterproductive strategies.
3. Approach-automatic involves an under-regulation of self-regulatory style and results in over-learned sexual scripts, as well as impulsive and poorly planned behavior.
4. Approach-explicit involves effective self-regulation and a desire to offend. The offender uses careful planning in offending.

TYPOLOGIES

Some attempts have been made to create typologies of sex offenders. These are presented here to enhance the understanding of sex offenders and not to encourage typing.

Groth's Typology for Child Sexual Abusers

- Fixated child sexual abusers have sexual desires and preferences that center around children. They are unlikely to have healthy sexual contacts with age-appropriate partners, and they tend to be emotionally immature, and are preoccupied with children. These individuals usually go to great lengths to establish "relationships" with more vulnerable children, often using extensive grooming and premeditation.

- Regressed child sexual abusers have "normal" sexual interests toward and encounters with appropriate partners. They do not tend to be interested sexually in children; however, they turn to sexual contact with children as a means of coping or as a substitute for an appropriate partner during times of considerable stress in their lives. Thus, their behaviors may be more situational, opportunistic, and impulsive (Groth, 1979).

Groth's Typology for Rapists

- Anger rapists commit rape in part as a means of expressing anger and hostility that has built up over time. They tend to have intimate relationships that are marked by conflict, and they discharge their hostility and resentment on the victims whom they target. They tend to use considerable force and are both physically and verbally aggressive toward their victims, often causing considerable physical injury.
- Power rapists are primarily motivated by power and are interested more in having control over their victims and "possessing" them than they are interested in causing physical harm. Power rapists typically feel inadequate or controlled by others, or they are insecure about their masculinity.
- Sadistic rapists are probably the most dangerous. They experience a great deal of pleasure and excitement from inflicting harm on their victims and enjoy watching the victim's suffering. They may restrain and torture their victims in idiosyncratic and bizarre ways, and, at the most extreme end, may even mutilate or kill their victims. These crimes tend to be the product of considerable planning and premeditation (Groth, 1979).

The FBI's Crime Classification Manual

- Felony rape (rape committed during the commission of a felony, such as robbery); the felony may be primary (intended to rob, rape was secondary) or primary (intended to rape, robbery was secondary).

- Personal cause sexual assault (interpersonal aggression that results in sexual assault).
- Nuisance offences (no physical contact).
- Domestic sexual assault (family, household member or former household member sexually assaults another household member; includes familial child sexual assault).
- Entitlement rape (forceful rape with power and control issues; includes social acquaintance rape).
- Anger rape (offenders who hate women and express their anger through rape).
- Sadistic rape (offender uses more violence than is necessary to control the victim and becomes aroused by the victim's pain).
- Child/adolescent pornography (collecting, maintaining, and prizing child pornography material).
- Historical child/adolescent sex rings (children are used to create pornographic material).
- Multidimensional sex rings (multiple young victims; multiple offenders; fear used as common tactic; bizarre or ritualistic activity).
- Abduction rape (person forcibly removed from one location and raped in another).
- Group cause sexual assault (multiple offenders, three or more) (if two offenders, they are each classified into a personal cause category); includes gang rapes.
- Informal gang sexual assault (loosely structured group that congregates, typically on the spur of the moment, with the common goal of engaging in an antisocial activity) (Douglas, Burgess, Burgess, & Ressler, 1992).

Rapists have two styles of attack—blitz and confidence.

- The blitz rape happens out of the blue. There is no prior interaction between the offender and victim. The victim may be attacked during normal daily activities or even in her sleep. Offenders jump, grab, push, or shove the victim, typically from behind. Some pull victims into cars.
- The confidence rape has a more subtle set-up. The offenders obtains sex under false pretenses using deceit, betrayal, and often

violence. There is interaction between the offender and victim prior to the assault. He may know the victim or have a relationship with her. Like the confidence man (con artist), he gains the victim's trust. Multiple offenders may be involved as either assailants or accomplices. Other women may act as accomplices, usually acting as decoys. Victims have also been made into victims of gang rape by being tricked into thinking they are going to a party.

Grooming describes the process of desensitizing and manipulating victims for the purpose of gaining an opportunity to commit a sexually deviant act. Child molesters spend a considerable amount of time on the grooming process to gain the child's trust and confidence, and to assume a position of power. Methods vary, but most are based on trickery and threats. Offenders use such methods as bribery; threats of harm to the child, siblings, parents, and even the offender ("You don't want me to go to jail, do you?"); threats to break up the family; withdrawal of affection; and taking advantage of the child's innocence ("Everybody does this"). Some offenders use pornography to desensitize the child. Offenders will also groom the parents or caregivers, and it is not unusual for a child molester to seek out and marry a vulnerable single-female with young children. By grooming the adult, the offender reinforces his position as a trusted member of the child's inner circle. Once the grooming process succeeds, the child may feel obligated to accept the abuse, which typically begins with sexual touch. Grooming is extremely effective and can keep children from disclosing abuse (King County Sexual Assault Resource Center, 2003).

Female Sex Offenders

Female sex offenders account for less than 10% of sex crimes. However, it is likely that sex crimes committed by females are underreported, probably even more so than male-perpetrated sex crimes. Female sex offenders are likely to have: a history of childhood maltreatment, including sexual victimization; mental health symptoms, personality disorders, and substance abuse problems; difficulties in intimate relationships, or an absence of intimate relationships; a propensity to primarily victimize children and adolescents (rarely adults); a tendency to commit offenses against persons who are related or otherwise well known to them; and an increased likelihood of perpetrating sex offenses in concert with a male intimate partner.

Matthews, Matthews, and Speltz (1989) identified three types of female sex offenders, based on clinical observation and not empirical methods. These are:

- Male-coerced offenders tend to be passive and dependent women with histories of sexual abuse and relationship difficulties. Fearing abandonment, they are pressured by their male partners to commit sex offenses, often against their own children.
- Predisposed offenders have histories of incestuous sexual victimization, psychological difficulties, and deviant sexual fantasies. They tend to act alone in their offending and often victimize their own children or other young children within their families.
- Teacher/lover offenders often struggle with peer relationships, seem to regress, and perceive themselves as having romantic or sexually mentoring "relationships" with under-aged adolescent victims of their sexual preference.

Internet Sex Offenders

Unfortunately, health care providers are usually unaware of their clients' Internet activities and interests. Online sexual activity (OSA), like real-world sexual activity, ranges from the normal to the highly deviant. Deviant online sexual behavior serves as: a mechanism for sexual arousal; a way to facilitate online social relationships in addition to existing, offline social relationships; a means of developing online relationships, including sexual relationships, as an alternative to offline, real-world relationships; an obsessive-compulsive process; an addiction; and a means of financial gain. When deviant online behavior involves minors, it becomes illegal. Most online sex offenders target teens and groom their victims into sexual relationships, usually under the guise of romance. Online offenders target vulnerable youths, those with histories of abuse, family problems, and high-risk behaviors.

PREVALENCE

A 2003 Bureau of Justice Statistics report by Langan, Schmitt, and Durose (2003) provided data that represents the largest follow-up study ever conducted of convicted sex offenders following their release from prison. According to this report, of the 9,691 sex offenders released in 1994, 67% were white males and 32% were black males. Of the 9,691, nearly 4,300 were identified as child molesters. Within 3 years following their release,

5.3% of sex offenders (men who committed rape or sexual assault) were rearrested for another sex crime. Sex offenders with the highest rate of rearrest for another sex offense were those who had a history of prior arrests for various crimes. While 3.3% of sex offenders with one prior arrest were arrested for another sex crime after their release, 7.4% of those with 16 or more prior arrests were arrested for sex crimes after release. Of the released sex offenders who allegedly committed another sex crime, 40% who reoffended sexually did so within a year or less from their prison discharge. An estimated 3.3% of the 4,300 released child molesters were rearrested for another sex crime against a child within three years, and most of their alleged victims were 13 years old or younger.

ETIOLOGY

The question of what causes an individual to become a sexual offender has attracted considerable scientific attention over the past several years. Theoretical models focus primarily on a single or small cluster of causal factors, including biological mechanisms in the onset of sexually deviant behavior, and postulating that genetic determinants, hormone imbalances, or both are responsible for sexual aggression. Other theorists point to brain abnormalities, as well as attachment disturbances suggesting that insecurely attached boys with emotionally unsupportive parents are more likely to become sexual predators later in life. Social learning theory notes that children learn from their social environments, and that if those childhood social environments include violence, abuse, and the degradation of women, the propensity to mimic those behaviors is strengthened. These reasons have led some theorists to suggest that the graphic violence on television, in conjunction with the portrayal of women as submissive and sexualized, desensitizes children to violence and promotes sexual aggression. Although these theories have supportive evidence, none of them can account for all instances of sexual violence. Etiological pathways to sexual offending are multiple and complex, and thus, more recent models have attempted to incorporate several or all of these individual factors.

ASSESSMENT

General Principles

Working with sex offenders means working with those already convicted of a sex crime, and thus, assessment focuses on treatment needs and recidivism risk. Risk assessment aids in many key decisions with sex offenders, such as disposition or sentencing, the type of placement or required level of care, release from facilities, and the application of registration and community notification policies. Assessing risk is also helpful for guiding decisions about which individuals will benefit most from interventions and strategies that are both time- and resource-intensive, such as prison-based or residential sex offender treatment, intensive supervision, and ancillary accountability measures such as electronic monitoring.

Risk assessment includes the identification of static and dynamic risk factors. Historical characteristics that cannot be altered, such as age of the offender, gender of the victims, relationship between the offender and the victims, and prior offense history, are referred to as static factors. Attitudes and characteristics that can change throughout a person's life are termed dynamic factors. Dynamic factors can be further categorized as stable or acute. Stable dynamic factors include deviant sexual preferences and practices and victim blaming, while acute dynamic factors include intoxication preceding the offense.

Risk Assessment

The two predominant methods of assessing risk of reoffending in adult male sex offenders are actuarial risk assessment and clinical judgment. Actuarial risk assessment involves the incorporation of risk factors that have been identified through scientific research and incorporated into an actuarial measure. Based on the individual's score on the measures, the probability of reoffending is calculated. These actuarial measures rely almost exclusively on static, or unchanging, factors, such as criminal history, the nature of the offense, age at time of offense, and so on. Examples of actuarial risk assessments are the Static-99, the Static 2002 (the one more recently utilized), and the Minnesota Sex Offender Screening Tool (MnSOST-R).

Static-99 is an instrument designed to assist in the prediction of sexual and violent recidivism for sexual offenders. The Static-99 consists of 10 items and produces estimates of future risk based upon the number of risk factors present in any one individual. The risk factors included in the risk assessment instrument are the presence of prior sexual offenses, having committed a current nonsexual violent offense, having a history of nonsexual violence, the number of previous sentencing dates, an age of less than 25 years old, having male victims, having never lived with a lover for two consecutive years, having a history of noncontact sex offenses, having unrelated victims, and having stranger victims. The recidivism estimates provided by the Static-99 are group estimates based upon reconvictions and were derived from groups of individuals with these characteristics. As such, these estimates do not directly correspond to the recidivism risk of an individual offender. The offender's risk may be higher or lower than the probabilities estimated in the Static-99 depending on other risk factors not measured by this instrument. The Static-99 Coding Rules Revised may be found at http://www.2.ps-sp.gc.ca/publications/corrections/pdf/Static-99-coding-Rules_e.pdf.

Static-2002 is an instrument designed to assist in the prediction of sexual and violent recidivism for sex offenders. Using eight replication samples from four countries (Canada, United Kingdom, United States, Denmark; n = 3,034), Static-2002 demonstrates moderate to large accuracy in the prediction of sexual, violent, and general recidivism. Static-2002 consists of 14 items and produces estimates of relative risk based upon the number of risk factors present in any one individual. The risk factors included in the risk assessment instrument are grouped into five domains: age, persistence of sex offending, deviant sexual interests, relationship to victims, and general criminality. Normative data for Static-2002 scores were based on a sample of Canadian sexual offenders (n = 2,507) that was reweighted according to type of sentence (federal prison, provincial prison, and noncustodial) in order to approximate the real distribution of Canadian sex offenders. The norms are presented as percentile ranges, reflecting the estimated percentage of offenders scoring at or below a specified score. In other words, percentiles provide a relative ranking. Relative rankings are thought to be most useful in situations where the allocation of limited resources must be made, such as for treatment or community supervision. Absolute degrees of recidivism risk cannot be directly inferred from these relative rankings. The appropriateness of applying the known Canadian distribution of Static-2002 scores to sexual offenders in other countries is not yet known. Under Static-2002, an offender can be placed in one of five risk categories based on his or her total score (ranging from 0–14): low (0–2), low-moderate (3, 4), moderate (5, 6), moderate-high (7, 8) and high (9+). Static 2002 coding rules may be found at http://www.static99.org/pdfdocs/static2002codingrules.pdf.

The Minnesota Sex Offender Screening Tool–Revised (MnSOST-R) consists of 16 items that measure dynamic, criminality/chronicity, offender-related, and unstable lifestyle variables. Two reliability studies attest to the reliability of raters using the MnSOST-R. A Minnesota study yielded a reliability coefficient of .76, while a Florida study yielded a reliability coefficient of .86. The validity indices for the MnSOST-R in a cross-validation study (r = .35, ROCAUC = .73) are comparable to ones reported for similar sex offender actuarial risk assessment tools (Epperson et al., 2000)

The risk factors included in this risk assessment instrument are number of sex-related convictions, length of sexual offending history, whether the offender was under any form of supervision when committing any sex offense for which the offender was eventually charged or convicted, whether the sex offense was committed in a public place, whether force or the threat of force was ever used to achieve compliance in any sex offense (charged or convicted), whether any sex offense (charged or convicted) involved multiple acts against a single victim within any single contact event, number of different age groups victimized across all sex/sex-related offenses (charged or convicted), whether the offense was against a 13- to 15-year-old victim and the offender was more than five years older than the victim at the time of the offense (charged or convicted), whether the victim was a stranger in any sex/sex-related offense (charged or convicted), evidence of adolescent antisocial behavior in the file, pattern of substantial drug or alcohol abuse (12 months prior to arrest for instant offense or revocation), employment history, discipline history while incarcerated (does not include discipline for failure to follow treatment directives), chemical dependency treatment while incarcerated, sex offender treatment history while incarcerated, and age of offender at time of release. Guidelines and further psychometric data for the MnSOST-R can be found at http://www.psychology.iastate.edu/~dle/mnsost_download.htm.

Other assessment tools include the Rapid Risk Assessment for Sex Offense Recidivism (RRASOR), which correlated at 0.27 with sexual recidivism; the Violence Risk Appraisal Guide (VRAG), which was developed to determine risk for violent recidivism for males who have committed a violent offense that was either sexual or nonsexual in nature; and the Sex Offender Risk Appraisal Guide (SORAG), which has 14 items in total (10 identical to VRAG items) and was developed to predict offenders' probability for committing sexually violent and sexual offenses. The Acute 2007 and the Stable 2007 are tools that can be utilized with the Static 99, thus combining dynamic and static risk factors. Tools used to measure dynamic risk factors can also be helpful for treatment purposes.

An alternative assessment method involves the use of clinical judgment through the collection of interview materials and offender criminal records, considering factors such as criminal history, psychiatric diagnosis, social supports, and relationship stability. Once the relevant information has been collected and reviewed, the clinician arrives at a judgment about the offender's likelihood of reoffending. However, research suggests that clinical judgments are subjective, lack reliability, and are often inferior to actuarial results. Thus the empirical and professional trend has been to integrate the clinical judgment and risk assessment tools to maximize predictive power and accuracy. Overall, the integration of actuarial and clinical approaches, static and dynamic factors, and dispositional and contextual factors appears to be the current trend. The ultimate goal, both empirically and clinically, is to achieve a comprehensive approach to risk assessment that will result in more accurate predictions and appropriate treatment methods.

There are other testing measures used in evaluation and treatment, all of which are used to determine whether a sex offender is at heightened risk of reoffending. The Abel Assessment for Sexual Interest (AASI-2), a screening tool for deviant sexual interests that measures visual reaction time, requires a test subject to view slides of clothed persons of varying ages and sexes, so that the person's level of sexual attraction can be rated. The length of time an individual views a particular slide determines the individual's sexual interest for different groups of people, both adults and children. The AASI-2 is widely mandated by U.S. courts as a condition of sex offender supervised release.

Penile plethysmography (PPG) measures increments of erection of the penis via a small device on the penis. The device is attached to a computer operated by an evaluator in another room. The offender listens to audiotape descriptions of various kinds of sexual behavior, or views slides that depict males and females of various ages, typically photographs of individual nudes, while the plethysmograph detects blood flow to his penis, a measure of his erotic arousal to these various stimuli. The test is intrusive and costly and not completely accurate because some offenders can distract themselves sufficiently so that they do not exhibit arousal in the laboratory when, in fact, they would otherwise have arousal in ordinary circumstances.

The polygraph assesses whether sex offenders are being deceptive, and this is regarded as a valuable tool in sex offender treatment. Determining whether an offender is being deceptive can be critically important in the treatment process. The polygraph assesses whether or not sex offenders have knowingly withheld any information from their sexual history. This can result in significantly increased disclosures of sexual misconduct, even prior to the actual administration of the polygraph examination.

Female Sex Offender Assessment

Little is known about female sex offenders. The literature notes that no risk measures have yet been developed for female sex offenders. The extremely low numbers of female sex offenders that come to the attention of the authorities and that are available for follow-up studies have significantly impeded researchers' attempts to identify specific risk factors associated with sexual recidivism with this population.

In terms of recidivism, female sex offenders, like male sex offenders, engage in a variety of recidivism behaviors (sexual, nonsexual violent, and others), but at lower levels than males. Recidivism characteristics include: previous violent partner; more than one victim in the index offense; being physically abused; having been bullied at school; prior drug arrests; prior violent felony offense arrests; prior incarceration; young age at the time of the offense; and prior child abuse. Like male sexual offenders, prior criminal history is the best predictor of future recidivism; however, no other systematic risk factor has been found among women. But one should account for the number of prior victims and prior child abuse history, as these may indicate higher propensity for sexual recidivism. Evaluation of female sex offenders should also take into consideration the dynamic risk factors related to general recidivism in women, which include: antisocial attitudes and associates; substance abuse as a precursor to offending; and problematic relationships, including especially the woman's stance toward her co-offender, and emotional dyscontrol.

INTERVENTION

The Center for Sex Offender Management (CSOM) notes that sex offender treatment is a field where the stakes are high, the dynamics are complex, the interventions are specialized, and the literature is evolving; therefore, it is essential that treatment providers be equipped with the necessary knowledge and skills to provide ethically sound and quality treatment. They strongly suggest specialized education, training, experience, and supervision, and note that some states (e.g., Colorado, Illinois, Texas, and Utah) require that those wishing to provide treatment for sex offenders meet established criteria or undergo a formal certification process. Many of the criteria used for these purposes are based on published practice standards from the Association for the Treatment of Sexual Abusers (ATSA).

Commonalities and Differences of Sex Offender Treatment

Sex offender treatment has similarities to other psychiatric treatments. Clients should understand the interventions and procedures that will be utilized, as well as any associated risks and benefits. Thus, informed consent should be provided. Interventions should be guided by formal assessments and appropriately individualized to the needs of each client. A therapeutic rapport must be established and maintained. Treatment goals should be specific and measurable, and progress (or lack of progress) must be accurately and thoroughly documented.

Some aspects of treatment are qualitatively different from approaches to intervention for other populations:

■ Treatment is defined as the delivery of prescribed interventions as a means of managing crime-producing factors and promoting positive and meaningful goal attainment for participants. This is in the interest of enhancing public safety.
■ Treatment is often involuntary. Sex offenders tend to enter specialized treatment as a result of external pressures or legal mandates, rather than being driven solely by internal motivation.
■ Treatment goals are not solely driven by the client's desires. Many of the broad goals of sex offender treatment are largely predetermined to include relatively standard goals, such as addressing denial, identifying and managing risk factors, enhancing empathy for victims, and developing prosocial skills.
■ Confidentiality is limited, because treatment takes place within the context of the justice system. The routine involvement of the courts and multiple agencies often necessitates collaboration and critical information sharing in order to support accountability, enhance management strategies, and ultimately promote public safety.
■ With treatment for those who commit sex offenses, the potential impact of failed interventions is more far-reaching than treatment failure in other venues. Besides the impact on the offender and the offender's family, public safety may be compromised. The

result of treatment failure can be additional sexual victimization and the associated impact on the victim, victim's family, and the community.

- Working with sex offenders increases the potential for vicarious trauma and burnout for treatment providers. Those who provide treatment to sex offenders are regularly exposed to very detailed descriptions of abusive sexual behaviors, the attitudes and statements that support or minimize these behaviors, and the readily apparent harm to victims. This cumulative exposure, especially when combined with other influences, such as professional isolation, a high volume of cases, intense public scrutiny, and limited healthy coping responses, can lead treatment providers to experience vicarious or secondary trauma.

Most convicted sex offenders reside at some point (on probation, parole, or release) in the community, thus requiring a comprehensive and collaborative sex offender management program that combines treatment with supervision to enable the offenders to control their sexually abusive behaviors. The desired outcome of treatment is the prevention of future sexual victimization. In general, most sex offender treatment has the following goals for the offender:

- Accept responsibility.
- Learn to understand their patterns (cycles) of criminal behavior.
- Modify cognitive distortions.
- Learn attitudes, cognitive skills, and behaviors needed to safely live in the community.
- Develop victim empathy.
- Control deviant sexual arousal, interests, preferences, and behaviors.
- Improve social competence.
- Reduce impulsivity and develop self-regulation.
- Manage negative emotions.
- Develop healthy relationships and correct intimacy deficits.
- Establish supervision conditions and networks.
- Develop an effective relapse prevention plan.

Treatment is also individualized and aimed at the underlying disorder (e.g., paraphilia or antisocial personality disorder) and associated problems (substance abuse, mood disorders, developmental disability, etc.). Treatment may take place in a correctional institution, forensic psychiatric unit, or the community. Offenders can be terminated from treatment for noncompliance or failure to make adequate progress in treatment, sexual behavior, assaults and fighting, violating confidentiality of others in the program, or being placed in a high security category.

Community Notification

As a result of federal legislation, all 50 states have enacted some type of sex offender community notification laws to ensure that the public can access information that will assist them in protecting themselves and their families from dangerous sex offenders who reside in their communities. Significant variation exists among jurisdictions in how these statutes have been implemented. Despite the intention of enhancing public safety, community notification laws can have negative effects on the criminal justice system, the community, victims, and offenders, and especially the offender's family members. Many programs throughout the country have made efforts to reduce these effects. Individual state registries and information may be found at the Federal Bureau of Investigations National/State Sex Offender Registry at http://www.fbi.gov/hq/cid/cac/registry.htm.

Civil Commitment

Many states have enacted what are termed "sexually violent predator" and/or "civil commitment" statutes that allow authorities to hold a sex offender after his or her criminal sentence has expired if the offender is deemed too dangerous to be released. These individuals will be confined to a treatment facility until such time as they are assessed to no longer pose an imminent risk to the community.

PREVENTION/PATIENT TEACHING

Primary Prevention

Most of the research on sexual offending centers on recidivism. However, health care providers can assess for risk factors and refer clients when appropriate. In a review and meta-analysis of risk factors for the perpetration of child sexual abuse, Whitaker et al. (2008) found general risk factors in the areas of family/parenting, externalizing behaviors, internalizing behaviors, social deficits, sexual behaviors, and attitudes/cognitions.

- Family/parenting risk factors: history of abuse; poor histories of family functioning, including harsh discipline; poor attachment or bonding; and generally poor functioning of their family of origin
- Externalizing behaviors: aggression and violence; nonviolent criminality; anger/hostility; substance abuse; paranoia/mistrust; and antisocial personality disorder
- Internalizing behaviors: anxiety, depression, external locus of control, and low self-esteem
- Social deficits: low social skills/competence; loneliness; and difficulties with intimate relationships
- Sexual behaviors: high sex drive and preoccupations; deviant sexual interests; and greater sexualized coping
- Attitudes/cognitions: more attitudes tolerant of adult–child sex; and cognitions that minimize the perpetrator's culpability

Secondary Prevention

Secondary prevention should focus on the identification of paraphilias and offending-related personality traits or disorders before they lead to sexual offending. This is difficult at best, as those affected may be resistant to seek help or discuss their problems due to shame or fear of criminal implications.

Tertiary Prevention

The goals of tertiary prevention are recidivism prevention and successful reentry back into society.

RESOURCES

Association for the Treatment of Sexual Abusers: http://www.atsa.com
Center for Sex Offender Management. http://www.csom.org
National Criminal Justice Reference Service Edition on Sex Offenders: http://www.ncjrs.gov/sexoffenders
National Institute of Justice (NIJ): Prison Rape: http://www.ojp.usdoj.gov/nij/topics/corrections/prison-rape/welcome.htm

REFERENCES

American Psychiatric Association. (2000). *Diagnostic and statistical manual of mental disorders* (4th ed., text revision). Washington, DC: American Psychiatric Association.

Brannon, G. (2005). Paraphilias. *Emedicine from WebMD.* Retrieved from http://www.emedicine.com/med/topic3127.htm

Center for Sex Offender Management (CSOM). (2004). *The comprehensive approach to adult and juvenile sex offender management: An overview.* U.S. Department of Justice, Office of Justice Programs, Bureau of Justice Assistance. Retrieved from http://www.csom.org/pubs/cap/overview.htm

Center for Sex Offender Management (CSOM). (2007). *Managing the challenges of sex offender re-entry.* U.S. Department of Justice, Office of Justice Programs. Retrieved from http://www.csom.org/pubs/reentry_brief.pdf

Douglas, J., Burgess, A., Burgess, A., & Ressler, R. (1992). *Crime classification manual: A standard system for investigating and classifying violent crimes.* Federal Bureau of Investigation (FBI) National Center for the Analysis of Violent Crime. San Francisco, CA: Jossey-Bass.

Epperson, D. L., Kaul, J. D., Huot, S. J., Hesselton, D., Alexander, W., & Goldman, R. (2000). *Minnesota Sex Offender Screening Tool—Revised (Mn-SOST-R): General instructions.* St. Paul, MN: Department of Corrections.

Groth, N. (1979). *Men who rape: The psychology of the offender.* New York: Plenum.

Hanson, R. K., & Harris, A. (1998). *Dynamic predictors of sexual recidivism.* Ottawa: Solicitor General of Canada. Retrieved from http://ww2.ps-sp.gc.ca/publications/corrections/199801b_e.pdf

Hanson, R. K., Lloyd, C. D., Helmus, L., & Thornton, D. (2008). Using multiple samples to estimate percentile ranks for actuarial risk tools: A Canadian example using Static-99 and Static-2002. Unpublished manuscript.

Hynes, F., Taylor, N., & Lenihan, F. (2007). The role of the mental health professional in cases of online sexual activity. *The British Journal of Forensic Practice, 9*(3), 19–24.

King County Sexual Assault Resource Center. (2003). *Sexual offender grooming techniques.* Retrieved from http://www.kcsarc.org/nForParentsAndCaregivers/Sex%20Offender%20Grooming%20Techniques.pdf

Langan, P., Schmitt, E., & Durose, M. (2003). *Recidivism of sex offenders released from prison in 1994.* U.S. Department of Justice Office of Justice Programs Bureau of Justice Statistics. NCJ 198281. Retrieved from http://www.ojp.usdoj.gov/bjs/pub/pdf/rsorp94.pdf

Mathews, R., Matthews, J., & Speltz, K. (1989). *Female sexual offenders: An exploratory study.* Brandon, VT: The Safer Society Press.

Singer, K. (2006). *Grooming or setting up your victim.* The Awareness Center. Retrieved from http://www.theawarenesscenter.org/offendersarticles.html#Grooming

Ward, T., & Hudson, S. (1998). A model of the relapse process in sexual offenders. *Journal of Interpersonal Violence, 13*(6), 700–725.

Ward, T., & Siegert, R. J. (2002). Toward a comprehensive theory of child sexual abuse: A theory knitting perspective. *Psychology, Crime, and Law, 9,* 125–143.

Whitaker, D., Le, B., Hanson, K., Baker, C., McMahon, P., Klien, A., et al. (2008). Risk factors for the perpetration of child sexual abuse: A review and meta-analysis. *Child Abuse & Neglect, 32,* 529–548.

34 Older Adult Perpetrators of Sexual Violence

DEFINITION

Once called "dirty old men," older men who commit nonconsensual sex acts are finding themselves labeled sex offenders. Elderly sex offenders is a new category of sex offenders recognized by law enforcement, psychology, psychiatry, and social work. People who commit sexual offenses and are over the age of 60 or 65 are placed into this category.

PREVALENCE AND ETIOLOGY

Very little research on this category of sex offenders has been conducted, and statistics on sexual offenses committed by a person over age 65 do not currently exist. However, two important studies have been completed related to this type of offender. Fazel, Hope, O'Donnell, and Jacoby (2002) interviewed 101 incarcerated sex offenders over the age of 59 years. They then compared the sex offender interviews to interviews of 102 incarcerated offenders who were not sex offenders. The findings about the sex offender group were as follows:

6% had a diagnosis of psychosis

7% had a diagnosis of severe depression

33% had a personality disorder

5% had dementia

This information was compared to the interview data of 102 incarcerated people who were not sex offenders. The data looked almost identical. The sex offenders and nonsex offenders had very similar mental health diagnoses. Both groups had more personality disorders than they had mental illnesses. However, on further analysis it was noted that the sex offender group had different personality disorders than the nonsex-offender group. The sex offender group was more schizoid, more obsessive-compulsive, and more avoidant than the nonsex-offender group. Another interesting finding was that those in the sex offender group had fewer antisocial personality traits than those in the nonsex-offender group.

Cross (2000) examined offenders in a maximum security forensic hospital. All of the offenders committed very serious violent crimes, and some of the offenders committed sexual offenses. Cross noted that 41% of the offenders were psychotic, 59% had a previous psychiatric hospital admission, and 45% had a history of head trauma. Cross's study noted that elderly offenders who commit violent sex crimes may be psychotic and have cognitive impairment.

ASSESSMENT

Specific assessment strategies of elderly sex offenders have yet to be designed. Beginning research has focused on incarcerated elderly sex offenders. However, sex offenders also reside at home and in long-term care facilities. Elderly sex offenders who reside in the community may have been offending for many years without consequence. Biological deficiencies in sexual performance can be compensated for via medication, so sex offending that includes penetration can continue into older age. Sex offenders can be residing in long-term care facilities. Sex offenders who have comorbid medical diagnoses that require nursing intervention are assigned to long-term care facilities by sex offender boards and judges. Placing an elderly sex offender in a long-term care facility can jeopardize the health and welfare of the residents in the facility.

INTERVENTION

Interventions for elderly sex offenders include treatment for any psychiatric disorders and treatment for personality disorders. Treatment of elderly sex offenders is complicated by multiple medical diagnoses that coexist with the mental health issues of the offender. Medication to reduce sexual aggression may be utilized.

PREVENTION/PATIENT TEACHING

Preventing elderly sexual offenders from offending requires careful monitoring of the offender. The offender residing in the community must be identified and treated in order to protect the community. Elderly sex offenders living in long-term care facilities must be isolated from the general population in the facility. Older sex offenders can and do assault elders in nursing homes.

REFERENCES

Burgess, A. (2007). Sex offenders of the elderly: Classification by motive, typology and predictors of severity of the crime. *Aggression and Violent Offenders, 12*(5), 582–597.

Cross, G. (2000). Clinical and demographic characteristics of elder offenders at a maximum security forensic hospital. *Journal of Forensic Science, 45*(6), 1193–1196.

Fazel, S., Hope, T., O'Donnell, I., & Jacoby, R. (2002). Psychiatric demographic and personality characteristics of elderly sex offenders. *Psychological Medicine, 32*(2), 219–226.

Ozkan, B. (2008). Older sex offender's pharmacotherapy for inappropriate sexual behaviors in dementia. *American Journal of Alzheimer's Diseases and Other Dementias, 23*(4), 344–354.

Rosen, T., & Lachs, M. (2008). Resident to resident aggression in long term care facilities. *Journal of the American Geriatric Society, 56*(8), 77–87.

35 Female Offenders

DEFINITION

Female offenders are those age 18 and older who have been arrested and convicted of a crime. The majority of their offenses are related to drugs and/or alcohol, either directly, as in the possession or sale of illegal substances, driving while intoxicated, or commercial sex work in exchange for drugs and/or money for drugs; or committed while the offender was under the influence of drugs and/or alcohol.

Prostitution

Prostitution is a widespread public health concern. Most prostitutes are women. Their clients, commonly called "johns," are their customers. Recent National Institute of Justice–funded research has disclosed information on this seriously under-researched population. This research reveals that many women enter prostitution as minors and use their income to support a drug habit or to stave off homelessness. Many prostitutes suffered abuse as children. They also have extremely high rates of on-the-job victimization and possibly the highest homicide rate of any group of women studied by the Institute of Justice. Researchers have also examined data from a study of prostitutes' clients to find out who they are, why they solicit sex from prostitutes, and what attitudes they hold toward violence against women. Male customers of prostitutes who commit acts of violence against the prostitutes are likely to have a criminal past and are likely to have a history of violent offenses, including rape.

Prostitution is an example of a blending of victim with offender. Selling sex for money is illegal in most areas of the United States. The person selling sex, male or female, is an offender in the eyes of the law. What minimal research has been conducted about prostitution primarily focuses on women. Many women are recruited into prostitution by force, fraud, or coercion. Some women need money to support themselves and their children; others need money to support their drug habits.

Abuse is a common theme in the lives of prostitutes. Many were abused as children, either physically or sexually or both. Many street prostitutes are running away from abusive situations when they are recruited into prostitution. Even when street prostitutes try to leave the streets, they often return to prostitution because their limited education and lack of skills make finding employment very difficult. Without a means to support themselves and perhaps their children, they think staying on the streets is less risky than leaving prostitution.

PREVALENCE

More than one million women are under some form of correctional supervision, and the majority of these women are mothers to an estimated 2 million minor children, 70% of whom were living with their mother at the time of arrest; 5% to 10% of women are pregnant at the time of arrest.

According to the Bureau of Justice Statistics (2002), there were 103,910 women in state and federal prison on June 30, 2004. On that same date, 86,999 women were incarcerated in jails. Women also represent a growing population in probation and parole since 1995. In 2004 females accounted for one in four probationers and about one in eight parolees.

In a Texas study of 471 female sex offenders, the majority (88%) were White, with ages that ranged from 18 to 77 (M = 32) (Vandiver & Kercher, 2007). The researchers also noted that the most common arrests for these female offenders were for indecency with a child (sexual contact, sexual assault on a child, and aggravated sexual assault on a child).

In a special report prepared for the Bureau of Justice in 1999, 14% of violent crime (2.1 million) was committed by females, and 28% of the

2.1 million females found guilty of a violent offense were juveniles. The population of female offenders in both prisons and jails has been increasing twice as fast as that of male offenders since 1990. Three out of four female offenders in 2002 were found guilty of simple assault. Males were more likely to use weapons in their offenses, but victims of male or female offenders have the same rate of hospitalization. Of felons who appeared before a state court in 2002, 16% were female. The most common felony offense noted in state courts was aggravated assault.

ETIOLOGY

Female offenders usually come from backgrounds of poverty, neglect, and abuse. They usually have histories of emotional problems linked with substance abuse, and have poor health in general. There are several risk factors associated with becoming a female offender.

> *Physical or sexual abuse in the past:* A 1999 Bureau of Justice Special Report showed that 6 out of 10 female offenders had a history of physical or sexual abuse in their past. In a 2002 report to the Justice Department, 36% of female offenders reported abuse in their past. In 2006, the Bureau of Justice reported a high incidence of previous victimization in female offenders (Rand & Catalano, 2007).

> *Use of drugs and alcohol:* In 2004, approximately 80% of state and federal inmates reported using drugs, with over half reporting using drugs in the month before arrest; 60% of female inmates were classified as meeting criteria for drug dependence or abuse. The risk factor for drug and alcohol abuse was noted in a Bureau of Justice Report in 2002; one-half of all female offenders in state prison used alcohol and drugs in 2002. In a report written for the Department of Justice, Leverentz (2006) reported a high use of drugs by female offenders.

> *Poverty:* Of female offenders, according to a Bureau of Justice Report (2002), 30% named government assistance as their only source of income.

> *Prior arrest:* According to the Department of Justice, 65% of female offenders had a prior conviction in 2006.

ASSESSMENT

General Principles

Female inmates report higher rates of medical and mental illness than males. Nearly 20% of female inmates reported having asthma, with other common ailments being diabetes, arthritis, and hypertension. Female jail inmates reported significantly higher rates of cervical cancer than the general female population. As with male offenders, female offenders also have high rates of infectious diseases, mental illness, and substance abuse.

The majority of incarcerated women are mothers, and many are pregnant at the time of their arrest. Pregnant inmates with underlying medical and psychiatric disorders need specialized prenatal and postnatal nursing care. They can also benefit from comprehensive prenatal education, including the health effects of drug, alcohol, and tobacco use, and parenting skills. Interventions to decrease their mental distress include self-help groups, stress management, and programs to enhance self-esteem. Increased contact between parents and their children contributes to an inmate's successful reintegration into the community and reduces recidivism. While the need for family-oriented programs for inmates is recognized, there is great variability among state departments of correction as to the provision of these programs. While some special programs are available to imprisoned mothers and their children, more than half of incarcerated parents do not have any visitation with their children while incarcerated; 40% of mothers report no contact of any kind. Mothers incarcerated before or soon after giving birth may not see their child again until after the period of mother–infant attachment is over. Communities of color have experienced a disproportionate burden of the adverse effects of governmental "zero-tolerance" drug policies. The impact continues from one generation to the next, as large numbers of children of color are raised with absent parents, and resources are diverted toward prison expansion rather than community services.

History and Physical Assessment

While incarcerated, female offenders undergo a detailed mental health evaluation, as well as a physical assessment with a gynecological examination. A treatment plan is devised for the offender and implemented by a health care team. Risk for suicide is carefully evaluated, and preventative measures put in place as needed. Female offenders are evaluated for sexually transmitted infections (STIs) and pregnancy while incarcerated. Female offenders are treated for any infection, including STIs. All female offenders are entitled to prenatal care.

Female offenders while incarcerated are evaluated for illicit drug and alcohol use. Treatment for drug addiction in incarceration is typically a 12-step group therapy program. The physical effects that result from drug withdrawal are handled via medication for physical symptoms. Methadone is used in very few incarceration facilities that hold females.

Most female offenders are not incarcerated. The majority of females are living in the community on probation and parole. Programming in jails and prisons does not extend to the community. Caseworkers assigned to the female offender assist in connecting the offender in the community to the services they require.

Diagnostic Testing

Routine testing for STIs and TB are warranted, as is a pelvic examination with screening for cervical cancer and pregnancy testing.

Assessment of Prostitutes

Prostitution is generally ignored in the United States. There is a generalized assumption by the public that people choose a life of prostitution. A history given to the health care provider on violence in the living arrangement, forced sex, drug addiction, dependency on others for necessities, and no form of income may indicate that the person giving the history is a prostitute. A red flag is that prostitutes are often estranged from family and have little or no contact with them. Prostitutes rarely present to a health care facility with a family member. An interview of any victim of violence should be conducted alone and in a clinical setting. People who work in the sex industry control the prostitute and the money she or he makes. Someone may be accompanying the prostitute to the health care setting in order to prevent an accurate history being given by the prostitute.

The most prevalent health consequences to women from prostitution are the same injuries and infections suffered by women who are subjected to any form of violence. The physical health consequences include: injury (head injury, fractures, bruises, and lacerations); STIs (including HIV/AIDS, chlamydia, gonorrhea, herpes, human papilloma virus, and syphilis); general gynecological problems, including chronic pelvic pain and pelvic inflammatory disease (PID); unwanted pregnancy and miscarriage; and positive cervical cancer screens. The emotional health consequences of prostitution include severe trauma, stress, depression, anxiety, self-medication through alcohol and drug abuse, and eating disorders.

INTERVENTION

Medical problems need to be addressed, as do routine wellness needs such as breast self-examination teaching. The American Diabetes Association has recently set general guidelines for diabetic care in correctional institutions, which address intake screening and management of diabetes (http://care.diabetesjournals.org/content/29/suppl_1/s59.full). Additionally, the guidelines recommend that correctional institutions identify particularly high-risk patients in need of more intensive evaluation and therapy, including pregnant inmates.

Women's Health

Female offenders require information and health assessment related to pregnancy, birth control, child placement, and abortion. Inmates are medically screened for pregnancy upon admission and instructed to inform medical staff as soon as they suspect they are pregnant. If necessary, the childbirth takes place at a hospital outside of the institution, and arrangements are made with outside social service agencies to aid the inmate in finding an appropriate placement for the child. Newborn children are not permitted to return to the institution with their mothers; however, they can accompany an adult visitor in accordance with visiting policy. Parenting classes are critical and should begin prior to childbirth whenever possible. Pregnant inmates receive medical, religious, and social counseling regarding their decision whether to carry the pregnancy to term or to have an elective abortion. If an inmate decides to have an abortion, arrangements are made for these medical services to be provided in an appropriate clinic outside the institution. Prenatal care must be provided to incarcerated women, but when the female offender is released into the community, access to prenatal care becomes a challenge. The provision of accessible and affordable prenatal care is a contribution to the health and well-being of the female offender and her unborn child.

Parenting programs are offered in jails and prisons. Community parenting programs that serve the population of female offenders on probation and parole are needed. Communities in which the children of female offenders reside assume the responsibility for caring for these children. Innovative programs that provide safe homes and promote visitation with incarcerated mothers have developed throughout American communities. Community development of safe homes and safe jobs for the female offender and her children living in the community is needed.

Intimate Partner Violence

Some female offenders are also victims of intimate partner violence (IPV). Interventions for partner abuse should be offered for female offenders (see chapter 12). Female batterers also require intervention, especially since this behavior is what may have caused their incarceration in the first place.

Mental Health and Substance Abuse

Mental illness and substance abuse treatment are critical. Female offenders are more likely than males to have used serious drugs, such as cocaine and heroin, to have used them intravenously, and to have used them more frequently prior to arrest. They are also more likely to have a coexisting psychiatric disorder and to have low self-esteem. Posttraumatic stress disorder (PTSD) is common among survivors of abuse. The combined effects of PTSD and substance abuse may exist with comorbid Axis I and II disorders, medical problems, psychological symptoms, in-patient admissions, interpersonal problems, lower levels of functioning and compliance with aftercare and motivation for treatment, and other significant life problems (such as homelessness, HIV, domestic violence, and loss of custody of children). PTSD and co-occurring substance-abuse disorders can have devastating effects on the female offender's ability to care for her children properly when in the community. The unpredictable, volatile, and depressive behaviors associated with PTSD may cause these women to be viewed as unfit or inadequate mothers, placing them at risk for removal of their children or loss of custody.

Substance abuse treatment programs for female offenders is needed during incarceration and while living in the community. Most correctional programs are designed for males but used for women. Effective drug treatment programs for women are difficult to locate in female incarceration sites. Keeping a connection to drug treatment after release from incarceration is a challenge for female and male offenders. Communities in which female offenders reside should create situations in which drug treatment, inpatient and outpatient, is readily accessible to female offenders.

PREVENTION/PATIENT TEACHING

Little is known about prevention for this population at this time. Primary prevention should focus on programming to reduce risk factors for offending in women, including substance abuse, poverty, and lack of education and employment. Secondary prevention that focuses on early identification, treatment, and social service referral of women at risk may aid in minimizing offending. Tertiary prevention focuses on recidivism prevention.

RESOURCES

Helping Individual Prostitutes Survive (HIPS): http://www.hips.org/
National Institute on Corrections: Women Offenders: http://www.nicic.org/Women Offenders
Prostitution Research & Education: http://www.prostitutionresearch.com/
Women's Prison Association: http://www.wpaonline.org

REFERENCES

Broidy, L., & Caufmann, E. (2006). Understanding female offenders. Department of Justice NCJ 216615. Retrieved from http://www.ncjrs.gov/pdffiles1/nij/grants/216615.pdf
Bureau of Justice Statistics. (2002). Profile of jail inmates in 2002. Bureau of Justice NCJ 201932. Retrieved from http://www.ojp.usdoj.gov/bjs/abstract/pji02.htm
Cecil, D., McHale, J., Strozier, A., & Pietsch, J. (2008). Female inmates, family caregivers and young children's adjustment: A research agenda and implications for corrections programming. *Journal of Criminal Justice, 36*(6), 513–521.
Cohan, D. (2006). Sex workers health. *Sexually Transmitted Infections, 82*(5), 418–422.
Covinton, S. (2001). A woman's journey home: Challenges for female offenders and their children. In *From Prison to Home: The Effect of Incarceration and Reentry on Children, Families, and Communities.* U.S. Department of Health and Human Services (HHS). Retrieved from http://aspe.hhs.gov/hsp/prison2home02/Covington.htm#Mental
Federal Bureau of Prisons. (n.d.) Female offender programs. Retrieved from http://www.bop.gov/inmate_programs/female.jsp

Goodyear, M., Lowman, J., Fischer, B., & Green, M. (2005). Prostitutes are people too. *The Lancet, 366*(9493), 1264–1265.

Greenfield, L., & Sneli, T. (1999). Special report: Women offenders. Bureau of Justice NCJ 175688. Retrieved from http://www.ojp.usdoj.gov/bjs/pub/pdf/wo.pdf

Johnson, C. (n.d.). Women in prison. *Nursing Spectrum.com.* Retrieved from http://ce.nurse.com/RetailCourseView.aspx?CourseNum=ce523&page=1&IsA=1

Leverentz, S. (2006). People places and things: The social process of reentry for female ex-offenders. NCJ 215178. Retrieved from http://www.ncjrs.gov/pdffiles1/nij/grants/215178.pdf

Mikulincer, M., & Shaver, P. (2007). *Attachment in adulthood: Structure, dynamics and changes.* New York: Guiford Press.

Moloney, K. P., & Moller, L. F. (2009). Good practice for mental health programs for women in prison: Reframing parameters. *Public Health, 123*(6), 431–432.

Rand, M., & Catalano, S. (2007). Crime victimization, 2006. Bureau of Justice Statistics Bulletin (NCJ 219413). Retrieved from http://www.rainn.org/pdf-files-and-other-documents/News-Room/press-releases/2006-ncvs-results/NCVS%202006-1.pdf

Richie, B., Tsenin, K., & Widom, C. (1999). Research on women and girls in the justice system: Plenary papers of the 1999 Conference on Criminal Justice Research and Evaluation—Enhancing Policy and Practice Through Research, Volume 3. National Institute of Justice (NIJ). Retrieved from http://www.ncjrs.gov/pdffiles1/nij/180973.pdf

Vandiver, D., & Kercher, G. (2007). Offender and victim characteristics of registered female sexual offenders in Texas: A proposed typology of female sexual offenders. *Sexual Abuse: A Journal of Research and Treatment, 16*(2), 121–137.

Wormer, K., & Kaplan, L. E. (2006). Results of a national survey of wardens in women's prisons: The case for gender specific treatment. *Women and Therapy, 29*(1/2), 133–151.

36   Animal Cruelty

DEFINITION

Companion animals are considered part of the family in the majority of American households, and nearly 75% of families with school-age children have at least one companion animal. Companion animals are often treated like members of the family, but they may become victims of abuse in violent households. Pets are often an important source of comfort and stability to abuse victims, especially children. But abusive family members may threaten, injure, or kill pets, often as a way of threatening or controlling others in the family. Animal abuse or cruelty is socially unacceptable behavior that intentionally causes unnecessary distress, suffering, or pain, and/or death of an animal. Animal cruelty is associated with other forms of violence including juvenile delinquency, child abuse, domestic violence, elder abuse and sexual violence.

All 50 states and the District of Columbia have anticruelty laws (http://www.animal-law.org/statutes), and more than 40 states currently have felony statutes for certain types of animal cruelty. Some felony statutes require psychiatric counseling for convicted abusers.

Animal cruelty is typically classified as follows:

1. Neglect occurs when a person deprives an animal of food, water, shelter, or veterinary care. It usually happens as a result of

ignorance on the owner's part and is typically handled by police or government officials, who require the owner to correct the situation. Neglect cases are acts of omission rather than commission and do not give satisfaction to the person whose animals are neglected. Nearly 90% percent of animal cruelty calls to animal control involve neglect.

2. Physical abuse results from malicious torturing, maiming, mutilation, or killing. These acts of intentional cruelty are often shocking and usually indicative of a serious human behavioral problem. Persons who commit these intentional acts of cruelty may derive satisfaction in causing harm.

3. Animal sexual abuse, or bestiality, is the sexual molestation of animals by humans and includes a wide range of behaviors, including: fondling; vaginal, anal, or oral penetration; oral-genital contact; penetration with an object; and injuring or killing an animal for sexual gratification. Like rape, this is an eroticization of violence, control, and exploitation. The animal may be severely injured or even killed in the encounter.

4. Hoarding, which is similar to neglect, occurs when a person accumulates a large number of animals, provides minimal standards of nutrition, sanitation, and veterinary care, and fails to act on the deteriorating condition of the animals and/or the environment. Unlike most other perpetrators of animal cruelty, the majority of hoarders are female. Hoarded animals often suffer extreme neglect, including lack of food, proper veterinary care, and sanitary conditions. Hoarding also creates hazards for the human occupants of the home. Unsanitary conditions attract disease vectors such as insects and rodents, which can also threaten neighboring households. Homes involved in hoarding usually must be condemned by the health department due to unlivable conditions. Hoarding also places a tremendous burden on already overburdened animal shelters, which lack the space or resources to deal with an influx of large numbers of animals, many of whom are usually in dire need of medical attention.

5. Cock fighting is the term used when two or more specialty birds, or gamecocks, are placed in an enclosure to fight to the death, sometimes of both birds. Cockfighting is illegal in the United States, and a felony in 39 states. It is closely connected to other

crimes, including gambling, drug dealing, illegal firearms sales, and even homicide.

6. Organized dog fighting is illegal in the United States and is a felony in all 50 states. Dog fighting is a contest between two specifically bred, conditioned, and trained-to-fight dogs that are placed in a pit to fight. Usually the loser dies, is left to die, or is killed by the owner. Both cock fighting and dog fighting are for the purposes of gambling or entertainment, and both, particularly dog fighting, may be associated with other criminal activity. The American Society for the Prevention of Cruelty to Animals (ASPCA) notes that police often categorize dog fighting into three groups: (a) *Street fighters* engage in informal dog fights, usually on a street corner, alley, or playground. They have no fight rules and pit fights are usually triggered by taunts, insults, or turf invasions. Street fights are associated with gang activity, and the fights may be associated with money, drugs, or bragging rights as the pay off. The dogs are bred to be threats to other dogs and usually also to people. (b) *Hobbyist fighters* are more organized and use fights for entertainment and/or supplemental income. They pay more attention to the care and breeding of their dogs. (c) *Professional dog fighters* have large numbers of animals and earn money from fighting, breeding, and dog sales. They dispose of dogs that do not perform through a variety of methods, including blunt force trauma and shooting. Recently, a group of wealthy fighters have emerged who may make up a fourth category because they have the financial resources of professional fighters but the philosophy of street fighters.

7. During a hog–dog fight ("hog-dog rodeo"), a trained dog attacks a trapped feral hog inside an enclosed pit from which there is no escape. Fight organizers give the advantage to the dog by either cutting off the hog's tusks or outfitting the dog in a Kevlar vest. The dog is timed to see how quickly he can pin down the hog by tearing into the hog's snout, ears, and eyes. Hog–dog fight promoters often bill these fights as "family entertainment"; however, they are closely connected to other crimes and forms of violence in addition to cruelty to animals. In some cases, the operator encourages children into a game of "catch the pig." The handler tapes the hog's snout closed and encourages children to chase the terrified animal around the pen.

PREVALENCE

A 2009 study showed that the lifetime prevalence of animal cruelty in U.S. adults was 1.8%. Males, African Americans, Native Americans/Asians, native-born Americans, persons with lower levels of income and education, and adults living in the western region of the United States reported comparatively high levels of cruelty to animals. Latinos reported comparatively low levels of such behavior. Animal cruelty was significantly associated with all assessed antisocial behaviors, and adjusted analyses revealed strong associations with lifetime alcohol use disorders; conduct disorder; antisocial, obsessive-compulsive, and histrionic personality disorders; pathological gambling; and family history of antisocial behavior.

In a 2007 survey of 1,869 perpetrators of animal cruelty, the Humane Society of the United States (HSUS, 2009) noted the following statistics:

- Intentional cruelty   66% male; 7% female
- Animal fighting: 79% male; 7% female
- Neglect: 58% male; 38% female
- Hoarding: 31% male; 66% female

The abuse of animals by humans for sexual gratification has been recorded for thousands of years and in many societies worldwide. It is usually condemned, often for religious or moral reasons, but also because many people appear to feel repulsion at the mere thought of someone having a sexual interest in animals. The prevalence is unknown at this time. However, the Vermont Animal Cruelty Task Force (http://www.vactf.org) notes that evidence of its occurrence is readily available on the Internet. A Web search can reveal very graphic and disturbing material describing and promoting the sexual abuse of animals, and photographs of this abuse are easily accessed by anyone on the Internet, even children. Detailed how-to guides for the sexual abuse of animals involving a variety of species can be found, along with information on laws, animal transmitted diseases, personal advertisements, "pro-zoophile" resources, and even a model letter for an animal abuser to use to " come out" to his or her friends and relatives.

ETIOLOGY: CONNECTION BETWEEN ANIMAL CRUELTY AND HUMAN VIOLENCE

Jeffrey Dahmer, who confessed to killing, dismembering, and occasionally cannibalizing 17 boys and men, impaled dogs and staked cats to trees as a child. "Boston Strangler" Albert DeSalvo trapped dogs and cats in orange crates and shot arrows through them. Columbine shooters Harris and Klebold frequently spoke of mutilating animals. All forms of violence share common characteristics—their victims are living creatures who can display signs of pain with which humans should empathize, and who may die as a result of their injuries. According to one study, individuals who abuse animals are five times more likely to abuse humans than those who do not abuse animals. It is unknown whether the relationship between animal abuse and other forms of human interpersonal violence is causal; however, some research has suggested a causal relationship.

Intimate Partner Violence

A survey of 38 women seeking shelter at a safe house in Utah for battered partners demonstrated that 71% reported that their partner had threatened and/or actually hurt or killed one or more of their pets Thirty-two percent reported that one or more of their children hurt or killed family pets (Ascione, 1998). Another study showed that 46.5% of the study population of 43 battered women in South Carolina reported threats or harm to their pets by their partners, but only 7% reported cruelty by their children (Flynn, 2000). The complex interconnections between animal and human violence have been further illustrated by findings that women in battered women's shelters often report worrying about family pets and have delayed their decision to leave a violent home environment because of concerns about their pets' well-being. The prevalence of this issue has prompted many shelters to provide foster care for the animals while women are in the shelters.

Child Abuse

One study followed 53 families that met New Jersey state criteria for child abuse and that had pets in their homes. The incidence of animal abuse was 88% higher among families in which physical child abuse occurred than in families in which other forms of child abuse occurred. Another study compared a sample of sexually abused children ($n = 276$) with a sample of nonabused children ($n = 880$) between the ages of 2 and 12 years and found that the abused children were significantly ($p < 0.001$) more likely to have abused animals than the nonabused group.

Elder Abuse

Although statistics are lacking, humane officers have found cases of elder abuse while responding to reports of animal cruelty—a dead dog in a dumpster led to their finding a neglected 90-year-old woman; whimpering from a closet proved to be a battered elder instead of suspected animal neglect. Abusive family members abuse an elder's pets for complex reasons. Perpetrators may abuse or neglect the elder's pet as a form of retaliation or control, a way to obtain the elder's financial assets, or as an act of frustration over their caretaking responsibilities. Extreme neglect can also indicate the elder's inability to provide self-care or care for the animal and thus indicate the need for assistance.

Other Violent Behavior

Animal cruelty has also been associated with violent criminal behavior. In a study of convicted male sexual homicide perpetrators, researchers found that 36% reported abusing animals as children, while 46% abused animals as adolescents. In a study of 299 inmates incarcerated for various felonies and 308 undergraduate students, researchers found higher percentages of animal abuse in the prison population compared to the college students: hurting animals—16.4% versus 9.7%; killing a stray—32.8% versus 14.3%, and killing a pet—12% versus 3.2%. A survey of 117 men incarcerated in a South African prison found that 65% of the men who committed aggressive crimes had committed animal cruelty as compared to only 10.5% of the nonaggressive inmates.

ASSESSMENT

General Principles

The abuse of a pet or any animal is an ominous sign for client functioning and is a means of identifying individuals at risk for committing other aggressive acts. Flynn (2000) argues that the maltreatment of animals by family members must be addressed for the following seven reasons: (a) it is disturbing, antisocial, and illegal behavior; (b) among children and adolescents, both witnessing and perpetrating animal cruelty are relatively common; (c) abusing animals, and possibly observing abuse by others, is likely to have negative developmental consequences for children; (d) perpetrating animal abuse is likely to lead to other forms of interpersonal aggression, both within and outside the family; (e) the presence of animal cruelty may be a marker of other forms of violence taking place in families; (f) the welfare of companion animals, most of whom are viewed as family members, is being neglected; and (g) addressing violence in all of its forms, including violence against animals, will help efforts to promote and achieve a more humane and less violent society for all beings—human and animal.

History, Physical Assessment, and Diagnostic Testing

Pets rarely survive past the age of 2 years in violent households, because they are either killed, die from neglect, or run away to escape the abuse. Interview questions to elicit animal cruelty histories (developed from the Boat Inventory, 1998) include:

- Do you have any pets or other animals in your house?
- Whose pets/animal are they?
- What kind? What are their names? How old are they?
- Who takes care of the pet/animal?
- Where does the pet sleep? What does the pet/animal eat?
- How is the pet/animal disciplined (trained)?
- Does anyone ever hurt the pet/animal? Who? How was the pet/animal hurt?
- Has anyone ever touched the pet/animal sexually or had sex with the pet/animal? Who? What did the person do to the pet/animal?
- Have you ever lost a pet/animal you cared about?
- Do you worry that something bad will happen to the pet/animal?

Compulsive hoarding may or may not be part of another psychiatric disorder. It is most often associated with obsessive-compulsive disorder (OCD), an anxiety disorder characterized by intrusive thoughts and compulsive behaviors. Hoarding has also been considered a symptom of an impulse-control disorder (ICD), such as compulsive shopping or gambling, and it may be symptomatic of a neurodegenerative disease. Since hoarding can appear in the absence of any other pathology and results in severe impairment, some believe that hoarding should be considered a syndrome or entity in its own right. However, neither the clinical community nor the standard nomenclature recognizes it as a diagnostic entity. Animal hoarding poses more human health and sanitation risks than other types of hoarding. Studies show that dead or sick animals were discovered in 80% of reported cases, and 69% of cases reveal fecal and urine accumulation (in over one-quarter of these cases feces and urine soiled the hoarder's bed). In 60% of cases, the hoarder would not acknowledge the problem. A significant number of hoarders had no functional utilities, including plumbing, electricity, or refrigeration. Hoarders justify their behaviors by claiming an intense love of animals, the feeling that animals are surrogate children, the belief that no one else would or could take care of them, and the fear that the animals would be euthanized.

Zoophilia, a sexual preference for animals, would come under the diagnostic category of paraphilia not otherwise specified in the *Diagnostic and Statistical Manual of Mental Disorders,* 4th Edition, Text Revision (*DSM-IV-TR*). The essential features of paraphilias are recurrent, intense sexually arousing fantasies, sexual urges or behaviors that involve nonhuman objects, the suffering or humiliation of oneself or one's partner, or sexual behavior with children or other nonconsenting partners (animals are nonconsenting partners), over a period of at least six months. Assessment of zoophilia typically involves a psychiatric interview and physiological testing, including penile plethysmography (PPG), a type of testing that measures changes in blood flow in the penis in response to sexual arousal to specific stimuli (different types of animals in zoophilia).

As noted in chapter 26, on risk assessment, it is not possible to predict dangerousness. However there are aggravating factors that suggest a person has been or will be involved in violence against people. Lockwood (2003) suggests that five or more of the following factors should cause serious concern:

- The victim is vulnerable (small, helpless, very young, or very old animal victims).
- There are multiple victims in the same cruelty event.
- There are numerous instances within a time frame (several instances in 24 hours suggests a premeditated and predatory attack).
- There is severe injury.
- The injury inflicted is intimate (beating, strangling, stabbing, etc.)
- The victim is incapacitated (caged, tied, boxed, incapable of escape).
- Fire is used (intended burning of a live animal is a significant indicator of potential violence against humans).
- There is prolonged maltreatment or torture.
- Other illegal acts are committed at the scene of the abuse (vandalism, theft)
- The individual was instigator of an act involving multiple persons.

- There was past history of positive interactions with the victim (such as own pet)
- The act was accompanied by sexual symbolism (viewed animal as person, "the pussy had to die").
- Perpetrator projected human characteristics on the victim.
- Animal victim was posed or displayed (wearing skin; leaving body on front steps); this should be considered a serious sign for escalated or repeated violence.
- There were ritualistic or satanic acts.
- The abuse involved staging for the media or fantasy sources (copying a news report or playing a video game).
- The perpetrator experienced strong positive affective changes during the attack (laughter, a "rush").
- The perpetrator lacks insight into cause or motivation for the abuse.
- The perpetrator sees himself as a victim.

Health care professionals who have the opportunity to observe their clients' pets (e.g., home health nurses), should observe them for signs of battered pet syndrome:

- Unusually subdued or fearful
- Openly frightened
- Fractures
- Bruising
- Eye injuries
- Burns and scalds
- Munchausen syndrome by proxy
- Signs of malnutrition

Other possible signs of abuse include head injury, paw injuries, blood in the stool, imbedded collar, ligature injuries, signs of gunshot wounds (abrasion rings, gunshot residue), signs of dog fighting (puncture wounds on face, neck, and legs; heavy chains used as collars).

INTERVENTION

Contact the local animal control agent or the police if an animal is in apparent danger. Do not attempt to aid an injured animal without professional (veterinary or animal control) assistance, since you may cause additional injury to the animal or incur bites and scratches from a frightened animal.

Specific treatment is preferred for animal abusers. The AniCare Model of Treatment for Animal Abuse (http://societyandanimalsforum. org/AniCare.html) is the first professional program for animal abusers over the age of 17. Since most of these individuals receiving treatment are referred by the courts, treatment may be relatively short-term and clients who are not entering treatment voluntarily may initially resist therapy. AniCare uses a cognitive-behavioral approach, with direct interventions emphasizing the client's need to acknowledge accountability for his or her behavior, similar to the approach used with batterers. The AniCare manual contains exercises that offer and explain to the clinician specific intervention strategies, as well as homework assignments to reinforce the particular intervention. AniCare identifies seven concepts—accountability, respect/freedom, reciprocity, accommodation, empathy, attachment, and nurturance—to address with clients.

Animal hoarders have poorer treatment outcomes than persons who hoarded only possessions. When clutter in a hoarder's home results in a health crisis or a complaint from neighbors, the health department or another state agency may visit to clear out the place. As soon as the authorities leave, however, the clutter will accumulate again; thus, treatment is warranted. Cognitive-behavioral therapy (CBT) is used to treat hoarding. Referral to a therapist is warranted, as is referral to a neurologist to rule out a neurodegenerative disorder. While hoarding does not respond to medications, medications are often used to treat comorbid conditions such as depression, psychosis, social phobia, and dementia. Medication may also help treat cognitive distortions and anxiety symptoms, making CBT more effective. A potential treatment may involve cholinesterase inhibitors such as donepezil hydrochloride (Aricept), used in treating memory problems, and stimulant medications used to improve attention in ADD/ADHD.

There is no cure for a paraphilia, and persons with zoophilia may be poorly motivated to undergo treatment. They may also have other paraphilias and/or psychiatric disorders. Those who are motivated (or court mandated) may benefit from psychological and pharmacological (medications) approaches. As with other psychiatric disorders, a combination of the two is usually more effective than either alone. While there are several possible psychotherapeutic techniques, cognitive behavioral methods, including relapse prevention strategies, appear the most effective. Pharmacological interventions may include sex-drive-reducing hormones such as Provera, Androcur, and Lupron, or selective serotonin reuptake inhibitors (SSRIs) such as Prozac and Paxil.

PREVENTION/PATIENT TEACHING

Primary Prevention

Humane education is not a panacea, but it helps. Therefore, policies should provide for humane education as part of school curricula to better enable all children to develop compassion for all living beings.

Secondary Prevention

The number of cruelty cases can only be estimated, because there is no nationwide reporting mechanism. An ideal policy would establish a national data bank that could track trends and serve as a baseline to measure the effectiveness of interventions. In the interim, forensic health care professionals can lobby for mandatory reporting by veterinarians and health care personnel. Veterinarians should be trained to recognize all forms of animal abuse and be mandated to report it. However, most states do not require such reporting. Veterinarians should also be educated on the connection between animal cruelty and human violence, as their animal clients may be part of an abusive system in which children may also be victims. Community nurses should be taught the signs of abuse pets and be responsible for reporting them. Forensic health care professionals can also encourage policy that would allow for anonymous reporting by the public, similar to what is done for child abuse.

Assessing for the presence of animal cruelty should be part of all routine health care visits and episodic visits for clients who present with behavioral problems or signs of abuse. Just asking the age of the household pets may prove significant, as abused pets rarely live past 2 years because they get killed, die of neglect, or run away to escape the abuse. Formal assessment protocols are in their formative stage of development. In the interim, forensic health care professionals can encourage other health care providers to utilize questions that can easily be integrated into their psychosocial histories. All episodes of abuse, even those done out of curiosity, warrant intervention with referral to a counselor, the criminal/juvenile justice system, or both.

Tertiary Prevention

Animal abusers should be referred for psychological evaluation and treatment. Hoarders should also have a neurological evaluation.

RESOURCES

American Humane Society: http://www.americanhumane.org
AniCare Model of Treatment for Animal Abuse. http://www.psyeta.org/AniCare.html.
American Society for the Prevention of Cruelty to Animals: http://www.aspca.org
Humane Society of the United States First Strike Program: http://www.hsus.org/firststrike
Latham Foundation: http://www.latham.org
National Association for Human and Environmental Education: http://nahee.org/
People for the Ethical Treatment of Animals: http://www.peta.com
Society and Animal Forum: http://www.psyeta.org

REFERENCES

American Psychiatric Association. (2000). Diagnostic and statistical manual of mental disorders, (4th ed., text revision). Washington, DC: American Psychiatric Association.

American Society for the Prevention of Cruelty to Animals (ASPCA). (2010). Dog fighting FAQ. Retrieved from http://www.aspca.org/fight-animal-cruelty/dog-fighting/dog-fighting-faq.html

Ascione, F. (2001). Animal abuse and youth violence. OJJDP Juvenile Justice Bulletin, NCJ 188677. Retrieved from http://www.ncjrs.org/html/ojjdp/jjbul2001_9_2/contents.html

Ascione F. (1998). Battered women's reports of their partners and their children's cruelty to animals. *Journal of Emotional Abuse, 1*(1), 119–133.

Ascione, F. R., Weber, C. V. Thompson, T. M., Heath, J., Maruyama, M., & Hayashi, K. (2007). Battered pets and domestic violence: Animal abuse reported by women experiencing intimate violence and by non-abused women. *Violence Against Women, 13*, 354–373.

Boat, B. (1998). Abuse of children and abuse of animals. In F. Ascione & P. Arkow (Eds.), *Child abuse, domestic violence, and animal abuse* (pp. 83–100). West Lafayette, IN: Purdue University Press.

Bohrer, G., & Haynes, L. (n.d.). Compulsive hoarding: Sign of a deeper disorder. Retrieved from http://www.nurse.com/ce/CE372–60/CoursePage

Colorado Veterinary Medical Association. (2007). Mandatory reporting of cruelty to animals and animal fighting. Retrieved from http://www.colovma.org/displaycommon.cfm?an=1&subarticlenbr=57

DeGue, S., & DiLillo, D. (2009). Is animal cruelty a "red flag" for family violence? Investigating co-occurring violence toward children, partners, and pets. *Journal of Interpersonal Violence, 24*(6), 1036–1056.

DeViney, L., Dickert, J., & Lockwood, R. (1983). The care of pets within child abusing families. *International Journal for the Study of Animal Problems, 4*(4), 321–336.

Flynn, C. (2000). Why family professionals can no longer ignore violence toward animals. *Family Relations, 49*(1), 87–95.

Freidrich, W. (1992). Child Sexual Behavior Inventory: Normative and clinical comparisons. *Psychological Assessment, 4*(3), 303–311.

Frost, R. (2000). People who hoard animals. *Psychiatric Times, 17*(4). Retrieved from http://www.psychiatrictimes.com/display/article/10168/54031?verify=0

Hensley, C., Tallichet, S., & Singer, S. (2006). Exploring the possible link between childhood and adolescent bestiality and interpersonal violence. *Journal of Interpersonal Violence, 21*(7), 910–923.

Humane Society of the United States (HSUS). (2009). Animal cruelty demographics. Retrieved from http://www.hsus.org/acf/cruelty/publiced/cruelty_demographics.html

Humane Society of the United States. (n.d.). First strike program. Retrieved from http://www.hsus2.org/firststrike

Lockwood, R. (2003). Animal abuse risk assessment. *Pet-abuse.com.* Retrieved from http://www.pet-abuse.com/pages/abuse_connection/risk_assessment.php

Munro, H. (2006). Animal sexual abuse: A veterinary taboo? *The Veterinary Journal, 172,* 195–197.

Munro H. (1999). The battered pet. In F. Ascione & P. Arkow (Eds.), *Child abuse, domestic violence, and animal abuse* (pp. 199–208). West Lafayette, IN: Purdue University Press.

Muscari, M. (2004). Four-legged forensics: What forensic nurses need to know and do about animal cruelty. *Forensic Nurse,* Jan/Feb, 10–12, 23–24.

Muscari, M. (2005). Animal cruelty as a predictor of human violence. *Advance for Nurse Practitioners, 13*(4), 55–59.

Schaefer, K., Hays, K., & Steiner, R. (2007). Animal abuse issues in therapy: A survey of therapists' attitudes. *Professional Psychology: Research and Practice, 38*(5), 530–537.

Vaughn, M., Fu, Q., DeLisi, M., Beaver, K., Perron, B. Terrell, K. et al. (2009). Correlates of cruelty to animals in the United States: Results from the National Epidemiologic Survey on Alcohol and Related Conditions. *Journal of Psychiatric Research.*

37 Parenting While Incarcerated

DEFINITION

Over 1.7 million children in this country have a parent serving a sentence in a state or federal prison. Prisoners' family networks are complex. Parents held in state prison are equally likely to report living with their children in a single-parent household as they are to report living with their children in a two-parent household. Many have parented children with more than one partner. Fathers' provider and nurturing roles vary. Some children live with them at the time of arrest, some were supported and visited regularly, and others were neither visited nor supported. Many mothers do not function in typical single-parent roles. Instead, prior to incarceration, many incarcerated mothers share caregiving responsibilities with the children's fathers, other family members, and/or close friends. Mothers are more likely than fathers to report homelessness, past physical or sexual abuse, and medical and mental health problems.

Inmates' own parents are assuming a considerable amount of care for children, especially for children whose mothers are in prison. Thus health care providers who care for older adults need to assess whether they have assumed primary care of their grandchildren, and they also need to appropriately assist these grandparents in caring for the children and themselves. One important issue in these types of kinship arrangements is legal custody. Legal custody allows the kinship caretaker to assume a guardian role and thus have the legal right to make decisions about the children, such as where they live. When incarcerated parents are not capable of making proper decisions for their children, caretakers should be encouraged to talk to a lawyer about obtaining legal custody.

PREVALENCE

Approximately 809,800 prisoners of the 1,518,535 held in the nation's prisons at midyear 2007 were parents of children under age 18. Incarcerated parents (52% of state inmates and 63% of federal inmates) reported having an estimated 1,706,600 minor children, accounting for 2.3% of the U.S. resident population under age 18. Hispanic children are three times more likely and African American children nine times more likely than white children to have a parent in prison. The number of children with a mother in prison has more than doubled since 1991.

ETIOLOGY

Incarcerated parents typically have a history of having been raised by adults who were chemically dependent, abusive, or both. They may have learned to cope and adapt to trauma by striking out at others and/or by self-medicating with drugs or alcohol. Incarcerated parents can lack the ability to attach to others and may not have internalized adequate or healthy models of child rearing. For many, rage, depression, and addiction have been a part of life, followed by the criminal activity related to substance abuse. Some perpetrators are incarcerated because of crimes against their family members, including parents imprisoned for domestic or sexual violence, or homicides involving their own children or partner. However, these are relatively rare cases and are not typical of incarcerated parents and their children.

ASSESSMENT

General Principles

Parental incarceration creates challenges for families that often result in: financial instability and material hardship, with financial problems the most severe for already vulnerable families and caregivers who support contact between the incarcerated parent and his or her child; instability in family structure and relationships, as well as residential mobility; school behavior and performance problems; loss of preincarceration support systems; and shame and stigma.

As parents struggle to make a fresh start upon reentry, they encounter an array of legal barriers that will make it very difficult for them to succeed in caring for their children, finding work, getting safe housing, going to school, accessing public benefits, or even, for immigrants, staying in the same country as their children. Some of the barriers can, singly and in combination, rip families apart, create unemployment and homelessness, and guarantee failure, thereby harming parents and children, families, and communities.

History and Physical Assessment

Health care providers should perform routine assessments but focus on issues related to parents who are incarcerated, on probation or parole, or who have been incarcerated in the past. These issues include: employment status, housing, substance abuse, health issues (particularly those related to substance abuse), financial stability, and child rearing. Health care providers can also play a key role in custody assessment to determine whether or not incarcerated parents should regain custody of their children upon release from prison.

INTERVENTION

Intervention should be tailored to meet the individual parent's needs, with focus on improvement and maintenance of physical health, substance abuse treatment, and treatment of mental health problems. Referrals may be warranted to parenting classes and social services, with the latter focusing on housing and financial needs.

- Incarcerated parents can benefit from strategies that reduce tension and conflict in their relationships and that help them develop positive, healthy ways of relating to others.
- Family members need support to reconcile their feelings about the offender's incarceration, and to heal the loss, hurt, confusion, and damage the incarceration has caused them.
- Health care providers should work with corrections to assure that the family is a central focus of corrections and reentry policies and

interventions, because children do best when their families do well. Policies should help to facilitate healthy connections among all family members, using safe and appropriate methods.

■ Visitation should be encouraged, since visitation and communication between the child and his or her incarcerated parent can strengthen the parent–child relationship, which can result in lower recidivism. Visitation can be costly, so health care providers may need to work with families to find alternatives for staying in contact.

■ Families benefit from services provided to parents before, during, and after incarceration that help them build stronger family relationships, constructively manage conflict, strengthen parenting skills, and prepare them to be responsible parents and members of their community.

An increasing number of children of incarcerated parents are being raised by their grandparents. These grandparents face a number of important challenges, beginning with how to help the children deal with the parent's incarceration. Health care providers can use these suggestions for grandparents, modified from AARP (2008):

■ Children want to know what happened, and it is best to tell them the truth. Grandparents should talk to their children in a developmentally appropriate manner. Give young children a simple explanation of what happened, and give older children the complete story. Most children can understand what you mean when you say that the parent did something wrong and is being punished.

■ Children feel many conflicting emotions when their parent is incarcerated. They may feel anger and shame, while still feeling very loyal to the parent. They may fear that they will never see the parent again and that you may leave them too. Let your grandchildren know that you love them and that you are not going anywhere. Listen, and let them know that it's okay to feel the way they do, even if their feelings are different from others'. Some children miss their parent and want to see the parent often, while their grandparents may be angry at the parent and want no contact. Respect the child's feelings and do not try to change those feelings.

■ Except in extreme circumstances, children should stay in touch with their parent. It gives them a chance to make peace and to adjust more easily when the parent comes home. Staying in touch could even help the parent turn his or her life around, since offenders with strong family ties usually do better after they leave prison. Children can talk with an incarcerated parent on the telephone or exchange letters with the parent. Mail cards on special holidays, send report cards and other school papers, and remind the parent to send cards on the children's birthdays. If possible, take the children to visit the parent in prison. The prison may be a distance away, travel may be costly, and the prison may not be child-friendly. However, talk to your health care provider to help you get assistance. Children do better at home if they can visit a parent in jail, since they tend to think that prison conditions are much worse than they really are. Seeing the parent in prison can set their minds at ease.

■ Some children don't want to have any contact with an incarcerated parent. Do not force the child to visit. Instead, try to gently convince the child to stay in touch by phone or mail. If this does not work, try to get the parent to contact the child.

■ Sometimes children are severely affected by their parent's incarceration. They may cry often, withdraw, or become aggressive. If this happens, talk to your health care provider.

Grandparents can also feel the same stressors as any parent, as well as stress from aging and chronic illnesses. Raising grandchildren can cause financial and social stress, as well as legal problems if the grandparents have not been made legal custodians. Therefore, referral to social and legal services, as well as other agencies, may be helpful.

PREVENTION/PATIENT TEACHING

Primary Prevention

Since many incarcerated parents are imprisoned because of drug offense, health care professionals can reduce this occurrence by utilizing preventive measures to prevent substance abuse.

Secondary Prevention

Health care providers can minimize the effects of incarceration on families by supporting policies and programs that:

■ Actively encouraging kinship care placements
■ Ensure that child welfare authorities remain in touch with incarcerated parents

- Facilitate visitation between children and incarcerated parents
- Make appropriate reunification services available to incarcerated parents
- Explore alternatives to incarceration that could make child welfare intervention and child removal unnecessary in many cases

Tertiary Prevention

Tertiary prevention involves recidivism prevention. Regular contact between incarcerated parents and their children can decrease the chances of the parent reoffending, as well as decreasing the chances of the children going to prison later in life.

RESOURCES

GrandCare Tool Kit: Resources for Grandparents Raising Children: http://www.aarp.org/family/grandparenting/articles/grandcare_toolkit.html

Incarcerated Parents Manual: http://www.prisonerswithchildren.org/pubs/ipm.pdf

National Resource Center on Children and Families of the Incarcerated (NRCCFI) at Family and Corrections Network (FCN): http://fcnetwork.org

REFERENCES

AARP. (2008). *Grandparent tool kit*. Retrieved from http://www.aarp.org/family/grandparenting/articles/grandcare_toolkit.html

Bouchet. S. (2008). Children and families with incarcerated parents: Exploring development in the field and opportunities for growth. A report prepared for the Annie E. Casey Foundation. Retrieved from http://www.aecf.org/~/media/Pubs/Topics/Child%20Welfare%20Permanence/Permanence/ChildrenandFamilieswithIncarceratedParentsExp/Children%20and%20families%20with%20incarcerated%20parents.pdf

Community Legal Services, Inc., and the Center for Law and Social Policy. (2002). Every door closed: Barriers facing parents with criminal records. Retrieved from http://www.clasp.org/admin/site/publications_archive/files/0092.pdf

Glaze, L., & Maruschak, L. (2008). Parents in prison and their minor children. Bureau of Justice Statistics Special Report NCJ 222984. Retrieved from http://www.ojp.usdoj.gov/bjs/pub/pdf/pptmc.pdf

Hairston, J. (2002). Prisoners and families: Parenting issues during incarceration. Retrieved from http://www.cpwdc.org/youthcouncil/forum%20materials/Prisoner%20and%20Families-%20Parenting%20Issues%20During%20Incarceration.pdf

Unnatural Deaths

38 Medicolegal Death Investigation

DEFINITIONS

The purpose of death investigation is to determine the cause and manner of death. The process involves the systematic collection and analysis of interview data and physical evidence. Not all deaths warrant investigation. Those that do include, but are not limited to: deaths in which there are unexplained, unusual or suspicious circumstances; homicides; deaths due to poisoning; accidents; suicides; maternal deaths due to abortion; deaths of inmates in public institutions; deaths of persons in custody of law enforcement; deaths associated with diagnostic, therapeutic, or anesthetic procedures; deaths from neglect; sudden unexpected infant death; and natural deaths in which the decedent does not have a physician familiar with the case, or when the decedent's physician refuses to sign the death certificate.

■ Cause of death is the injury, disease, or combination of the two responsible for initiating the sequence of disturbances that produce the fatal termination. The term "initiating" is critical, because causes may not be immediately fatal, such as carcinoma or gunshot wounds.

■ Manner of death is the circumstance in which the cause of death arose.

■ Natural: Death is directly related to a natural disease (cancer, arteriosclerotic heart disease)
■ Accident: Death is the result of the unintentional actions of the decedent or another person (motor vehicle accident, drowning)
■ Homicide: Death results from the intentional act of another, whether lawfully or unlawfully (intentional gunshot, death penalty)
■ Suicide: Death results from an intentional act by the decedent, who anticipates dying (self-inflicted gunshot, intentional drug overdose)
■ Undetermined: Circumstances surrounding the death cannot be determined with reasonable certainty (cannot tell if overdose was accidental or suicide)

■ Mechanism of death is the physiologic change or biochemical disturbance incompatible with life initiated by the cause of death.

Families may be unsure as to why an investigation is needed, especially when a loved one dies of natural causes, so it helps to know the benefits of death investigation: obtaining life insurance benefits, discovery of genetic/inherited disorders, providing evidence for prosecution or exoneration, providing evidence for civil matters, identifying infectious diseases, identifying defective products, identifying medical errors, and evaluating transplant donors.

CORONER AND MEDICAL EXAMINER SYSTEMS

Deaths are investigated by coroners, medical examiners, and/or death investigators. Death investigation varies among jurisdictions (state, county, district, or city). The most noticeable difference is that some jurisdictions use the medical examiner system and others use the coroner system. Medical examiners are usually appointed and usually must be licensed physicians. Coroners are usually elected, may not need to be physicians, and usually only have to be of a minimum age (often 18) and a resident of the county or district. There are approximately 2,000 medical examiners and coroners' offices in the United States. These offices are responsible for the medicolegal investigation of death: conducting death scene investigations, performing autopsies, and determining the cause and manner of death when a person has died as a result of violence, under suspicious circumstances, without a physician in attendance, or for other reasons. States function differently when it comes to having coroner- or medical-examiner-based systems. Each state has one of the following: centralized statewide medical examiner system, county coroner system, county medical examiner system, mixed county medical examiner and coroner system, or decentralized death investigation systems.

Medical examiners and coroners are responsible for investigating sudden, unexpected, and violent deaths and for providing accurate, legally defensible determinations of the causes of these deaths. Information provided by medical examiners and coroners plays a critical role in the judicial system and in decisions made by public safety and public health agencies. Coroner and medical examiner records provide vital information about patterns and trends of mortality in the United States and are excellent sources of data for public health studies and surveillance.

SIGNS OF DEATH

When a person dies, the pupils dilate and become unresponsive. The corneal reflexes are absent and the cornea becomes cloudy. Other changes include the following:

Rigor mortis: The muscles become flaccid after death, but within one to three hours, they become increasingly rigid and the joints freeze. Rigor is affected by body temperature—the higher the temperature, the faster rigor occurs. Thus, someone with a fever or who exercised vigorously before death will develop rigor faster. Conversely, rigor is slowed by cooling, as in death from exposure in winter. The body appears to stiffen from the head down, from the jaws to the elbows and then to the knees. A body is in complete rigor when the jaw, elbows, and knees are immovable, a process that takes 10 to 12 hours in an environmental temperature of 70 to 75 degrees F. A body remains rigid for 24 to 36 hours before muscles start to loosen in the same order they stiffened.

Livor mortis: This discoloration is due to the settling of blood no longer being circulated through the body. Blood settles in vessels by gravity in dependent areas and colors the skin purple-red; however, the skin may not discolor if it is pressed against a bony prominence. Livor is noticeable one hour after death. The color increases intensity and becomes fixed (does not blanche under pressure) in eight hours. Fixed blood in nondependent areas means the body was moved after death. Color variations may occur, depending on the cause of death. Carbon monoxide or cyanide poisoning may cause bright cherry red livor, while extensive blood loss may have a very light or nonexistent livor. Livor can be difficult to determine in dark-skinned persons.

Algor mortis: The body cools after death to the surrounding environmental temperature. Liver temperature and environmental temperature can give a very crude estimate of the time of death.

Decomposition: As rigor passes, the body first turns green in the abdomen, and the color spreads to the rest of the trunk. The body swells due to bacterial methane gas production. Rates and types of decomposition depend on the environment. Bodies buried in dirt, submerged in water, left in the hot sun, or placed in a cool basement all look different after the same postmortem period.

SCENE INVESTIGATION

The sudden or unexplained death of a loved one has a profound impact on families and friends and places significant responsibility on the agencies tasked with determining the cause of death. Adherence to clear and well-grounded protocols aids investigators in carefully assessing and analyzing the death. The following is adapted from the National Institute of Justice (1999) document, *Death Investigation: A Guide for the Scene Investigator.*

Arriving at the Scene

1. Introduce and identify self and role: Introductions aid in establishing a collaborative investigative effort.
2. Exercise scene safety: The safety of all investigative personnel is essential to the investigative process. Risks of environmental and physical injury (e.g., hostile crowds, collapsing structures, traffic, and environmental and chemical threats) must be removed prior to initiating a scene investigation.

3. Confirm or pronounce death: Appropriate personnel must make a determination of death prior to the initiation of the death investigation. Confirmation determines jurisdictional responsibilities.

4. Participate in scene briefing with attending agency representatives: Scene investigators must recognize jurisdictional and statutory responsibilities that apply to each agency representatives (e.g., law enforcement, fire, EMT, death investigator). Determining each agency's responsibility is essential in planning the scope and depth of each scene investigation and the release of information to the public.

5. Conduct scene "walk through": The walk through provides an overview of the entire scene and gives the investigator the first opportunity to locate and view the body, identify valuable and fragile evidence, and determine initial investigative procedures that will allow for systematic examination and documentation of the scene and body.

6. Establish chain of custody: This ensures the integrity of the evidence and safeguards against subsequent allegations of tampering, theft, planting, and contamination of evidence.

7. Follow laws of evidence: All agencies must follow local, state, and federal laws for the collection of evidence to ensure its admissibility. The death investigator works with law enforcement and the legal authorities to determine laws regarding collection of evidence.

Documenting and Evaluating the Scene

1. Photograph the scene: Photographic documentation creates a permanent historical record of the scene. Photographs provide detailed corroborating evidence that constructs a system of redundancy should questions arise concerning the report, witness statements, or position of evidence at the scene.

2. Develop descriptive documentation of the scene: The narrative report provides a permanent record that may be used to correlate with and enhance photographic documentation, refresh recollections, and record observations.

3. Establish probable location of injury or illness: The death scene may not be the actual location where the injury/illness

that contributed to the death occurred. It is imperative that the investigator attempt to determine the locations of any and all injuries/illnesses that may have contributed to the death. Physical evidence at these locations may be pertinent in establishing the cause, manner, and circumstances of death.

4. Collect, inventory, and safeguard property and evidence: The investigator must safeguard the decedent's valuables/property to ensure proper processing and eventual return to next of kin.

5. Interview witnesses at the scene: Documented comments of witnesses allow the investigator to obtain primary source data regarding discovery of the body, witness corroboration, and terminal history.

Documenting and Evaluating the Body

1. Photograph the body: Photographic documentation of the body creates a permanent record that preserves essential details of body position, appearance, identity, and final movements. Photographs also allow sharing of information with other agencies investigating the death.

2. Conduct superficial external body examination: This provides the investigator with objective data regarding the single most important piece of evidence at the scene, the body, by giving detailed information regarding the decedent's physical attributes, the person's relationship to the scene, and possible cause, manner, and circumstances of death. This examination is performed in a manner that does not contaminate or destroy evidence.

3. Preserve evidence on the body: Photographic and narrative documentation of evidence on the body allows the investigator to obtain a permanent historical record of that evidence. Evidence must be collected, preserved, and transported properly, and the chain of custody maintained. All of the physical evidence visible on the body (such as blood and other body fluids) must be photographed and documented prior to collection and transport. Fragile evidence (that which can be easily contaminated, lost, or altered) must also be collected and preserved, and the chain of custody maintained.

4. Establish decedent identification: Confirmation of the decedent's identity is paramount to the death investigation to allow notification of next of kin, settlement of estates, resolution of criminal and civil litigation, and the proper completion of the death certificate.

5. Document postmortem changes: Documenting postmortem changes assists the investigator in explaining body appearance in the interval following death. Inconsistencies between postmortem changes and body location may indicate movement of the body and validate or invalidate witness statements. Postmortem changes to the body, when correlated with circumstantial information, can also assist the investigators in estimating the approximate time of death.

6. Participate in scene debriefing: Scene debriefing helps investigators from all agencies to establish postscene responsibilities. Scene debriefing provides each agency the opportunity for input regarding special requests for assistance, additional information, special examinations, and other requests requiring interagency communication, cooperation, and education.

7. Determine notification procedures (next of kin): Every reasonable effort should be made to notify the next of kin as soon as possible. This helps initiate closure for the family and disposition of remains, and facilitates the collection of additional information relative to the case.

8. Ensure security of the remains: Ensuring security of the body requires the investigator to supervise the labeling, packaging, and removal of the remains. An appropriate identification tag is placed on the body to preclude misidentification upon receipt at the examining agency. This function also includes safeguarding all potential physical evidence and/or property and clothing that remains on the body.

Establishing and Recording Decedent Profile Information

1. Document the discovery history: The decedent profile includes documenting a discovery history and circumstances surrounding the discovery. The basic profile will dictate

subsequent levels of investigation, jurisdiction, and authority, as well as the focus (breadth/depth) of further investigation.

2. Determine terminal episode history: Preterminal circumstances play a significant role in determining cause and manner of death. Documentation of medical intervention and/or procurement of antemortem specimens help to establish the decedent's condition prior to death.

3. Document decedent medical history: Most deaths referred to the medical examiner/coroner are natural deaths. Establishing the decedent's medical history helps focus the investigation. Documenting the decedent's medical signs or symptoms prior to death determines the need for subsequent examinations, since the relationship between disease and injury may play a role in the cause, manner, and circumstances of death.

4. Document decedent mental health history: The decedent's mental health history can provide insight into his or her behavior/state of mind. That insight may produce clues that will aid in establishing the cause, manner, and circumstances of the death.

5. Document social history: Social history includes marital, family, sexual, educational, employment, and financial information, just as it does in the social history of the living. Daily routines, habits and activities, and friends and associates of the decedent help develop the decedent's profile and aid in establishing the cause, manner, and circumstances of death.

Completing the Scene Investigation

1. Maintain jurisdiction over the body: This helps the investigator to protect the chain of custody as the body is transported from the scene for autopsy, specimen collection, or storage.

2. Release jurisdiction of the body: Prior to releasing jurisdiction of the body to an authorized receiving agent or funeral director, it is necessary to determine the person responsible for certification of the death. Information to complete the death certificate includes demographic information and the date, time, and location of death.

3. Perform exit procedures: Bringing closure to the scene investigation ensures that important evidence has been collected and the scene has been fully processed. A systematic review of the scene ensures that artifacts or equipment are not inadvertently left behind and that any dangerous materials or conditions have been reported.

4. Assist the family: The death investigator provides the family with a timetable so they can arrange for final disposition. The death investigator also provides information on available community and professional resources that may assist the family.

THE FORENSIC AUTOPSY

The forensic autopsy, which should be performed by a forensic pathologist, is performed chiefly for legal purposes, to determine the cause and manner of death. Forensic autopsies protect the public interest and provide the information necessary to address legal, public health, and public safety issues in each case. The forensic autopsy is key to both finding forensic evidence and identifying the cause, mechanism, and manner of death. The forensic autopsy is typically handled by the Office of the Medical Examiner or a coroner's office, with the exact system for handling forensic autopsies varying from state to state and often by county within a state.

CULTURE AND DEATH RITUALS

Death rituals vary across cultures and are frequently influenced by religion, the country of origin, and the level of acculturation. The duration, frequency, and intensity of the grief process may also vary based on the manner of death and the individual family's cultural beliefs. Rituals may be performed so that family members can be with the body and prepare the body for viewing. These rituals are critical and in many cases provide closure for the family. Some religions require that the body be buried on the day of death, which is not feasible in many cases when the death is being investigated. This and other beliefs may warrant certain considerations in the investigative process. Other beliefs may include:

- Many Native American cultures are not concerned with body preservation, so embalming is not common. Dismemberment and mutilation outside the natural deterioration of the body is taboo, which may be impacted by the need for autopsy.
- Muslims require that the body be washed with certain rituals before the funeral ceremony begins. This typically takes place at a special section of the mosque or in the morgue.
- In Catholicism, the Sacraments of the Sick are performed as the person is dying. However, if a person dies before the sacraments are given, the priest will anoint the deceased conditionally within three hours of the time of death.

FAMILY NOTIFICATION

The office of the coroner or medical examiner is responsible for family notification of the death. Sudden, unexpected, or violent death creates significant stress for the families of the decedent. Homicide bereavement is typically intense, persistent, and inescapable, and the cruel and purposeful nature of murder compounds the rage, grief, and despair of the survivors. Unlike the loss of a relative with a progressive illness, bereavement by homicide does not allow anticipatory psychological inoculation to soften the traumatic impact. Survivors are also confronted with their own mortality and vulnerability as their vision of safety and order in the world is shattered. Therefore it is critical that the death investigator be well educated in bereavement and crisis intervention.

- Preparation
  - Obtain specialized training to perform death notification.
  - Assure that you have the correct name of the decedent, as well as the correct name and address of the family members who are being notified.
  - Rehearse what will be said and discuss anticipated reactions and problems with your team; create a sample script of what to say.
  - Talk about your reactions to the death with your team to enhance your focusing on the family when you arrive.

■ Initial contact

- Go in person. If there is no alternative to a phone call, arrange for a professional, neighbor, or friend to be with the next of kin at the time of your call.
- Do not take any possessions of the victim to the notification.
- Take someone who is experienced in dealing with shock and/or trained in CPR/medical emergency (next of kin have been known to suffer heart attacks when notified). The additional person may also be needed to create a diversions for children when they are present.
- If a large group is to be notified, bring a team of notifiers.
- Identify yourself, present credentials, and ask for permission to enter.
- Ask if there are any other family members in the house that need to hear this information. Conversely, ascertain if some family members (e.g., young children, frail elderly) may be better off not being present during the notification.
- Sit down, ask them to sit down, and be sure you have the nearest next of kin—do not notify siblings before notifying parents or spouse; do not notify a minor child, and do not use a child as a translator.
- Be compassionate but direct with your notification; avoid euphemisms.
- Use the victim's name.
- Allow time for the family to comprehend the news; repeat information as necessary.
- Answer all questions tactfully and truthfully, but do not reveal more information than is necessary during initial contact; if the family member requests more information, provide it at an appropriate pace and level.
- Do not give unsolicited and unnecessary advice, and do not encourage a quick recovery from their grief.
- Encourage them to verbalize their feelings, but do not attempt to falsely identify with them.
- Offer to make phone calls to family, friends, neighbors, employers, clergy, doctors, child care, and so on. Provide them with a list of the calls you make, as they will have difficulty remembering what you have told them.
- Ask family members if they want you to get someone to stay with them.

- Respect the family's privacy, but do not leave a family member alone unless you are sure they're safe.
- High emotionality can impair memory, so give pertinent information and instructions in writing.
- Provide family members with the names and telephone numbers of appropriate agency contacts: a victim advocate, prosecutor, medical examiner, social service agency, and/or hospital. It helps to have preprinted cards with this information.
- Determine if the family members require some means of traveling to the coroner/medical examiner's office, hospital, or police station. Offer to drive them or arrange for a ride if they have no transportation, but be sure to arrange for a ride back home.

- Follow-up

  - When leaving, let them know you will check back the next day to see how they are doing and if there is anything else you can do for them.
  - Call and visit again the next day.
  - If the family does not want you to visit, spend some time on the phone and again express willingness to answer all questions.
  - Ask the family if they are ready to receive their loved one's possessions (if appropriate); honor their wishes.
  - Debrief your personal reactions with your team after the notification and with qualified mental health personnel on a frequent and regular basis.

BODY IDENTIFICATION

Bodies are identified through DNA and possibly dental records. But families may be asked to identify the bodies of their deceased loved one (or the family members may ask to view the body). The finality of identifying the deceased's body can have a paradoxical effect. Viewing the body shatters any hope that the decedent may still be alive, but it also often provides a strange sort of reassuring confirmation that the decedent's death agonies may have fallen short of the survivor's imagined horrors or that the decedent's suffering is finally over. Families may want to touch the decedent to say a final good-bye. Allow them time to do so, unless there is a reason the body is not to be disturbed, such as when further evidence is being collected. This is a difficult time, so provide appropriate support.

When the victim's body is significantly mutilated, dismembered, burned, decomposed, or disintegrated, try to arrange to have the viewing area as clean as possible before identification. Major wounds should be dressed or covered, and the viewing area should be reasonably free of blood spills, body fluids, and other debris. However, law enforcement may insist on keeping the body as it was found if evidence is yet to be collected, and the family should be notified of this for these cases. At times the visual sight of something as small as a finger or a relatively intact portion of the face can solidify the reality of the death for the family member and allow a final goodbye.

DEATH REVIEW TEAMS

Adult fatality review teams began operating in the early 1990s. There are several teams currently operating in many areas around the United States, most of which focus on deaths of older adults or deaths from intimate partner violence. Fatality review teams are multiagency, multidisciplinary groups that systematically review fatalities at a regional, county, or state level. The ultimate goal of fatality review is to gain a better understanding of the circumstances surrounding the deaths in order to more efficiently target funding and prevention efforts.

RESOURCES

American Board of Medicolegal Death Investigators: http://medschool.slu.edu/abmdi/index.php
International Association of Coroners and Medical Examiners: http://theiacme.com/iacme/index.aspx
Medline Bereavement: http://www.nlm.nih.gov/medlineplus/bereavement.html
National Association of Medical Examiners: http://thename.org/
National Association of Medical Examiners Forensic Autopsy Performance Standards (2006): http://thename.org/index2.php?option=com_docman&task=doc_view&gid=18&Itemid=26

REFERENCES

Hanson, D. (2008). *Forensic autopsy: A body of clues*. Retrieved from http://www.officer.com/web/online/Investigation/Forensic-Autopsy--A-Body-of-Clues/18$37565

Hickman, M., Hughes, K., Strom, K., & Ropero-Miller, J. (2007). Medical examiners and coroners' offices, 2004. Bureau of Justice Statistics NCJ 216756. Retrieved from http://www.ojp.usdoj.gov/bjs/pub/pdf/meco04.pdf

Miller, L. (2008). Death investigation for families of homicide victims: Healing dimensions of a complex process. *Omega, 57*(4), 367–380.

U.S. Department of Justice Office of Justice Programs National Institute of Justice. (1999). *Death investigation: A guide for the scene investigator.* Retrieved from http://www.ncjrs.gov/pdffiles/167568.pdf

Deaths of Elders in Long-Term Care Facilities

DEFINITION

One typically thinks of death investigation as necessary and needed in cases of unexpected death. Death of a resident in a long-term care facility is an expected event and is therefore unlikely, in most jurisdictions, to trigger a death investigation process. However, death investigation in a nursing home population can be appropriate and necessary; there are indeed cases in which suspicious deaths occur in long-term care facilities. When a death that could have been prevented occurs in a long-term care facility, investigation should take place. Elders with medical diagnoses and younger people with chronic illnesses who reside in long-term care facilities can die of neglect or abuse.

PREVALENCE

According to the Federal Interagency Forum on Ageing Statistics (2008), the top eight causes of death in 2004, were, in order: heart disease, malignant neoplasms, cerebrovascular diseases, chronic lower respiratory diseases, Alzheimer's disease, diabetes mellitus, influenza, and pneumonia. Heart disease and cancer were the leading causes of death regardless of gender, race, or presence or absence of Hispanic origin; however, for other causes of death, these factors were significant. Males had higher suicide rates than females at all ages in the geriatric spectrum, with the largest difference occurring for those age 85 and older. Non-Hispanic White males age 85 and older have the highest rate of suicide overall.

ETIOLOGY

Deaths occur in long-term care facilities for natural reasons on a regular basis. Distinguishing death from neglect and abuse in an elderly population versus death from natural causes requires a careful screening process. It is required that death investigation determine the cause of death. Cause of death in a long-term care facility may be natural, accident, homicide, suicide, or undetermined.

ASSESSMENT

General Principles

Some states have a state-wide system for investigation of all deaths in long-term care facilities. A screening tool is utilized every time an elder dies in a facility. Everyone is inspected for signs of abuse and neglect. Every death in a nursing facility is *not* assumed to be natural.

History and Physical Assessment

Abuse and neglect in long-term care facilities most frequently occurs to people who cannot speak for themselves. Victims in nursing facilities often suffer from dementia and cannot give a coherent history of abuse or neglect. However, medical and health care provider records may indicate abuse and/or neglect. Physical findings that may indicate abuse should be searched for in the patient's records. Records of bruising, fractures, or burns may indicate abuse. In many cases, what is not recorded is what is important. The absence of dental care, the absence of range-of-motion exercising and turning, resulting in decubiti, the absence of indication of the time taken to feed, the absence of indicators of good skin care, and the absence of good health care for incontinent people may indicate neglect.

Death investigation includes examining the living arrangement of the deceased. Detectives and health care personnel routinely examine the area of the long-term care facility in which the deceased resided. Signs of neglect and/or abuse may be detected upon visual inspection of the sleeping, bathing, and toileting physical spaces. Death investigation also includes interviews. Interviews may be conducted of staff in the long-term care facility and of the family of the deceased.

INTERVENTION

Routine investigation of each and every death that occurs in a long-term care facility can lead to prosecution of facilities in which neglect and abuse occur. Death investigation does not undo the death of the deceased person whose case is being investigated. Rather it holds the offenders accountable for their behavior. Every elder deserves to be safe and secure in his or her long-term care facility. Routine death investigation of elders in a facility also leads to the determination of patterns of death in long-term care facilities. The office of the medical examiner becomes aware of how many deaths are occurring in each facility and the cause and manner of each death.

PREVENTION/PATIENT TEACHING

Primary Prevention

Simply stated, making facilities accountable for their actions via a death review team investigation for every elder who dies under the charge of the facility appears to be a good idea. Knowledge of upcoming review and investigation acts as primary prevention. There is an overall expectation that elders residing in a nursing care facility will die there. However, there should be an enforced standard of care for how and when and under what circumstances the elder dies. Elders in facilities should be treated with respect and dignity and should receive the best possible physical care via a care plan that is tailor-made to each person's needs.

Secondary Prevention

Health care providers who work as death investigators are in a unique circumstance. They can assist in the process of speaking for vulnerable elders and in helping to assure that the end-of-life care for every elder in an institution is humane, appropriate, and relevant.

Tertiary Prevention

Record review and physical examination of every elder who dies in a long-term care facility establishes a database that can be used to develop standards for prevention of elder abuse in facilities. Elder death review teams can also examine the cause and manner of deaths in long-term care facilities to determine which are preventable and to suggest prevention mechanisms.

RESOURCES

Center for Excellence in Elder Abuse and Neglect: http://www.centeronelderabuse.org/page.cfm
Elder Abuse Fatality Review: http://ican-ncfr.org/hmElderAbuseFatality.asp
Elder Abuse Fatality Review Teams: A Replication Manual: http://www.abanet.org/aging/fatalitymanual.pdf

REFERENCES

Alzheimer's Association. (2009). Alzheimer's disease facts and figures. *Journal of the Alzheimer's Association, 5*(3), 234–270.
Federal Interagency Forum on Ageing Statistics. (2008). Mortality indicators. Retrieved from http://www.aoa.gov/agingstatsdotnet/Main_Site/Data/2008_Documents/Health_Status.aspx
Feldkamp, J. (2006). Medical directors are key in abuse prevention: Open lines of communication can help leaders identify a facility's areas of vulnerability. *Caring for the Ages, 7*(8), 17–18.
Godwin, T. (2005). End of life: Natural or unnatural: Death investigation and certification. *Disease-A-Month, 5*(14), 218–277.

40 Suicide

DEFINITION

Suicide describes the destructive, self-inflicted actions that result in actual or attempted self-harm or death, the intentional ending of one's life. Suicidal ideation is defined as having thoughts of wanting to end one's own life. Clinicians usually view the severity of suicide risk along a continuum, ranging from suicidal ideation alone (relatively less severe) to suicidal ideation with a plan (highest severity). The latter is a significant risk factor for suicide attempts. Suicide attempts are the self-initiated acts with the intention of ending one's own life and are less frequent than suicidal ideation. In adolescents, overdose is the most common method of attempt, whereas firearms, jumping, and hanging are the more common methods in completed suicides.

Suicide is a major public health problem. Besides the tragic loss of a life, suicide may also mean the sudden loss of the breadwinner for the family, long-lasting psychological trauma for the family, and loss of economic productivity.

PREVALENCE

According to the Centers for Disease Control and Prevention (2007), suicide was the eleventh leading cause of death in the United States in 2006, accounting for 33,300 deaths. The overall rate was 10.9 suicide deaths per 100,000 people, and an estimated 12 to 25 attempted suicides occur per every suicide death.

- Males take their own lives at nearly four times the rate of females and represent 79.0% of all U.S. suicides.
- During their lifetime, women attempt suicide about two to three times as often as men.
- Suicide is the seventh leading cause of death for males and the sixteenth leading cause for females.
- Suicide rates for males are highest among those aged 75 and older (rate 35.7 per 100,000).
- Suicide rates for females are highest among those aged 45–54 (rate 8.4 per 100,000 population).
- Firearms are the most commonly used method of suicide among males (56.0%).
- Poisoning is the most common method of suicide for females (40.3%).
- Suicide is the second leading cause of death among 25- to 34-year-olds and the third leading cause of death among 15- to 24-year-olds.
- The rate of suicide for adults aged 75 years and older was 15.9 per 100,000.

The National Violent Death Reporting System (http://www.cdc.gov/NCIPC/profiles/nvdrs/default.htm) includes information on the presence of alcohol and other substances at the time of death. For those tested for substances, the findings from the 16 states involved revealed that one-third of those who died by suicide were positive for alcohol at the time of death, and nearly one in five had evidence of opiates, including heroin and prescription painkillers.

Suicide is the thirteenth leading cause of death in persons age 65 years or older. Older adults have the highest risk of suicide in the United States. Risk factors for this group include psychiatric disorders, physical health problems, life events, and social stressors such as financial strain during retirement, and disability.

ETIOLOGY

Undiagnosed or undertreated mental health problems, such as depression, bipolar disorder, and psychosis are the most common reasons for suicide. Suicide.org (n.d.) lists several triggers and other factors that may correlate with suicide, including the following:

- The death of a loved one
- A divorce, separation, or breakup of a relationship
- Losing custody of children, or feeling that a child custody decision is not fair
- A serious loss, such as a loss of a job, house, or money
- A serious illness
- A terminal illness
- A serious accident
- Chronic physical pain
- Intense emotional pain
- Loss of hope
- Being victimized (domestic violence, rape, assault, etc.)
- A loved one being victimized (child murder, child molestation, kidnapping, murder, rape, assault, etc.)
- Physical abuse
- Verbal abuse
- Sexual abuse
- Unresolved abuse (of any kind) from the past
- Feeling trapped in a situation perceived as negative
- Feeling that things will never get better
- Feeling helpless
- Serious legal problems, such as criminal prosecution or incarceration
- Feeling taken advantage of
- Inability to deal with a perceived humiliating situation
- Inability to deal with a perceived failure
- Alcohol and/or drug abuse
- A feeling of not being accepted by family, friends, or society
- Experiencing a horrible disappointment
- Feeling like one has not lived up to his or her high expectations or those of another
- Experiencing bullying (adults, as well as children, can be bullied)
- Low self-esteem

ASSESSMENT

General Principles

Suicide risk often goes undetected in health care settings. Unrecognized suicidality in emergency departments (EDs) is a important problem for several reasons: increasing numbers of clients now present to hospital EDs with mental health concerns; ED staff are increasingly being given the responsibility of triaging clients with mental health problems to crisis intervention and appropriate follow-up treatments; and unrecognized suicidality in the ED is associated with substantial morbidity, possible mortality, and increased health care utilization and costs. Approximately one-half to two-thirds of individuals who commit suicide visit health care providers less than 1 month before taking their lives; 10% to 40% visit in the week before. Yet, despite the substantial proportion of primary care providers who encounter suicidal patients, most providers do not routinely screen their patients for suicidality or associated risk factors.

History and Physical Assessment

In taking the history, assess for risk factors:

- Family history of suicide
- Family history of child maltreatment
- Previous suicide attempt(s)
- History of mental disorders, particularly depression
- History of alcohol and substance abuse
- Feelings of hopelessness
- Impulsive or aggressive tendencies
- Cultural and religious beliefs (e.g., belief that suicide is a noble resolution of a personal dilemma)
- Local epidemics of suicide
- Isolation, a feeling of being cut off from other people
- Barriers to accessing mental health treatment
- Loss (relational, social, work, or financial)
- Physical illness
- Easy access to lethal methods
- Unwillingness to seek help because of the stigma attached to mental health and substance abuse disorders or to suicidal thoughts

Assess for warning signs, per the Substance Abuse and Mental Health Services Administration (2007):

- Threatens to hurt or kill himself or herself or talks about wanting to hurt or kill himself or herself
- Looks for ways to kill himself or herself by seeking access to firearms, pills, or other means
- Talks or writes about death, dying, or suicide when these actions are out of the ordinary for the individual
- Feels hopeless
- Feels rage or uncontrolled anger or is seeking revenge
- Acts recklessly or engages in risky activities—seemingly without thinking
- Feels trapped—like there is no way out
- Increasing alcohol or drug use
- Withdraws from friends, family, and society
- Feels anxious, agitated, or unable to sleep, or sleeps all the time
- Experiences dramatic mood changes
- Sees no reason for living or has no sense of purpose in life

Explore suicidal ideation.

- Ask if they ever thought of hurting or killing themselves (hurting is different than killing).
- If the answer is yes, ask when they thought of killing themselves.
- Ask how they planned to kill themselves.
- Ask if they ever tried to kill themselves before and if they received help that time.
- Ask if they believe that they have any other options besides suicide to resolve their problems.

Persons who verbalize planned, lethal means to commit suicide and who feel that they do not have any other options are at extreme risk of carrying out their plan, especially if they have attempted it in the past.

In physical examination check for the following:

- Assess for signs of underlying medical disorders.
- Inspect for signs of self-abusive behaviors (unusual scars, death-themed body art).

Diagnostic Testing

The U.S. Preventive Services Task Force (USPSTF, 2004) found no evidence that screening for suicide risk reduces suicide attempts or mortality and that there is limited evidence on the accuracy of screening tools to identify suicide risk in the primary care setting, including tools to identify those at high risk. As a result, the USPSTF could not determine the balance of benefits and harms of screening for suicide risk in the primary care setting.

INTERVENTION

Suicidal clients should be referred for appropriate evaluation and treatment. Those who verbalize significant ideation or other high risk should be transferred to mental health treatment immediately.

PREVENTION/PATIENT TEACHING

Primary Prevention

Promote overall mental health by reducing early risk factors such as depression and substance abuse, and building resiliency. Promote protective factors:

- Effective clinical care for mental, physical, and substance abuse disorders
- Easy access to a variety of clinical interventions and support for help seeking
- Family and community support (connectedness)
- Support from ongoing medical and mental health care relationships
- Skills in problem solving, conflict resolution, and nonviolent ways of handling disputes
- Cultural and religious beliefs that discourage suicide and support instincts for self-preservation
- National suicide prevention strategies include:
- Public education
- Responsible media reporting

- School-based programs
- Detection and treatment of depression and other mental disorders
- Attention to those abusing alcohol and drugs
- Attention to individuals experiencing somatic illness
- Enhanced access to mental health services
- Improvement in assessment of attempted suicide
- Postvention (aftermath)
- Crisis intervention
- Work and unemployment policy
- Training of health professionals
- Reduced access to lethal methods

Secondary Prevention

There are many paths to suicide; thus, prevention must address psychological, biological, and social factors if it is to be effective. Collaboration across a broad array of agencies, institutions, and groups—from faith-based organizations to health care associations—is a way to ensure that prevention efforts are comprehensive. Collaboration can also generate greater and more effective attention to suicide prevention than can these groups working alone. Primary care–based collaborative care programs for depression represent one strategy to reduce suicidal ideation and potentially the risk of suicide in older primary-care patients.

Tertiary Prevention

Assure that suicidal clients have access to adequate mental health and substance abuse treatment programs that can decrease suicidality and its underlying factors.

RESOURCES

National Institute for Mental Health: http://www.nimh.nih.gov
National Suicide Prevention Lifeline: http://www.suicidepreventionlifeline.org (or call 1-800-273-TALK)
Substance Abuse and Mental Health Services Administration: http://www.samhsa.gov
Suicide Prevention Resource Center: http://www.sprc.org
Surgeon General's Call to Action to Prevent Suicide: http://www.surgeongeneral.gov/library/calltoaction/default.htm

REFERENCES

Anderson, M., & Jenkins, R. (2005). The challenge of suicide prevention: An overview of national strategies. *Disease Management & Health Outcomes, 13*(4), 245–253.

Caruso, K. (n.d.). Suicide causes. Retrieved from http://www.suicide.org/suicide-causes.html

Centers for Disease Control and Prevention (CDC). (2007). Web-based injury statistics query and reporting system (WISQARS). National Center for Injury Prevention and Control, CDC (producer). Retrieved from http://www.cdc.gov/injury/wisqars/index.html

Centers for Disease Control and Prevention (CDC). (2009). Suicide risk and protective factors. Retrieved from http://www.cdc.gov/ViolencePrevention/suicide/riskprotectivefactors.html

Karch, D., Dahlberg, L., Patel, N., Davis, T., Logan, J, Hill, H., et al. (2006). Surveillance for violent deaths—National violent death reporting system, 16 states. *Morbidity and Mortality Weekly (MMWR), 58*(ss01), 1–44.

Mezuk, B., Prescott, M., Tardiff, K., Vlahov, D., & Galea, S. (2008). Suicide in older adults in long-term care: 1990 to 2005. *Journal of the American Geriatrics Society, 56*(11), 2107–2111.

Substance Abuse and Mental Health Services Administration (SAMHSA). (2007). Suicide causes. *SAMSHA Newsletter, 15*(6), 1. Retrieved from http://www.samhsa.gov/SAMHSA_News/VolumeXV_6/article6.htm

Suicide.org. (n.d.). *Suicide causes.* Retrieved from http://suicide.org/suicide-causes.html

Unützer, J., Tang, L., Oishi, S., Katon, W., Williams, J. W., Hunkeler, E., et al. (2006). Reducing suicidal ideation in depressed older primary care patients. *Journal of the American Geriatric Society, 54,* 1550–1556.

U.S. Preventive Services Task Force (USPSTF). (2004). Screening for suicide risk: Recommendation and rationale. Retrieved from http://www.ahrq.gov/clinic/3rduspstf/suicide/suiciderr.htm

41 Autoerotic Asphyxia

DEFINITION

Autoerotic asphyxia involves choking oneself during sexual stimulation to heighten sexual pleasure. Sometimes referred to as scarfing, bagging, or breath play, autoerotic asphyxia may involve elaborate bindings, sophisticated escape mechanisms, sexual images, or cross-dressing, although these are said to be more common in adults than adolescents. Death can occur if loss of consciousness leads to inability to reverse or stop the means of strangulation. Autoerotic death is usually associated with a constrictive cervical ligature tied to either other parts of the victim's body or to an inanimate object such as a door. Other modalities include ligature around the thorax or abdomen, plastic bags covering the face, electrical current, inhalation of a toxic gas or chemicals, or partial or total submersion, known as aquaerotic asphyxiation. Sexual asphyxia can also be practiced as part of a consensual sadomasochistic activity between two or more people and can still result in fatality.

Persistent autoerotic asphyxia is classified as a paraphilia in the *Diagnostic and Statistical Manual of Mental Disorders,* 4th edition, text revision *(DSM-IV-TR)*. Hypoxyphilia or asphyxiophilia is a form of sexual masochism that involves sexual arousal by oxygen deprivation via strangulation, chest compression, plastic bag, mask, or chemicals (typically a volatile nitrate). Paraphilias are disorders characterized by recurrent, intense, sexually arousing fantasies, sexual urges, or behaviors that generally involve nonhuman objects; the suffering or humiliation of oneself or one's partner; or children or other nonconsenting persons, over a period of at least 6 months. Participants of asphyxia activities are at risk for short-term memory loss, hemorrhage, and retinal damage, as well as head injuries from falling when unconscious, stroke, seizures, permanent brain damage, coma, and death. Death can be caused by prolonged asphyxia or nerve pressure that causes the heart to stop.

PREVALENCE

Most participants are older adolescent and adult males under age 30. The exact number of deaths from autoerotic asphyxia is unknown since it is most often practiced in secrecy and solitude. Most cases become apparent when the results are fatal. Approximately 500 to 1,000 autoerotic fatalities are reported each year in the United States and Canada. Adolescents are especially vulnerable to a fatal outcome because they often do not understand the risks associated with this behavior.

Although this behavior is mostly a male activity, women do engage in sexual asphyxia. However, a male-to-female ratio is greater than 50:1. Currently, there is no typical or predominant profile of someone who engages in any kind of sexual asphyxia. It is known to be practiced by both sexes and across many cultures going back hundreds of years.

The number of fatalities attributed to hypoxyphilia are probably under-reported. The most common reasons for under-reporting are unfamiliarity with this mode of death on the part of the investigating officials, and the well-meaning interference in the scene by loved ones, who remove embarrassing items that would otherwise make determination less complex.

ETIOLOGY

Deaths from autoerotic asphyxia often occur when their rescue method/mechanism fails. Loss of consciousness caused by partial asphyxia leads to loss of control over the means of strangulation, resulting in continued asphyxia and death. In some cases, the body is discovered naked, surrounded by signs of masturbatory activity and/or sexual paraphernalia, which can include pornography, fetishistic materials, bondage materials, sex toys, and other equipment. However, family members often clean up the death scene to preserve the victim's dignity and/or minimize their own embarrassment. This can lead death investigators to suspect suicide unless they perform a careful history and assessment.

There are no overt signs of either predisposition to this behavior or the existence of this paraphilia. People who practice this behavior may be involved in healthy relationships, sexual and otherwise, and be committed partners and spouses. Autoerotic asphyxia is usually solitary, and the individual usually chooses a private or secluded place. The individual intends to control the degree of hypoxia and plans to escape from the situation. The intention is to survive the ritual, not die from it. When death occurs it is almost always due to the failure of a strategy intended to ensure release. Ejaculation may have occurred, although ejaculation can occur in other types of death and is not a conclusive sign. Cross-dressing in female clothing is a feature in some of the of the cases, and pornography and other sexual paraphernalia (mirrors, self-photography, bondage, hoods, and blindfolds) are found at many scenes or among the deceased's personal possessions. Often the elaborate nature of the equipment used in these cases makes it clear that the behavior has been carried out many times before. People who die from this autoerotic practice reportedly have concurrent paraphilias, including other forms of masochism, sadism, transvestic fetishism, and other fetishes.

ASSESSMENT

General Principles

Death investigators should consider autoerotic asphyxia activities when investigating asphyxia deaths, particularly those that appear to be suicide. Health care providers should assess for signs of autoerotic activities in their clients.

History and Physical Assessment

Asphyxial activities should also be added to the differential diagnosis in the assessment of headaches, behavior changes, head injuries, or abnormal marks around the neck or neck area.

The following signs indicate a client may be involved in asphyxia activities:

- Bloodshot eyes
- Marks on the neck
- Wearing high-necked shirts, even in warm weather
- Frequent, severe headaches
- Disorientation after spending time alone
- Increased and uncharacteristic irritability or hostility
- Ropes, scarves, and belts tied to bedroom furniture or doorknobs or found knotted on the floor
- Wear marks on furniture (bunk beds, curtain rods) from previous incidences
- The unexplained presence of dog leashes, choke collars, bungee cords, and the like.
- Petechiae under the skin of the face, especially the eyelids, or the conjunctiva

Health care professionals may become involved in the death investigation of a client who had been participating in autoerotic asphyxia, unknown to other investigators. Health care professionals can assist the investigation in determining the manner of death. Hazelwood, Burgess, and Groth (1981) have developed five criteria for determining an autoerotic death:

Presence of a well-defined self-rescue mechanism

Has a penchant for solitary activity

Employment of sexual fantasy aids

Previous autoerotic behavior

No suicidal ideation

Protective padding around the neck to prevent ligature marks and a distinct release mechanism may confirm the accidental and typical nature of this activity. However, these findings may be lacking at the scene. Investigators should also realize that most of what is known about autoerotic asphyxia is known about adult victims.

Male victims are more likely to be involved in atypical autoerotic asphyxia, resorting to gas masks, plastic bags, anesthetic gases, and binding the body with plastic or chains. Males often engage in cross-dressing and enjoy pornographic materials such as videos, magazines, or mirrors to a greater extent during their autoerotic experience.

Females are more inclined to use a ligature about the neck, which is controlled by movements of body position. They tend to be found naked without excessive paraphernalia. Female autoerotic death poses a greater challenge to investigators, usually because of the subtle findings at the scene, which may create an appearance of suicide. This subtleness may suggest that women are more cautious in their secretive behavior. Their deaths may also be misinterpreted as sexual homicides if the female utilized elaborate bondage mechanisms during the activity.

INTERVENTION

Intervention focuses on consequences of the asphyxia injuries and on preventative teaching. Clients who participate in autoerotic asphyxia are usually experimenting and have few if any paraphilic behaviors. Thus, those suspected of having paraphilic behavior should be referred to an appropriate therapist. Most persons with paraphilias have multiple paraphilias, and asphyxiophilia can be deadly.

PREVENTION/PATIENT TEACHING

Research is not available on the best strategies to prevent asphyxia activities. Clients and health care providers should be made aware of this public health threat and the warning signs that loved ones may be involved in asphyxial games.

RESOURCES

Forensic Science: An Objective Overview of Autoerotic Fatalities: http://cienciaforense. com/Pages/Psychology/AutoeroticFatalities.htm

REFERENCES

American Psychiatric Association. (2000). *Diagnostic and statistical manual of mental disorders* (4th ed., text rev.). Washington, DC: American Psychiatric Association.

Hazelwood R., Burgess, A., & Groth, A. (1981). Death during dangerous autoerotic practice. *Social Science Medicine, 15E,* 129–133.

Shields, L., Hunsaker, D., Hunsaker, J., Wetli, C., Hutchins, K., & Holmes, R. (2005). Atypical autoerotic death: Part II. *The American Journal of Forensic Medicine and Pathology, 26*(1), 53–62.

42 Homicide Survivors

DEFINITION

Losing a family member to homicide is one of the most traumatic experiences that a person can live through. There is no way to prepare for this tragic event, which leaves tremendous pain and upheaval in its wake. The impact crosses all cultures, races, and genders. Homicide grief experts estimate that there are 7 to 10 close relatives for each victim, and this does not count significant others, friends, neighbors and coworkers. Those left behind after homicide are called homicide survivors. No amount of justice, restitution, prayer, or compassion will bring their loved one back. However, health care professionals need to assist these survivors in moving through the grieving process so that they do not succumb to complications.

When a person is murdered, the death is sudden, violent, final, and completely incomprehensible. Shared plans and dreams are suddenly shattered and no longer possible. The loss will be grieved in different ways by all those who felt close to the victim, and grief reactions may be manifested long after the incident. Family members may have had a conflicted relationship with the victim, and the death means that these issues or bad feelings will remain unresolved, leaving the survivor with the additional loss of hope that things could have been worked out while the victim lived. The turmoil is manifested by an array of emotional reactions to trauma, including shock, anger, grief, and guilt. Homicide survivors often experience financial hardship due to expenses related to funerals, medical fees, and mental health counseling. They may feel loss of self, helplessness, loss of control, loss of religion, and loss of safety and security, because homicide leaves survivors feeling victimized physically, socially, and spiritually.

ETIOLOGY

The concept of stages of grief is no longer accepted; however, grief reactions and the tasks of grieving have been identified. Homicide survivors may also experience symptoms of posttraumatic stress disorder (PTSD). Grief usually follows any loss. The violence, suddenness, unexpectedness, and sometimes randomness of death by homicide create anger, self-blame, and guilt that may place family members at risk for what has been termed "complicated mourning."

Grief Reactions

Redmond (1989) described factors that may affect the grieving process for homicide survivors: the ages of the survivors and the victim at the time of the homicide; the survivors' physical and/or emotional state before the murder; their prior history of trauma; the way in which their loved one died; and whether or not the survivor has, and can make use of, social support systems. Social and cultural factors can also have great impact on the grieving process.

Initially homicide survivors may experience shock and disbelief, numbness, changes in appetite or sleeping patterns, difficulty concentrating, confusion, anger, fear, and anxiety. In cases where family members have not been able to view the deceased's body (either because it was not permitted or they felt unable to do so) it is often difficult for them to accept the reality of the death. Some urge that family members be permitted to go through this viewing process, as painful as it may be at the time. Homicide survivors sometimes feel like the whole world has stopped, and they cannot understand how everyone else is able to go on about their daily routine.

Later reactions usually include feelings of isolation, helplessness, fear and vulnerability, guilt or self-blame, nightmares, and a desire for revenge. Survivors may experience heightened anxiety or phobic reactions. Their anguish may seem intense and sometimes overwhelming. Some describe a physical pain (lump in the throat) that they could feel for several years after the murder.

It is not unusual for homicide survivors to have tremendous feelings of rage toward the perpetrator, and some experience anger toward the victim for getting killed. Depression and hopelessness can lead some to feel that they will never be happy again. Some may experience suicidal ideation, which warrants immediate attention.

Survivors may find themselves suddenly crying over their loss years after the event. These feelings reflect the depth of the pain of the loss. Many say that they know they are doing better when they begin to have more good days than bad days.

Tasks of Grieving

Worden (1991) described four "tasks" of grieving: accepting the reality of the loss, feeling the grief, adjusting to a life in which the deceased is no longer present, and emotionally relocating the deceased so that life can go on.

First task: The survivor acknowledges and accepts the reality that the loved one is dead. Some survivors often report a sense that they will still see the deceased; others report feeling compelled to follow someone who looked like the deceased. It is difficult for homicide survivors who have not viewed the body to know that their loved one is really dead.

Second task: Survivors must acknowledge and experience the physical and/or emotional pain associated with losing their loved one. This is a difficult task, even under the most supportive of circumstances. Homicide survivors may have to put their feelings on hold through court hearings, trials, and numerous appeals. However, no matter how much the pain is put aside, survivors must experience these feelings, or they may carry the pain of the loss for the rest of their lives.

Third task: Survivors must adjust to life without the deceased. They must begin to make personal or lifestyle changes that might take them in a very different direction than that planned while their loved one was still alive. Survivors may feel some guilt around these decisions and may feel they are being disloyal to the deceased; however, it is important for survivors to recognize and come to terms with these reactions and feelings.

Last task: Survivors must somehow find a place for their loved one within their emotional life and still realize that their lives can and do go on.

Posttraumatic Stress Reactions

Families of homicide victims may be at risk for developing posttraumatic stress disorder (PTSD). When a family member is murdered, the survivors often react with intense feelings of helplessness, fear, and horror.

PARENTS WHO LOSE THEIR CHILD TO HOMICIDE

Parents may find that they reexperience feelings of loss many years later, such as when they see friends of their murdered child graduate from high school or college, get a job, or start a family. Parents may have believed that, in the natural order of life, the older generation should die first; if so, they may have great difficulty with the fact that their young or grown children were killed while they themselves still live, thus violating this expectation. Compassionate Friends (2008), a group that assists families dealing with grief following the death of a child, notes that there are several unique issues that may complicate the grief process for the parents and family left behind. These may include:

- The child's body may be evidence, and the investigation and autopsy may cause a lengthy delay in the release of the child's body to the parents.
- The child's body may not be found.
- The child's body may not be viewable.
- The family may be viewed as suspects, creating a revictimization of those very survivors feeling the most acute pain.
- The child may have been killed by one of the family members, possibly one of the parents.
- Information on new developments may come slowly, and sometimes weeks and months may pass without contact from the authorities unless initiated by the family.

- If the child was murdered in another country, the family may be forced to deal with that country's law enforcement and legal system. They may also need to deal with language and communication barriers and numerous costly and frustrating trips.
- The child may seem dehumanized as the police, the press, prosecutors, and others refer to "the victim," "the body," and "the deceased."
- The perpetrator may never be caught or may choose suicide or death rather than capture.
- The perpetrator may go free for any number of reasons or receive a sentence far lighter than the family expected.
- The child may be blamed by some for contributing to the murder.
- The media may take away any hopes of privacy the family members may normally value.

Posttraumatic stress disorder (PTSD) often presents in primary and community care but may go unrecognized. Failure to identify and treat PTSD has adverse effects on client health, since PTSD is associated with increased health complaints, health services utilization, morbidity, and mortality. Persons with PTSD have persistent frightening thoughts and memories of the incident and feel emotionally numb, especially with people they were once close to. They may experience sleep disturbances, feel numb or detached, or be easily startled.

INTERVENTIONS

Grief work can be complicated for family members of homicide victims. Family survivors can distance themselves mentally from the grief process for a short time after the homicide but then find the grief flooding their emotions at a later date. Family survivors may become distracted by necessary tasks after the homicide but find when those tasks are complete that they are emotionally overwhelmed. Families consistently report intense emotional grief that is complicated by the intentionality of the homicide, the fact that the loved one was taken from them by another person.

Psychological and physical symptoms of grieving are determined by the coping skills of the survivor, the family support system, and support by the community. The pattern of communication utilized by the survivor also impacts the person's ability to grieve and accept support for the grieving process. Previous patterns of behavior and role functioning impact the grieving process. Self-blame and somatization of psychological symptoms is common during grieving after homicide. If the survivor is a child, the process of grieving is complicated by the developmental phase of the child. Regression is a common childhood response to grief after a homicide.

The appropriate health care intervention surrounding homicide involves recognizing the tremendous stress placed upon family members and making appropriate referrals to counseling services. Both individual and group counseling have been shown to be effective in facilitating the grieving process after homicide. Persons well trained to support the families of homicide victims are employed in the criminal justice system. In addition to counseling services located within the community, the justice system should support the families through the homicide investigation and prosecution. The justice system provides services that include accompaniment during court proceedings and notification of any legal activities involving the suspect.

RESOURCES

Compassionate Friends: http://www.compassionatefriends.org
Murder Victims' Families for Reconciliation: http://www.mvfr.org/
National Center for Victims of Crime: Homicide Survivors: http://www.ncvc.org/ncvc/
main.aspx?dbName=DocumentViewer&DocumentID=32358#1
Parents of Murdered Children: http://www.pomc.com
Safehorizon: http://www.safehorizon.org/page.php?page=homicide

REFERENCES

Armour, M. (2003). Meaning making in the aftermath of homicide. *Death Studies, 27,* 519–540.

Clements, P., Faulkner, M., & Manno, M. (2003). Family-member homicide: A grave situation for children. *Topics in Advanced Practice Nursing eJournal.* Retrieved from http://www.medscape.com/viewarticle/458064

Compassionate Friends. (2008). When your child dies by homicide. Retrieved from http://www.compassionatefriends.org/Brochures/when_your_child_dies_by_homicide.aspx

Hatton, R. (2003). Homicide bereavement counseling: A survey of providers. *Death Studies, 27,* 427–448.

MacLeod, M. (1999). Why did it happen to me? Social cognition processes in adjustment and recovery from criminal victimization and illness. *Current Psychology, 18,* 18–31.

McFarlane, A., Atchison, M., Rafalowicz, E., & Papay, P. (1994). Physical symptoms in posttraumatic stress disorder. *Journal of Psychosomatic Research, 38,* 715–726.

Miller, L. (2009). Family survivors of homicide. *American Journal of Family Therapy,* *37*(1), 67–79.

Niemeyer, R. A. (2000). Searching for the meaning of meaning: Grief therapy and the process of reconstruction. *Death Studies, 24,* 541–550.

Redmond, L. (1989). *Surviving: When someone you love was murdered.* Clearwater, FL: Psychological Consultation and Education Services.

Vigil G., & Clements P. (2003). Child and adolescent homicide survivors: Complicated grief and altered worldviews. *Journal of Psychosocial Nursing & Mental Health Services, 41*(1), 30–41.

Worden, J. W. (1991). *Grief counseling and grief therapy.* New York: Springer.

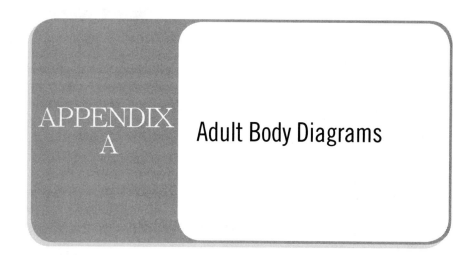

APPENDIX
A

Adult Body Diagrams

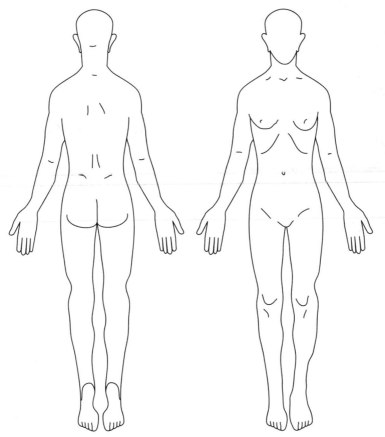

Figure Appendix A Adult body diagrams.

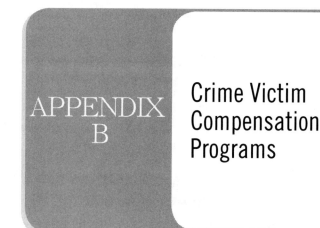

APPENDIX
B

Crime Victim Compensation Programs

National Association of Crime Victim Compensation Boards (NACVCB)
P.O. Box 16003
Alexandria, VA 22302
(703) 313-9500
http://www.nacvcb.org

Alabama
(334) 242-4007

Alaska
(907) 465-3040

Arizona
(602) 364-1155

Arkansas
(501) 682-1020

California
(916) 323-3432

Colorado
(303) 239-4493

Connecticut
(860) 747-4501

Delaware
(302) 995-8383

District of Columbia
(202) 879-4216

Florida
(850) 414-3300

Georgia
(404) 559-4949

Guam
(671) 475-3324

Hawaii
(808) 587-1143

Idaho
(208) 334-6080

Developed from the Office for Victims of Crime, Crime Victim Compensation Directory: http://www.ojp.usdoj.gov/ovc/help/progdir.htm.

415

Illinois
(217) 782-7101/
(312) 814-2581

Indiana
(317) 232-1295

Iowa
(515) 281-5044

Kansas
(785) 296-2359

Kentucky
(502) 573-2290

Louisiana
(225) 925-4437

Maine
(207) 624-7882

Maryland
(410) 585-3010

Massachusetts
(617) 727-2200

Michigan
(517) 373-7373

Minnesota
(651) 282-6256

Mississippi
(601) 359-6766

Missouri
(573) 526-6006

Montana
(406) 444-3653

Nebraska
(402) 471-2828

Nevada
(702) 486-2740/
(775) 688-2900

New Hampshire
(603) 271-1284

New Jersey
(973) 648-2107

New Mexico
(505) 841-9432

New York
(518) 457-8727/
(718) 923-4325

North Carolina
(919) 733-7974

North Dakota
(701) 328-6195

Ohio
(614) 466-5610

Oklahoma
(405) 264-5006

Oregon
(503) 378-5348

Pennsylvania
(717) 783-5153

Puerto Rico
(787) 641-7480

Rhode Island
(401) 222-8590

South Carolina
(803) 734-1900

South Dakota
(605) 773-6317

Tennessee
(615) 741-2734

Texas
(512) 936-1200

Utah
(801) 238-2360

Vermont
(802) 241-1250

Virgin Islands
(340) 774-1166

Virginia
(804) 378-3434

Washington
(360) 902-5355

West Virginia
(304) 347-4850

Wisconsin
(608) 266-6470

Wyoming
(307) 777-7200

Forensic Glossary

Acquittal: A jury verdict that a criminal defendant is not guilty; also the finding of a judge that the evidence is insufficient to support a conviction.

Actuarial risk assessment: A risk assessment based upon specific factors that have been researched and demonstrated to be statistically significant in the prediction of risk.

Actus reus: Latin for a "guilty act," the actus reus is the act that, in combination with a certain mental state, such as intent or recklessness, constitutes a crime.

Aftercare/Reentry: Activities and tasks that prepare adjudicated offenders for reentry into the specific communities to which they will return. Aftercare/reentry establishes the necessary arrangements with a range of public- and private-sector organizations and individuals in the community that can address known risk and protective factors,

The glossary was compiled from Center for Sex Offender Management Glossary of Terms Used in the Management and Treatment of Sexual Offenders: http://www.csom.org/pubs/glossary.pdf; Garner, B. (2004). *Black's law dictionary* (8th ed.). St. Paul, MN: Thomas West Group; and Merriam-Webster Online: http://www.merriam-webster.com.

419

and it ensures the delivery of prescribed services and supervision in the community.

Affidavit: A written document sworn under oath (e.g., Affidavit of Probable Cause)

Aggravated assault: A crime of physically attacking another person and causing serious bodily harm or assaulting another person with a deadly weapon such as a gun or knife.

Appeal: A formal request to a superior (appellate) court or administrative agency to review the decision of an inferior (trial or lower appellate) court or administrative agency.

Arraignment: An early step in the criminal process in which a defendant is formally charged with an offense and informed of his or her constitutional rights.

Assault: A crime that occurs when one person tries to physically harm another; actual physical contact is not necessary.

Bail: Release, prior to trial, of a person accused of a crime, with specified conditions designed to assure that the person will appear in court when required; also the amount of bond money posted as a financial condition of pretrial release.

Bench trial: Trial by a judge without a jury.

Best interest of the child: A standard used by child welfare agencies and child welfare courts when determining whether to undertake specific acts regarding a child.

Beyond a reasonable doubt: The amount of probability required to find a criminal defendant guilty.

Blunt force trauma: Injury caused by force from a blunt object, such as a baseball bat.

Bruise: An injury that causes ruptures of the small underlying vessels with resultant discoloration of tissues but that does not break the skin.

Case law: Law based on judicial opinions (including decisions that interpret statutes), as opposed to law based on statutes, regulations, or other sources. Also the collection of reported judicial decisions within a particular jurisdiction dealing with a specific issue or topic.

Child Abuse Prevention and Treatment Act (CAPTA). CAPTA was signed into law on January 31, 1974. The act emphasizes multidisciplinary approaches to child abuse and neglect.

Child Protective Services (CPS): The child welfare department/social service system designed to protect children. Usually the entity that receives and investigates reports of suspected child maltreatment and provides services to children and families to manage past maltreatment and prevent future maltreatment.

Child Welfare and Adoption Assistance Act (Public Law 96-272): A federal law passed in 1980 intended to prevent multiple foster care placements and increase effective permanency planning for children in foster care.

Child welfare court: The court that hears child welfare cases, including emergency removal, adjudication, disposition, review and termination of parental rights. States have different names for this court, including family court, juvenile court, and dependency court.

Circumstantial evidence: Evidence of a fact from which another fact can reasonably be inferred.

Civil commitment: Civil commitment is a process whereby a judge decides whether a person who is alleged to be mentally ill should be required to go to a psychiatric hospital or accept other mental health treatment.

Clear and convincing evidence: An amount of probability less than beyond a reasonable doubt but more than probable cause. It is used in some civil cases, including termination of parental rights cases and sex offender civil commitment hearings.

Collateral contacts: Contacts with significant others involved in a case or involved with the offender's life (family, teachers, etc.), to improve the effectiveness and quality of community supervision or for the purpose of completing an evaluation.

Commitment: Placement of a youth under the supervision of the juvenile justice system. Commitment dispositions range from low-risk nonresidential commitment to maximum residential commitment.

Common law: The system of jurisprudence (the form of law) that developed in England and came to the American colonies. Common law is derived and developed from the decisions of judges instead of statutes or constitutions.

Community notification: Laws that allow or mandate posting publicly accessible information, or actively informing the public about the identity and other personal information of an adjudicated sex offender.

Community service: A probation requirement that an offender perform some specific service to the community for a specified period of time.

Contempt of court: Behavior that violates a court order or otherwise disrupts or shows disregard for the court.

Coroner: A jurisdictional official, who is usually elected and whose duty it is to determine the cause and manner of sudden, unexpected, suspicious, or violent deaths. Education requirements vary by jurisdiction.

Coroner's inquest: An inquiry into the manner and cause of an individual's death, conducted by the coroner or deputy coroner.

Crime scene: The physical site where a crime may have occurred.

Culpable: Responsible for a wrong or error; accountable and liable.

Custody: Legal right to care and control of a child and the duty to provide that child's food, clothing, shelter, ordinary medical care, education, and discipline. Parents are the natural custodians of their child, but a court may grant temporary custody to someone other than a parent, pending further action or review by the court.

Defendant: In criminal proceedings, the person accused of a crime; synonymous with the accused. In civil proceedings, the party responding to the complaint brought by the plaintiff.

Dependency court: Specialized civil court designated to hear matters pertaining to child abuse/neglect.

Direct evidence: Evidence presented in the testimony of a witness who has direct knowledge of the fact being proved.

Disposition: The court's final determination in a case.

Disposition: In Child Protective Services, the finding of the validity of a report of child maltreatment that is made by the caseworker after investigation. Disposition categories vary from state to state.

Dispositional hearing: A juvenile case hearing at which the court determines the appropriate sanctions, such as probation, or commitment to the custody of the agency responsible for juvenile justice. It is analogous to a sentencing hearing in criminal court.

Disposition hearing: A court hearing that determines whether a child needs or requires the court's assistance, guidance, treatment or rehabilitation and, if so, the nature of that assistance, guidance, treatment, or rehabilitation.

Disposition review: A hearing in which the court reviews the child's case to ensure that a permanency plan is being implemented in the child's best interest.

Docket: Court calendar.

Due process of law: Peoples' rights under the 5th and 14th Amendments to the U.S. Constitution to procedural and substantive fairness in situations in which the government would deprive the person of life, liberty, or property.

Electronic monitoring: An automated method of determining compliance with community supervision restrictions through the use of electronic devices.

Evidence: Something that proves or disproves a fact.

Examination: The questioning of a witness.

Expungement: Destruction of records. Expungement may be ordered by a court after a specified number of years or when the juvenile, parent, or defendant applies for expungement and shows that his or her conduct has improved. Expungement also means the removal from the Central Registry of certain reports of abuse or neglect.

Family court: Court designated to hear matters pertaining to family law, such as child custody cases.

Family reunification: The process of reintroducing a youth back into the home after removal, preferably as part of the youth's treatment program.

Felony: Typically, any criminal offence for which the penalty is imprisonment for more than one year. Examples include murder, rape, and armed robbery (usually).

Felony murder: The unintentional killing of a human being during the commission of a felony, such as an armed robbery.

Forensic pathologist: A pathologist (physician) with training in criminal pathology.

Foster care: Placement for children under dependency court jurisdiction.

Guardian: An adult who is legally responsible for a child.

Guardian ad lItem: A person who has the legal authority (and the corresponding duty) to care for the personal and property interests of another person (often a child), called a ward.

Guilty: Responsible for a crime or a civil wrong.

Hearsay: Unverified information from a third party. Hearsay evidence is usually excluded from court proceedings, because it is considered unreliable and because the person making the original statement cannot be cross-examined.

Homicide: Death at the hands of another.

Hospital shopping: The use of different medical facilities so that each individual medical facility's sole contact with the person or family is involved with a single presenting injury.

Incarceration: Confinement in a secure correctional facility.

Incest: Sexual intercourse between persons who are closely related. This also includes other relatives, step-children, and children of common-law marriages.

Independent living: A permanent placement plan for a child in foster care in which the goal is self-sufficiency after discharge from foster care.

Indian Child Welfare Act (ICWA): A federal law that specifies the manner in which child welfare agencies and child welfare courts must handle cases involving Native American and Alaska Native Children.

Infanticide: The killing of one or more infants.

Investigation: The process of actively seeking facts. Investigations are typically conducted by law enforcement and/or child protective services in order to determine whether or not an offense was committed, but they can also be conducted by death investigators.

Involuntary manslaughter: Criminally negligent homicide.

Judgment: A court's final decision.

Jurisdiction: An agency's authority over an incident, investigation, and/or prosecution.

Juvenile: A youth who has not yet attained the age at which he or she should be treated us an adult for purposes of criminal law. Under the federal Juvenile Justice Delinquency Prevention Act, a "juvenile" means an individual who is 17 years of age or younger.

Kinship care (relative placement): Residential care-giving provided to children by nonparental relatives.

Laceration: A torn or jagged wound causing a splitting or tearing in the external skin surface that is caused by blunt trauma.

Late effects: Conditions or outcomes that may occur at any time after an acute intentional or unintentional injury.

Malice aforethought: The conscious intent to cause death or great bodily harm to another person before committing the offense.

Mandated agency: Agency designated by state law to receive and investigate reports of suspected child abuse and neglect.

Mandated reporters: Persons designated by state law who are legally responsible for reporting suspected child abuse and neglect to the mandated agency within their state. Mandated reporters are usually professionals who have frequent contact with children, such as physicians, nurses, school personnel, and social workers.

Manner of death: The official vital statistics classification: natural, suicide, homicide, accident, and undetermined.

Manslaughter: Unlawful killing of a person without malice aforethought.

Master: A person appointed by a court in certain cases to hear testimony and make reports that, if approved by the court, become the decision of the court. Masters may hear child welfare court cases. Also called referee or commissioner.

Mechanism of death: The process that causes one or more vital organs or organ systems to fail when a fatal disease, injury, abnormality, or chemical insult occurs; brain function that causes the heart and/or lungs to stop functioning. Examples include hemorrhage and hypovolemic shock.

Medical examiner: An official, usually a physician, whose duty it is to investigate sudden, suspicious, or violent death to determine the cause.

Megan's Law: The first amendment to the Jacob Wetterling Crimes Against Children and Sexually Violent Offenders Act. Megan's Law requires states to allow public access to information about sex offenders in the community. This law was named after Megan Kanka, a 7-year-old girl who was raped and murdered by a twice-convicted child molester in her New Jersey neighborhood.

Minimization: An attempt by the offender to downplay the extent and effect of his or her illegal behavior.

Misdemeanor: Criminal offenses that are less severe than felonies and generally punished by jail terms that do not exceed a year, or by lesser fines.

Murder: The unlawful killing of a human being with malice aforethought.

National Crime Information Center (NCIC): Criminal justice information systems operated by the Federal Bureau of Investigation in Washington, D.C.

Natural cause: Death resulting from inherent, existing conditions, including congenital anomalies, disease, sudden infant death syndrome (SIDS), and other medical causes.

Negligence: Doing something that a person of ordinary prudence would not do, or the failure to do something that a person of ordinary prudence would do, under given circumstances.

Noncontact offense: Sexual offenses that do not involve physical contact with the victim, such as indecent exposure, making obscene phone calls, and voyeurism.

Offense: A violation of federal, state, tribal, or municipal law, statute, or ordinance.

Parens patriae: "Parent of the country." The role of the state as sovereign and the guardian of persons under legal disability. Parens patriae allows the state to investigate possible child abuse and neglect, and to place a child in foster care.

Perjury: Knowingly and willfully giving false testimony under oath.

Perpetrator: Person who commits an act (usually a crime) against another.

Petition: A formal, written request to the court that it do something.

Physical evidence: Any tangible piece of proof. Physical evidence usually must be authenticated by a witness who testifies to the connection of the evidence (called an exhibit) with other facts of the case.

Plaintiff: In a civil case, the person who files a lawsuit.

Plea bargain: The negotiation of charges or dispositions in order to avoid trial on the original charge(s) in return for a guilty plea.

Pleadings: Formal allegations of the claim and defenses raised by the parties to the court case.

Preponderance of evidence: The proof must be more likely than not. The amount of proof required in most civil cases, including child welfare cases (except for termination of parental rights proceedings).

Prima facie: Evidence that will suffice as proof of the fact in issue until its effect is overcome by other evidence.

Probable cause: A requisite element of a valid search and seizure or of an arrest, which consists of the existence of facts and circumstances within one's knowledge that are sufficient to warrant the belief that a crime has been committed (in the context of an arrest).

Probation: A court-ordered disposition through which an adjudicated youth is placed under the control, supervision, and care of a probation field staff member in lieu of confinement, as long as the youth meets certain standards of conduct.

Prosecution: The act of pursuing a lawsuit or criminal trial, and the party initiating a criminal suit.

Recidivism: An officially detected recurrence of illegal behavior after a previous adjudication. Detections may include arrests, charges, convictions, child protection reports, and so on. There is no widely accepted definition of recidivism.

Reintegration: The gradual reentry from a restricted, highly supervised environment to a less structured environment.

Relapse: Complete or nearly complete return to a former problematic or illegal behavior. Distinguished from reoffense in that it involves both illegal and inappropriate events, and from recidivism in that it involves both detected and undetected events.

Relapse prevention: A cognitive-behavioral intervention model for risk management that considers internal self-management and external supervision in regard to precipitating and perpetuating factors such as risk situations and risk-related cognitions. This treatment program teaches clients to identify chains of risk factors, thinking patterns, and behavioral and cognitive sequences in order to identify and disrupt offense patterns.

Restitution: Repairing harm caused by a behavior. Restitution may be to the victim (apology, small monetary amount) or community (community service).

Restorative justice: Focuses on the repair of the harm to the victim and the community, as well as the improvement of prosocial competencies of the offender, as a result of a damaging act. Dispositions are focused on restitution and competency development rather than being exclusively punitive.

Reunification: A well-supervised, gradual procedure in which an adolescent sex offender is reintegrated back into the home where children are present.

Risk assessment: The process of assigning a probability for a future behavior, such as a sexual offense, to an individual.

Sanctions: Penalty, punishment, loss of reward, or coercive intervention connected to a violation of a law or rule as a means of enforcement.

Search warrant: An order issued by a judge and directing certain law enforcement officers to conduct a search of specified premises for specified things or persons and to bring them before the court. Search warrants are required by the 4th and 14th Amendments to the U.S. Constitution.

Sex offender registration: Laws requiring sex offenders to submit and keep current certain personal identifying information, such as photographs and current addresses, for purposes of maintaining a list of registered sex offenders in the community. Sex offender registration laws may or may not apply to adolescents, and different states have different inclusion criteria and provisions for adolescents. Registration may or may not involve public notification or public access, depending upon the jurisdiction.

Standard of proof: An amount of probability necessary for the court to render a decision regarding the evidence presented to it. There are three different standards: (a) Beyond a reasonable doubt, (b) Preponderance of the evidence, and (c) Reasonable degree of certainty.

Status offense: Acts that violate the law but only for individuals with juvenile status, such as underage drinking.

Statute: A law passed by a legislative body.

Subpoena: A command to appear at a certain time and place, on a certain date, and give testimony on a certain matter.

Summons: A document used to commence a civil action or special processing. A summons is issued by a court to the sheriff (or other designated official), requiring them to notify the person named that an action has been commenced against the person and that the person is required to appear on a day named and answer the complaint.

Termination of parental rights (TPR): A legal process that severs the legal relationship between parents and the child and vests authority in the child welfare agency.

Testimony: Evidence given by a competent witness under oath or affirmation, as distinguished from evidence derived from written or other sources.

Venue: Locality of the court or courts that possess jurisdiction.

Victims of crime fund: Money available to serve crime victims through a federal and/or state program.

Voluntary manslaughter: An intentional killing committed under circumstances that, although they do not justify the homicide, mitigate it.

Index

A

AARP. *See* American Association of Retired Persons
AAS. *See* Abuse Assessment Screen
AAS-D. *See* Abuse Assessment Screen-Disability
AASI-2. *See* Abel Assessment for Sexual Interest
Abel Assessment for Sexual Interest (AASI-2), 329
Abrasions, 24, 25, 134
Abuse Assessment Screen (AAS), 127
Abuse Assessment Screen-Disability (AAS-D), 127
Abusive parents, 297–304
  assessment of, 299–302
  CAPTA and, 297
  child abuse fatalities and, 299, 300
  etiology of, 299
  history/physical assessment/diagnostic testing of, 301–302
  intervention, 302
  PP and, 300–301
  prevalence of, 298–299
  prevention, 302–304
Abusive Relationships Inventory (ARI), 291–292
Actual Abuse Tool, 156
Actuarial risk assessments, 257
  MnSOST-R, 326, 327–328
  RRASOR/VRAG/SORAG/Acute 2007/Stable 2007, 328
  Static-99, 326–327
  Static 2002, 326, 327
Acute 2007 risk assessment, 328
Acute Stress Disorder (ASD), 89–90, 98

Acute Stress Disorder Interview (ASDI), 90
Acute Stress Disorder Scale (ASDS), 90
ADA. *See* Americans with Disabilities Act
ADHD. *See* Attention deficit hyperactivity disorder
Adult
  disabled, victimization of, 103–116
  forensics, 3–4
  IPV in, 4–6, 16–17, 87–88, 94, 99, 117–129, 237, 285–295, 347, 355
  survivors, of child sexual abuse, 4
  victimization effect on, 85–101
Adult perpetrators, of sexual violence, 315–335
  assessment of, 325–330
  etiology of, 325
  intervention, 330–333
  prevalence of, 324–325
  prevention, 333–334
  risk assessment of, 326–330
  sexual offense pathways, 315–320
  theories on reasons for, 325
Adult Protective Services (APS)
  mandatory reporting of elder abuse to, 135, 155, 163, 195, 310
  sexual assault of elder and, 192, 195
Advocacy
  for elder victims, of sexual assault, 196
  for male victims, of sexual assault, 186
  persons with disabilities, limited, 105
  for rape care, 178
  victim center for, 126
Aggravated Sexual Assault, 168

Alaskan Native, 10, 231
Alcohol
    CAGE questionnaire for use of,
      240–241
    IPV and, 287
Alcohol abuse, 236. *See also* Substance
    abuse
    of adult survivors of child sexual
      abuse, 4
    driving skills influence by, 238
    legal limit and, 238
Alcohol Use Disorders Identification
    (AUDIT) screening tool, 240
Alio, A., 88
Alzheimer's Association, 107, 108
Alzheimer's disease, 62
    Safe Return Program for, 107
    victims with, responding to, 107–108
Amar, A., 176
American Association of Retired Persons
    (AARP), 155, 163
American Disabilities Act, 103
American Indian, 10, 231
American Psychiatric Association (APA)
    DSM-IV-TR of, 89–90, 91, 245,
      247, 248, 316–319, 358, 360,
      399–404
    Practice Guideline for the Treatment
      of Patients with Acute Stress
      Disorder and Posttraumatic
      Stress Disorder of, 98
    PTSD revision, in *DSM-IV-TR*, 91
American Sign Language (ASL), 112,
    114
American Society of Addiction Medicine,
    240
Americans with Disabilities Act (ADA)
    (1990), 105, 111, 114
Anderson, L., 189
Angott, D., 88
AniCare Model of Treatment for Animal
    Abuse, 360
Animal cruelty, 351–363
    animal sexual abuse, 352, 354
    child abuse connection with, 355
    cock fighting, 352–353
    elder abuse connection with, 355–356

etiology, 354–356
    history/physical assessment/diagnostic
      testing of, 357–359
    hoarding, 352, 357, 360
    hog-dog fight, 353
    human violence v., 354–356
    intervention, 359–361
    in IPV, 118, 355
    mandatory reporting, lack of, 125
    need to address, 356–357
    neglect, 351–352
    organized dog fighting, 353
    prevalence of, 354
    prevention, 361
    zoophilia, 358
Antisocial pathway, to sexual offending,
    319
Antisocial personality disorder, 4, 248,
    256, 319, 338
APA. *See* American Psychiatric
    Association
APS. *See* Adult Protective Services
ARI. *See* Abusive Relationships
    Inventory
Arrest
    female offender prior, 343
    Miranda warning, 44–45
    postarrest and, 45–46
    probable cause and, 44
    sex offender rearrest, 324
ASDI. *See* Acute Stress Disorder
    Interview
ASDS. *See* Acute Stress Disorder Scale
ASL. *See* American Sign Language
Association for the Treatment of Sexual
    Abusers (ATSA), 331
ATSA. *See* Association for the Treatment
    of Sexual Abusers
Attention deficit hyperactivity disorder
    (ADHD), 256
AUDIT. *See* Alcohol Use Disorders
    Identification
Autoerotic Asphyxia, 399–404
    assessment of, 401–403
    criteria for death determination, 402
    death, 399
    etiology, 400–401

history/physical assessment of, 401–403
intervention, 403
physical signs of, 402
prevalence, 400
prevention, 403
Avoidant personality disorder, 338

B
Baker, T., 192, 195
Bartholomew, K., 140, 144
BASE. *See* Brief Abuse Screen for the Elderly
Battering. *See* Intimate Partner Violence, of adults
Baum, K., 218
Beck, A.J., 183
Behavioral Risk Factor Surveillance System (BRFSS), 131
Bipolar disorder, 249, 303
Birnbaum, B., 185
Bite marks, 28–29, 41
BLS. *See* Bureau of Labor Statistics
Blunt force trauma, 124
    abrasions, 24, 25, 134
    contusions, 24, 25–27
    lacerations, 24, 27–28, 87, 134
Body identification, 384–385
Body injury. *See also* Personal injury victim
    bite marks, 28–29
    blunt force trauma and, 24, 25, 124, 134
    gunshot wounds, 29–30, 39
    morphology/severity/mechanism classifications of, 210
    patterned injury and, 24, 124
    penetrating, 212
    types of, 24–25
Bonomi, A., 131
BOP. *See* Bureau of Prisons
Borderline personality disorder, 249, 256
BRFSS. *See* Behavioral Risk Factor Surveillance System
Brief Abuse Screen for the Elderly (BASE), 156
Bryant, R. A., 90

Btoush, R., 122, 128
Bureau of Justice Statistics, 254
    on convicted sex offenders, 324
    on IPV, 120, 286
    on prisoners, 266
    prison inmate crimes for drugs, 236
    on recidivism rates, of prisoners, 260
    on women prisoners, 342
Bureau of Labor Statistics (BLS), on homicides in health services, 66
Bureau of Prisons (BOP), Federal, 265, 270, 276
Burgess, A. W., 171, 192, 195, 402
Burnout, 76, 332

C
CAGE questionnaire, for alcohol use, 240–241
CAI. *See* Competency Assessment Instrument
Campbell, J., 87–88, 122, 128, 170
CAPTA. *See* Child Abuse Prevention and Treatment Act
Caregiver Abuse Screen (CASE), 156
Caregiver stress, 310, 319
    elder abuse, by family member and, 148–149, 150
    respite care for, 114
CASE. *See* Caregiver Abuse Screen
Catalano, S., 218
CBOs. *See* Community-based organizations
CBT. *See* Cognitive-behavioral therapy
CDC. *See* Centers for Disease Control and Prevention
Center for Sex Offender Management (CSOM), 330–331
    ABC approach to individual stress management, 78–80
Centers for Disease Control and Prevention (CDC), 3, 210
    IPV definition by, 117–118
    on post-sexual assault medications, 178
    on suicide, 392
Chain of custody, 178
    evidence and, 37–38

Locard's Exchange Principle, 38
   photography and, 33
   rules of evidence and, 37–38
Child abuse/neglect, 4
   adult survivors of sexual, 4
   animal cruelty connection with, 355
   CAPTA definition of, 297
   fatalities, 299, 300
   mandatory reporting for, 125, 302
   prevention, 7
   sexual abuser and, 320–321, 323
   substance abuse consequence of, 85
Child Abuse Prevention and Treatment
   Act (CAPTA), 297
Child Maltreatment 2007, 298–299
Children
   with disabilities, 104
   of incarcerated female offenders, 344
   IPV exposure to, 118–119
   violence exposure to, 5
Circumstantial evidence, 36
Civil commitment, 59, 333
CJ. *See* Criminal justice system
Class evidence, 35
Clinical assessments, 21, 257
Clinical judgment, for reoffending of sex
   offenders, 328–330
   AASI-2/PPG, 329
   polygraph, 329–330
Coalition to Eliminate the Abuse of
   Seniors, 6
Cock fighting, 352–353
Cognitive-behavioral therapy (CBT), for
   hoarding, 360
Cognitive dysfunction/impairment, 77
   MMSE to screen for, 149
   MR/learning disorders/organic brain
     syndrome, 250
   offenders with, 245–252
   sexual assault of elders and, 193
Collateral evidence, 36
Commission on Safety and Abuse in
   America's Prisons, 268
The Commonwealth of Pennsylvania v.
   John Smith, 47
Community-based organizations (CBOs),
   228–229

Community notification laws, on sex
   offender, 333
Community nursing, for older adults, 136
Compassionate Friends, 408
Compassion fatigue, 75
Competency, 59
   cultural, 18–20
   evaluation, 62–64
   fiduciary/tetamentary/criminal, 59–60
   of offender, 245
   to proceed, 245–246
   restoration of, 64
Competency Assessment Instrument
   (CAI), 246
Competency Screening Test (CST), 246
Competency to stand trial (CST),
   245–246
Complicated mourning, 406
Comprehensive National Survey, on chil-
   dren's exposure to violence, 5
Confidentiality, 21, 95, 208, 331
Conflict management, nonviolent strategies for, 7
Consent
   to collect forensic evidence, 24
   for photography, 31
Control tactics, of IPV perpetrators,
   287–288
Contusions, 24, 25–27
Coroner/medical examiner systems,
   374–375
Correctional facilities. *See also* Incar-
   ceration; Prisoner
   BOP operation of, 265
   offenders in, 265–273
Corso, P., 99
Counseling
   elder victims of sexual assault referral
     to, 196
   homicide survivor referrals to, 410
   male victims of sexual assault referral
     to, 189
   reasons for, 227–228
Court appearances, tips for, 57
Court appointed experts, 53
Crime, persons with disabilities underreporting of, 105

Crime laboratory, specimen analysis
by, 35
Criminal acts
animal cruelty and, 356
disability resulting from, 104, 106
Criminal competency, 21, 59–60
Criminal justice-based services, 229–231
Criminal justice (CJ) system
elder sexual abuse cases and, 195
juvenile, 7
navigation of, 43–48
offender path in, 43–47
substance abuse screening in,
241–242
victim path of, 47–48
victim services through, 227
Cross-contamination, of evidence, 178
CSOM. *See* Center for Sex Offender
Management
CST. *See* Competency Screening Test;
Competency to stand trial
Cultural aspects, of forensics, 9–20
female reproduction and, 13–15
grieving process and, 406
illness treatment practices, 15–16
immigration status, 10–11
Cultural competency, of health care
providers, 18–20
Culture
death rituals of, 381–382
human trafficking and, 17–18
IPV and, 16–17
Culture-bound syndromes, 11–13
Curriculum vitas (CVs), 50–51
CVs. *See* Curriculum vitas
Cycle of violence, 3–8
interventions, 7
in IPV, of adults, 120–121

D
Damages, compensatory/punitive,
209–210
DAST. *See* Drug Abuse Screening Test
"Date rape," 23, 179–180
Daubert test, for scientific evidence, 54
*Daubert v. Merrell Dow Pharmaceuti-
cals*, 54

Dauvergne, M., 5
Day treatment programs, for older
adults, 136
Death. *See also* Deaths of elders, in
LTC facility; Medicolegal death
investigation
of elder, in LTC facility, 387–390
investigation, 374–375
review teams, 385
rituals, 381–382
signs of, 375–376
*Death Investigation: A Guide for the
Scene Investigator*, 376
Deaths of elders, in LTC facility,
387–390
assessment of, 388–389
etiology of, 388
intervention, 389
prevalence of, 387–388
prevention, 389–390
Decedent profile information, 379–380
Dementia, 255
IPV, of older adults and, 132, 136–137
sexual assault of elders and, 193
Department of Health and Human
Services Administration of Children,
Youth and Families, 298
Department of Health and Human Services National Human Trafficking
Resource Center, 205
Department of Justice (DOJ)
Bureau of Justice Statistics of, 120, 236,
254, 260, 266, 286, 324, 342
National Crime Victimization Survey
of, 67
on parole/probation, 276
Depression, 77
adult survivors, of child sexual abuse
and, 4
of male victim, 4, 6
recent abuse influence on, 86
Developmental disabilities, 104
offenders with, 248
victims with, responding to, 109–114
*Diagnostic and Statistical Manual of
Mental Disorders (DSM-IV-TR)*,
245, 247

ASD criteria of, 89–90, 98
autoerotic asphyxia, 399–404
culture-bound syndromes in, 11–13
paraphilias criteria of, 316–319,
   399–404
psychopathology, 248
PTSD criteria of, 91
Diagrams, documentation and, 30
Differential diagnosis, elder abuse and,
   154
Direct evidence, 36
Direct examination, in trial, 56
Disabled adults, victimization of,
   103–116
DNA analysis, 35, 41, 188–189
   for body identification, 384
   in sexual assaults, 177–178
Documentation, 174–175
   diagrams in, 30
   forensic assessment and, 30–34
   of injury, in sexual assault, 178, 188
   narrative report, 30
   photography and, 31–33
   in stalking, 223–224
   of trauma, 210
Dog fighting, organized, 353
DOJ. *See* Department of Justice
Domestic violence. *See* Intimate Partner
   Violence
Draper, B., 85
Driving under the influence (DUI), 237
   alcohol legal limit and, 238
   mandatory screening/assessment of, 241
Driving while intoxicated (DWI), 236
Drug Abuse Screening Test (DAST), 241
"Druggist-style" envelope, for evidence
   collection, 41
*DSM-IV-TR. See Diagnostic and Statistical
   Manual of Mental Disorders*
DUI. *See* Driving under the influence
Durose, M., 324
Dusky v. U.S., 246
DWI. *See* Driving while intoxicated

E

EAI. *See* Elder Assessment Instrument
EAP. *See* Employee Assistance Program

Edinburgh Postnatal Depression Scale
   (EPDS), 301
Eighth Amendment, 265
Elder. *See also* Older adult
   death of, in LTC facility, 387–390
   incestuous abuse of, 192
   sexual assault of, 191–198
   suicide of, 392
Elder abuse, 4–5
   animal cruelty connection with,
     355–356
   by caregivers, 308
   caregiver stress and, 114, 310, 319
   etiology of, 148–149
   forensic assessment for, 22, 161
   legal assistance for, 155
   mandatory reporting of, 135, 155, 163,
     195, 310
   mortality rates of, 6
   perpetrators of, 305–313
   physical/mental impairment of patient
     and, 148
   as public health issue, 6
   RRA, 192, 308–309
Elder abuse, by family members,
     147–157, 307–308
   abuser psychopathology and, 148
   assessment of, 149–154
   caregiver stress and, 148–149, 150
   diagnostic testing, 154
   differential diagnosis and, 154
   financial exploitation, 148, 153–154
   history/physical assessment in, 149–151
   intervention, 155
   neglect/self-neglect, 147, 152–153
   physical abuse, 147, 151–152
   prevalence of, 148
   prevention, 155–156
   psychological/emotional abuse, 147,
     150–151
   sexual abuse, 148, 152, 192
   transgenerational violence and, 148,
     149
   types of, 147–148
Elder abuse, by health care workers,
     159–166
   assessment of, 161–162

etiology of, 160–161
facility characteristics, 161, 162
intervention, 162–163
physical condition of patient,
      161–162
prevalence of, 160
prevention, 163–165
specific markers for elder abuse in
      facilities, 161
types of, 159–161
Elder Assessment Instrument (EAI),
      156
Emergency Department (ED), 394
IPV code of, 122, 128
practitioners, forensic science and, 4
Emotional abuse
of elder, by family member, 147,
      150–151
in IPV, 99, 118
Emotional dysregulation pathway, to
      sexual offending, 316
Employee Assistance Program (EAP),
      for stress management, 80
EPDS. *See* Edinburgh Postnatal Depres-
      sion Scale
Estelle v. Gamble, 265
Evidence, 24, 31, 35–42. *See also*
      Scientific evidence; Trace
      evidence
chain of custody and, 37–38
circumstantial, 36
class, 35
collateral, 36
collection, 38–41, 177–178, 188–189,
      223–224
cross-contamination of, 178
eyewitness testimony, 36
observation and, 37
preservation of, 4
principles of, 36–38
Exhibitionism, 316, 317–318
Expert witness testimony, 49–57
qualifications for, 50–51
rules of evidence for, 52–53
subpoena for, 49
Exposure to violence, of children, 5
Eyewitness testimony, 36, 49

F
Faith-based organizations (FBOs), 229,
      262
Family members, elder abuse by,
      147–157, 307–308
Family Violence Prevention Fund, on
      IPV assessment, 124, 134
Fazel, S., 337
FBI. *See* Federal Bureau of Investigation
FBI's Crime Classification Manual, rape
      classifications of, 321–322
FBOs. *See* Faith-based organizations
Federal Bureau of Investigation (FBI)
background checks by, 164
Identification Record, 165
National/State Sex Offender Registry,
      333
Federal Bureau of Prisons Clinical
      Practice Guidelines for the Man-
      agement of Methicillin-Resistant
      Staphylococcus aureus (MRSA)
      Infections, 270
Federal Interagency Forum on Ageing
      Statistics, 387
Federal Rules of Evidence, 31, 52
Felony conviction, 277–278
Female Genital Mutilation (FGM),
      13–14
Female offenders, 341–349
children of incarcerated, 344
diagnostic testing of, 345
etiology of, 343
history/physical assessment of,
      344–345
intervention, 346–348
IPV and, 4–6, 288–289, 347
mental health/substance abuse of,
      347–348
past physical/sexual abuse of, 343
poverty/prior arrest of, 343
prevalence of, 342–343
prevention, 348
probation/parole of, 345
prostitution and, 341–453
PTSD of, 347
substance abuse and, 343, 347–348
women's health of, 346

Female perpetrators, of IPV, 288–289
Female reproduction, cultural customs
    related to, 13–15
Female sex offender, 323–324, 330
Female victims, of sexual assault,
    167–182
Fetal development, physical effects of
    violence on, 88
Fetishism, 316
FGM. *See* Female Genital Mutilation
Fiduciary competency, 59–60
Fifth Amendment, 44, 45
Financial abuse
    of elder, by family member, 148,
       153–154
    in IPV, 99, 118
Finkelstein, E., 99
Flinck, A., 142
Flynn, C., 356
Force amount, in body injury, 24
Foreign body ingestions, by prisoners,
    270–271
Forensic assessment
    autopsy in, 381
    confidentiality, lack of, 21
    consent and, 24
    documentation and, 30–34
    for elder abuse, by health care
       providers, 161
    etiology of, 22
    general principles of, 22
    interview, 22–24
    objectivity of, 21
    physical examination for, 24–30,
       124, 142–143, 149–152, 187–188,
       194–195, 204, 210–211, 239, 291,
       301–302, 309–310, 344–346,
       357–359, 367, 394–396, 401–403
    toxicology screening in, 177, 188
Forensics
    adult/older adult, 3–4
    cultural aspects of, 9–20, 406
Fourteenth Amendment right to due
    process, 246
Fourth Amendment, 44
Frotteurism, 316, 318
Frye rule, for scientific evidence, 54

G
Garza, V., 203
Gay Men's Domestic Violence Project,
    on IPV of LGBT, 140–141
General Duty Clause, of OSH Act, 66
Gennaro, S., 176
Gilmer, T., 94
Grandparents, raising children of incar-
    cerated parents, 368–369
Grieving
    family member grief work and,
       409–410
    grief reactions, of homicide survivor,
       406–407
    psychological/physical symptoms of, 410
    Worden tasks of, 407–408
Groth, N., 185, 402
Groth's Typology for Child Sexual Abus-
    ers (1979), 320–321
Groth's Typology for Rapists (1978),
    321
Guardianship, 59
    court appointed, 61
    guardian ad litem/guardian of the
       person/conservator, 60
    power of attorney and, 61
Gunshot wounds, 29–30, 39
Gynecological problems, from IPV,
    87–88

H
HALF. *See* Health, Attitudes Toward
    Aging, Living Arrangements, and
    Finances
Hall, R., 88
Hanrahan, N.P., 192, 195
Harrison, P.M., 183
Harvey, A. G., 90
Hazelwood, B., 402
HCR-20. *See* Historical, Clinical, and
    Risk Management checklist
Health, Attitudes Toward Aging, Living
    Arrangements, and Finances
    (HALF), 156
Health care
    of offender, in community, 277
    for prisoner, 265–266

Health care providers
  assault injury rates of, 66–67
  burnout of, 76, 332
  compassion fatigue of, 75
  cultural competency of, 18–20
  elder development of trust by, 194
  as expert witness, 49
  role of, 7–8
  traditional stress of, 74–75
  vicarious traumatization of, 75–76
Health care settings
  assessment of violence in, 68
  BLS on homicides in, 66
  IPV offenders and, 70
  prevention/patient teaching on violence in, 69–70
  substance abuse screening in, 240–241
  violence in, 65–71, 74
Health problem
  of violence, 3, 4–7
  of women victims, 6
Health problem, of prisoner, 4
  foreign body ingestions, 270–271
  infectious disease, 268–270
  reproductive problems, 271
  TBI, 267–268
Healthy People 2010, 140
Helping Patients Who Drink Too Much: A Clinician's Guide, 241–242
  AUDIT screening tool, 240
Hepatitis, 4
  B vaccine, post-sexual assault and, 178–179
Hewlett, J.B., 67
Historical, Clinical, and Risk Management checklist (HCR-20), 258
Histrionic personality disorder, 249, 256
HITS Domestic Violence Screening Tool, 127
HIV. *See* Human immunodeficiency virus
Hoarding, animal cruelty and, 352, 357, 360
Holstrom, L.L., 171
Homicide, 3
  bereavement, 382
  female, IPV and, 4–6
  intent, 246
  IPV and, 120, 286
  males as victims of, 6
  mercy/hero of elderly, 160
Homicide survivors, 405–411
  etiology, 406
  grief reactions of, 406–407
  intervention, 409–410
  parents of children, 408–409
  PTSD of, 406, 408, 409
  suicidal ideation of, 407
Hope, T., 337
H-S/EAST. *See* Hwalek-Sengstock Elder Abuse Screening Test
Hudson, S., 319
Humane Society of the United States, 354
Human immunodeficiency virus (HIV), 4, 6, 62, 268–269, 271
  from IPV, 87
  post-sexual assault treatment, 178
  sexual assault and, 189
Human trafficking, victims of, 199–207
  assessment, 201–204
  culture and, 17–18
  diagnostic testing, 204
  etiology of, 200–201
  force/fraud/coercion in, 201
  general principles of, 201–202
  health issues in, 202
  history, 202–204
  intervention, 204–205
  physical assessment, 204
  prevalence of, 200
  prevention, 205
  screening questions for, 203–204
  sex/labor, 199
  STI screening for, 204
  victim identification and, 203
Hwalek-Sengstock Elder Abuse Screening Test (H-S/EAST), 156
Hybrid test, for scientific evidence, 54
Hynes, P., 204

I

ICD. *See* Impulse-control disorder
Identification Record, of FBI, 165

Illness treatment, 15–16
Immigration
  consultant fraud, 18
  human trafficking and, 204
Immigration and Naturalization Service
  (INS), 18
Immigration status
  culture and, 10–11
  deportation fear and, 16–17
  IPV and, 17
  VAWA and, 17
Impairment, conditions of, 61–62
  mental retardation/autism, 62
  progressive diseases, 62, 63
  sudden-onset diseases/abrupt impair-
    ments, 62
Impulse-control disorder (ICD), 357
Incarceration. *See also* Correctional
    facilities; Offender; Prisoner
  parenting programs for females, 347
  parenting while, 365–370
  poverty correlation with, 277
  of pregnant inmates, 346
Incestuous abuse, of elders, 148, 152,
  192
Incremental Risk Reduction, for released
  prisoners, 272
Indecent Assault/Contact/Exposure, 168
Indicators of Abuse (IOA) Screen, 156
Individual evidence, of fingerprints/
  DNA/tool marks/footprints, 35, 41,
  177–178, 188–189, 384
Individual stress management, 78–79.
  See also Professional stress
  COSM ABC approach to, 78–80
Infection of offender, in community, 280
Infectious diseases, of prisoners, 4,
  268–270
  HIV, 268–269
  MRSA, 270
  respiratory-borne diseases, 270
  STIs, 269
  TB, 269
Informed consent, 331
INS. *See* Immigration and Naturalization
  Service
Insanity defense, *DSM-IV-TR* and, 247

Interpersonal violence offenders (IPV).
  See Intimate Partner Violence
Intervention
  for cycle of violence, 7
  psychotherapeutic/psychoeducational,
    106
Intimacy deficits pathway, to sexual
  offending, 316
Intimate Partner Violence (IPV), of
    adults. *See also* Perpetrators, of IPV
  alcohol, 287
  animal cruelty connection with, 118,
    355
  assessment of, 121–124
  CDC definition of, 117–118
  children exposed to, 118–119
  control of partner and, 287
  culture and, 16–17
  cycle of violence and, 120–121
  diagnostic testing in, 124
  ED code for, 122, 128
  emotional/financial/physical/verbal
    abuse, 99, 117, 118
  etiology of, 120–121
  Family Violence Prevention Fund for,
    124
  female and, 4–6, 288–289, 347
  general principles for, 121–122
  gynecological problems from, 87–88
  history of, 122–123
  HIV from, 87
  homicide and, 4–6, 120, 286
  intervention, 125–126
  JCAHO hospital requirements on, 125
  against males, 6, 120
  mandatory reporting in, 122, 135
  offenders, health care settings and, 70
  perpetrators of, 285–295
  physical assessment during, 124
  physical effects, on women, 87–88
  prevalence of, 119–120
  prevention, 126–128
  property destruction, 118
  PTSD and, 88
  SAFE screening tool for, 127
  safety plan for, 122, 125, 135
  screening methods for, 127–128

stalking as feature of, 118, 221–222
substance abuse and, 132, 136–137, 237
theories of, 286–287
violence of both partners in, 120
WHO on social/economic costs of, 94
Intimate Partner Violence (IPV), of
LGBT, 139–145, 289
assessment of, 141–143
etiology of, 140–141
intervention, 143–144
perpetrators abuse forms in, 143
physical assessment of, 142–143
power/control and, 140
prevalence of, 139–140
prevention, 144
Intimate Partner Violence (IPV), of older
adults, 131–138
assessment for, 133–134
dementia/substance abuse and, 132,
136–137
diagnostic testing of, 134
etiology of, 132
intervention, 134–136
mandatory reporting of, 135
mental capacity and, 136
prevalence of, 131–132
prevention, 136–137
skin/mucous membranes and,
133–134
Involuntary Deviant Sexual Intercourse,
167, 168
IOA. *See* Indicators of Abuse Screen
IPV. *See* Interpersonal violence offenders;
Intimate partner violence
Isolation, of persons with disabilities, 105

J
Jacoby, R., 337
Joint Commission on Accreditation
of Healthcare Organizations
(JCAHO), on IPV hospital policies,
125

K
Kangaspunta, K., 200–201
Keeping Children and Families Safe Act
(2003), 297

Kothari, C.L., 128
Kuffner, C.A., 189

L
Labor trafficking, 199
Lacerations, 24, 27–28, 87, 134
Lachs, M., 308, 309
Langan, P., 324
Lascivious Acts, 168
Law enforcement professional
evidence and, 37
forensic interview and, 23
Learned behavior, violence as, 5, 7
Legal assistance, for abused elders, 155
Legal proceedings. *See also* Trial
CST for, 246
health care sciences and, 3
Lesbian/gay/bisexual/transsexual
(LGBT), 10
IPV of, 139–145, 289
Levin, P.F., 67
Levine, J., 86
LGBT. *See* Lesbian/gay/bisexual/transsexual
Lindbloom, E., 161
Litigation, personal injury, 208
Locard, Edmund, 38
Locard's Exchange Principle, 38
Lockwood, R., 358
Logan, T., 126
Long-term care (LTC) facility, 159
deaths of elders in, 387–390
RRA and, 308–309
selection of, 163–164
sexual assault, of elders, 192
Long-term offenders, 259–263
intervention, 261–262
prevalence of, 260
recidivism of, 260–261
Long-term problems, of children exposed
to IPV, 119
LTC. *See* Long-term care
Lussler, R., 67

M
MacArthur Violence Risk Assessment
Study, 255
Maladaptive behaviors, 77

Male
gang violence and, 86
suicide rates of, 6
survivors of violence, 6
violence effect, against adult, 86
Male victims
depression/antisocial personality
disorder of, 4
of homicide, 6
of IPV, 6, 120
National Center for Victims of Crime
on, 86
of sexual assault, 183–190
Mandatory reporting
animal cruelty, lack of, 125
of child abuse, 125, 302
of elder abuse, 135, 155, 163, 195,
310
of IPV, 122, 135
sexual assault, female victims of, lack
of, 177
Manic-depressive disorder, 249
Masho, S., 189
MAST. *See* Michigan Alcohol Screening
Test
Matthews, J., 324
Matthews, R., 324
McCann, J., 219
McMann v. Richardson, 46
MDQ. *See* Mood Disorder Questionnaire
Measurement tools, for ASD, 90
Mechanism of injury (MOI), 210
Medicolegal death investigation,
373–385
body identification and, 384–385
cause of death and, 373
coroner/medical examiner systems,
374–375
culture/death rituals, 381–382
death, signs of, 375–376
death review teams, 385
family notification, 382–384
forensic autopsy, 381
manner of death and, 374
mechanism of death, 374
scene investigation, 376–381

Meiz, K., 144
Menstruation, cultural practices and, 15
Mental capacity in IPV, of older adults,
136
Mental illness. *See also Diagnostic
and Statistical Manual of Mental
Disorders*
crime victim and, 247
dementia, 132, 136–137, 193, 255
depression, 4, 6, 77, 86
ODD, 256
of offender, in community, 278–279
offender with, 245–252
personality disorders, 4, 248, 249,
255–256, 319, 338
of victims/prisoners, 4
victim with, responding to, 108–109
Mental retardation (MR), 62, 250, 256
Mental state at the time of the offense
(MSO), 245
Mental status exam (MSE), 246, 247
Mercy, J., 99
Mercy/hero homicides, 160
Methicillin-resistant staphylococcus
aureus (MRSA), 270
Michigan Alcohol Screening Test
(MAST), 241
Mini-Mental Status Examination
(MMSE), 149
Minnesota Sex Offender Screening Tool
(MnSOST-R), 326, 327–328
Miranda v. Arizona, 45
Miranda warning, 44–45, 245
MMSE. *See* Mini-Mental Status
Examination
MnSOST-R. *See* Minnesota Sex
Offender Screening Tool
MOI. *See* Mechanism of injury
Monahan, J., 255
Mood Disorder Questionnaire (MDQ),
301
Morphology of injury, 210
Mortality rates, of physically abused
elders, 6, 148
MR. *See* Mental retardation
MRSA. *See* Methicillin-resistant staphy-
lococcus aureus

MSE. *See* Mental status exam
MSO. *See* Mental state at the time of the offense
Mullen, P., 219–220
Multiple dysfunctional mechanism pathway, to sexual offending, 315–316
Murder. *See* Homicide

N

Nana, P., 88
Narcissistic personality disorder, 249, 256
Narrative report, 30
National Association of Crime Victim Compensation Boards, on state eligibility requirements, 100
National Center for PTSD, on PTSD screening tools, 91–93
National Center for Victims of Crime
on male victims, 86
on sexual assault, 167–168
simple obsessional/love obsessional/erotomanic stalkers typology of, 218
on stalking behaviors, 221
National Child Abuse and Neglect Data System (NCANDS), 298
National Child Abuse Hotline, 205
National Clearinghouse on Abuse in Later Life, 131
National Coalition of Anti-Violence Programs (NCAVP), 140, 142
National Crime Victimization Survey (NCVS), of DOJ, 67, 236, 254–255
National Domestic Violence Hotline, 205
National Institute for Occupational Safety and Health (NIOSH), 65, 74
National Institute of Alcohol Abuse and Alcoholism (NIAAA), *Helping Patients Who Drink Too Much: A Clinician's Guide* of, 240, 241–242
National Institute of Justice
on elder mistreatment, 161–162
on prisoner reentry, 261–262
on prostitution, 341
National Protocol for Sexual Assault Medical Forensic Examinations, 168–169

injury documentation/evidence collection in, 174–175
male victims guidelines of, 186
on physical examination of male victims, of sexual assault, 187–188
sexual assault information of, 172–174
National Respite Locator, 115
National Sexual Assault Hotline, 205
National/State Sex Offender Registry, of FBI, 333
National Survey on Drug Use and Health, on DUI, 237
National Violence Against Women Survey (NVAWS), 168
National Violent Death Reporting System, 392
NCANDS. *See* National Child Abuse and Neglect Data System
NCAVP. *See* National Coalition of Anti-Violence Programs
NCVS. *See* National Crime Victimization Survey
Neglect
of animals, 351–352
of elder, by family member, 147, 152–153
of elder person, 152–153
signs of, 152–153
Negligence, 209–210
NGRI. *See* "Not guilty by reason of insanity"
NIAAA. *See* National Institute of Alcohol Abuse and Alcoholism
NIOSH. *See* National Institute for Occupational Safety and Health
Nonviolence strategies, for conflict management, 7
"Not guilty by reason of insanity" (NGRI), 246
Nursing home. *See* Long-term care facility
Nursing Home Abuse Prevention Profile & Checklist, 310
Nursing Home Evaluation Checklist, of AARP, 163
NVAWS. *See* National Violence Against Women Survey

O

Objectivity, of forensic assessments, 21
Obsessive-compulsive disorder (OCD), 357
Obsessive-compulsive personality disorder, 338
Occupational Safety and Health Act (OSH Act) (1970), 66
Occupational Safety and Health Administration (OSHA), 66
OCD. *See* Obsessive-compulsive disorder
ODD. *See* Oppositional defiant disorder
O'Donnell, I., 337
Offender. *See also* Long-term offenders; Perpetrators; Sex offender
 with dual diagnosis, 248
 path in CJ system, 43–47
 psychopathology of, 148
 stalking behaviors, 220–221
Offender, in community, 274–283
 assessment of, 277–281
 etiology of, 276–277
 infection and, 280
 intervention, 281
 mental illness and, 278–279
 nutrition and, 280
 parole/probation of, 21, 275, 276, 278, 345
 prevalence of, 276
 prevention, 281–282
 substance abuse of, 279
 violence of, 279
 women's health and, 280–281
Offender, in correctional facilities, 265–273
 prevalence of, 266–267
 prevention, 271–272
Offender, with mental illness/cognitive impairment, 245–252
 assessment of, 250
 etiology of, 248–250
 intervention, 250–251
 prevalence of, 247–248
 prevention, 251–252
Office for Victims of Crime (OVC), 16, 19–20
 first responders tips for victims with disabilities, 106
 on victim needs, 95–97
 Victims Assistance Training Program of, 228
Office of Juvenile Justice and Delinquency Prevention, on abusive parent patterns, 299–301
Office of National Drug Control Policy, U.S., 235, 236–237
Older adult
 abuse/mistreatment of, 4–5
 with disabilities, victimization of, 103–116
 forensics, 3–4
 IPV in, 131–138
 victimization effect on, 85–101
 violence effect on, 86
Older adult perpetrators of sexual violence, 337–339
 assessment of, 338
 intervention, 338–339
 personality disorders of, 338
 prevalence/etiology of, 337–338
 prevention, 339
Older American's Act, 155
Online sexual activity (OSA), 324
Oppositional defiant disorder (ODD), 256
Oram, 140, 144
Order of protection, 98–99, 126
 for elder abuse, 155
 stalking and, 223
OSA. *See* Online sexual activity
OSHA. *See* Occupational Safety and Health Administration
OSH Act. *See* Occupational Safety and Health Act
OVC. *See* Office for Victims of Crime

P

Paavilainen, E., 142
Paraphilias, *DSM-IV-TR*
 autocratic asphyxia, 399–404
 exhibitionism, 316, 317–318
 fetishism, 316
 frotteurism, 316, 318

NOS types, 316
pedophilia, 316–317
sexual masochism, 316, 399–400
sexual sadism, 316, 318–319
transvestic fetishism, 316
voyeurism, 316, 317
zoophilia, 358, 360
Parenting, incarceration and, 365–370
assessment of, 366–367
etiology of, 366
grandparents and, 368–369
history/physical assessment of, 367
intervention, 367–369
parenting programs for females, 347
prevalence of, 366
prevention, 369–370
Parole, 275, 276
conditions of, 278
evaluation, 21
of female offenders, 345
Patterned injury, 24, 124
PCL-R. *See* Psychopathy Checklist—
Revised (PCL-R)
PC-PTSD. *See* Primary Care PTSD
Screen
Pediatric sexual assault nurse examiner
(PSANE), 50
Pedophilia, 316–317
Penetrating injury, 212
Penile plethysmography (PPG), 329, 358
Perpetrators. *See also* Adult perpetrators, of sexual violence; Older adult
perpetrators of sexual violence
of abuse/violence/criminal activity, 3
homicide survivor rage toward, 407
of persons with disabilities, 105
prevalence of, 286
Perpetrators, of elder abuse, 305–313
assessment of, 309–310
diagnostic testing and, 310
domineering, 306–307
etiology of, 305–309
history/physical assessment of,
309–310
impaired, 306
narcissistic, 306
overwhelmed, 305–306

prevention, 311–312
sadistic, 307
types of, 305–307
Perpetrators, of IPV, 285–295
assessment of, 289–292
behaviors of, 290
control tactics of, 287–288
diagnostic testing of, 291–292
etiology of, 286–289
female, 288–289
general principles, of assessment of,
289–290
intervention, 292
partner control an d, 287
physical assessment of, 291
prevention, 293–294
psychological assessment of, 290–291
same-sex, 289
therapy phases for, 292–293
Personal injury victim, 207–215
assessment of, 210–213
collisions and, 211
documentation for, 210
history/physical assessment of,
210–211
impact types, 210
intervention, 213–214
negligence, 208–210
prevalence/etiology, 210
restraint systems and, 211–212
torts, 208
Personality disorders, 248, 249, 255–256,
319
of adult survivors of child sexual abuse, 4
of older adult perpetrators of sexual
violence, 338
Persons with disabilities
assessment of, 105–106
children, 104
developmental, 104, 109–114, 248
etiology of, 104
obstacles of, 105–106
prevalence of victimization of, 103–104
prevention methods for victims of,
114–115
victimization of, 103–116
WHO definition of, 103

Pesola, G. R., 189
Pew's Public Safety Performance Project, 266
PFAs. *See* Protection from abuse orders
Photography, 31–33
Physical abuse
  of animals, 352
  of elder, by family member, 147
  history assessment, for elder, 151
  in IPV, 117
  physical examination, of elder for, 151–152
  during pregnancy, 88
Physical effects of violence
  on fetal development, 88
  IPV on women, 87–88
  sexual assault and, 88–89
Pillemer, K., 308, 309
Polygraph, 329–330
Postarrest, 45–46
Postpartum psychosis (PP), 303
  child abuse risk from, 300–301
  treatment, lack of, 302
Post-sexual assault
  Hepatitis B vaccination and, 178–179
  HIV diagnosis/treatment and, 178
  medications given at, 178
  pregnancy test, of female victim of, 176
Posttraumatic stress disorder (PTSD), 75, 76, 77, 256
  DSM-IV-TR criteria for, 91
  of female offenders, 347
  of homicide survivor, 406, 408, 409
  from IPV, 88
  as psychological effect of violence, 90–93
  screening tools for, 91–93
  treatment of, 98
Poverty
  of female offenders, 343
  incarceration correlation with, 277
Power of attorney, 61
PP. *See* Postpartum psychosis
PPG. *See* Penile plethysmography
Practice Guideline for the Treatment of Patients with Acute Stress Disorder

and Posttraumatic Stress Disorder, of APA, 98
Pregnancy
  of female prisoners, 271, 346
  physical assault during, 88, 124
  test, for sexual assault, of female victim, 176
  unwanted, from sexual assault, 89
Prevention methods, primary/secondary/tertiary
  for abusive parents, 302–304
  of adult perpetrator of sexual violence, 333–334
  for animal cruelty, 361–362
  child abuse prevention, 7
  for conflict management, 7
  for death of elders, in LTC facility, 389–390
  for elder abuse, by family member, 155–156
  of elder abuse, by health care workers, 163–165
  for elder victim, of sexual assault, 196–198
  for female victims, of sexual assault, 179–180
  for incarcerated parents, 369–370
  of infectious disease transmission, 271–272
  for IPV, for adults, 126–128
  in IPV, in older adults, 136–137
  juvenile justice system and, 7
  for offender, in community, 281–282
  for offender, in correctional facility, 272
  for offender, with mental illness/cognitive impairment, 251–252
  for perpetrators, of elder abuse, 311–312
  for perpetrators, of IPV, 293–294
  for personal injury victim, 213–214
  for persons with disabilities, 114–115
  for substance abuse, 242–243
  for suicide, 397–398
  for workplace violence reduction, 69–70

Preventive Services Task Force, U.S., 126
Primary Care PTSD Screen (PC-PTSD), 92
Prisoner
  crime for drugs, 236
  FBOs for released, 162
  health care of, 265–266
  health problems of, 4, 267–271
  infectious diseases of, 4
  mental illness of, 4, 247–248
  pregnancy among female, 271
  recidivism rates of, 260
  reentry, 261–262
  released, 272
  sexual assault, of male, 183–184
  weapon creation by, 266
  women, 342
Probable cause, 43, 44
Probation, 275
  conditions of, 278
  of female offenders, 345
Professional stress, 73–81
  burnout, 76, 332
  compassion fatigue, 75
  management of, 78–80
  signs of, 76–78
  traditional stress and, 74–75
  types of stressors for, 73–76
  vicarious traumatization, 75–76
Project START, for released prisoners, 272
Property destruction, in IPV, 118
Prophylactic treatment, for STIs, 189
Prostitutes
  abuse of, 342
  assessment of, 345–346
  physical health assessment of, 345–346
Prostitution, of female offenders, 341–342
Protection from abuse orders (PFAs), 98
PSANE. See Pediatric sexual assault nurse examiner
Psychiatric disorders, 255
Psychoeducational intervention, 106
Psychological disorders, 77
Psychological effects, of violence, 89–96
  ASD, 89–90
  on children exposed to IPV, 118–119
  PTSD, 90–93
  Stockholm syndrome, 93–94
Psychopathology, of abuser, 148, 248, 257
Psychopathy Checklist—Revised (PCL-R), 258
Psychosexual dysfunctions, of adult survivors of child sexual abuse, 4
Psychotherapeutic intervention, 106
PTSD. See Posttraumatic stress disorder
Punitive damages, 209–210

Q
Qualifications, for expert witness, 50–51
Quotations
  forensic interview recording of, 23
  in trauma documentation, 210

R
Ramsey-Klawsnik, H., 192, 305
Rand, M., 218
Rape, 167
  anger/power/sadism in, 321
  blitz/confidence, 322–323
  care advocacy, 178
  classifications of FBI's Crime Classification Manual, 321–322
  "Date rape," 23, 179–180
  prevalence of, 169–170
  -related trauma symptoms of elder victim, 193–194
  statutory, 167
  underreporting of, 170
Rapid Risk Assessment for Sex Offense Recidivism (RRASOR), 328
Raymond, J., 204
R-CRAS. See Rogers Criminal Responsibility Assessment Scales
Recidivism, 260–261, 370
  of female sex offender, 330
  prevention, 334
  programs for, 282
Red flag signs, of substance abuse, 239
Redmond, L., 406
Reentry programs, for prisoners, 261–262

Regan, K., 140, 144
Registry of Interpreters for the Deaf, 114
Reproductive problems, of prisoners, 271
Resident-to-resident aggression (RRA),
    elder abuse and, 192, 308–309
Respite care, 114
Rhodes, K.V., 128
Risk
    factors for health care workers, 67–68
    mental illness and, 254–256
    psychopathology and, 257
    substance abuse and, 256–257
Risk assessment for reoffending, of
    sexual offenders, 326–330. *See also*
    Violence risk assessment
    actuarial, 257, 326–328
    clinical judgment for, 326, 328–330
Risk of Abuse Tool, 156
Rogers Criminal Responsibility Assess-
    ment Scales (R-CRAS), 247
Rose, K., 218
Rosen, T., 308, 309
RRA. *See* Resident-to-resident aggres-
    sion
RRASOR. *See* Rapid Risk Assessment
    for Sex Offense Recidivism
Rules of evidence, 37–38, 52–53

S
Safe Return Program, of Alzheimer's
    Association, 107
SAFE screening tool, for IPV, 127
Safety plan, 126, 135
    development of, 96
    in IPV, 122, 125, 135
Saltzman, L., 94
Same-sex perpetrators, of IPV, 289
SANE. *See* Sexual assault nurse
    examiners
Sanity evaluations, 246–247
SART. *See* Sexual assault response team
Scene investigation, 376–381
    body, documenting/evaluating of,
    378–379
    completion of, 380–381
    decedent profile information, estab-
    lishing/recording, 379–380

scene, arrival at, 376–377
scene, documenting/evaluating of,
    377–378
Schizoid personality disorder, 338
Schizophrenia, 249, 255
Schmitt, E., 324
Scientific evidence
    admissibility of, 54
    Frye/Daubert/hybrid tests for, 54
Sebastian, S., 127
Secrecy of assault, by victim, 4
Self-neglect, of elder, 147, 152–153
Self-regulation model pathway, of Ward/
    Hudson, 319–320
Severity, of injury, 210
Sex offender. *See also* Adult perpetrators,
    of sexual violence
    anger/power/sexuality components
    of, 171
    civil commitment of, 333
    clinical judgment, for reoffending of,
    328–330
    community notification laws, 333
    female, 323–324, 330
    internet, 324
    management program, 332
    opportunistic/pervasively angry/sexual
    type, against elders, 193
    rearrest of, 324
    treatment commonalities/differences,
    331–333
Sex Offender Risk Appraisal Guide
    (SORAG), 328
Sex trafficking. *See* Human trafficking
Sexual abuse/assault, 3, 5–6, 124,
    167–168. *See also* Post-sexual
    assault
    animal, 352, 354
    bite marks and, 28
    CAPTA definition of, 297–298
    of child, 320–321, 323
    criminal charges of, 168
    DNA analysis in, 177–178
    documentation of injury in, 178, 188
    of elder, by family member, 148, 152,
    192
    evaluations, 21

examples of, 168
follow-up photographs of, 33
forensic interview for, 23
in IPV, 118
past, of female offenders, 343
physical effects of, 88–89
signs of elder, 152
STIs/HIV and, 89
unwanted pregnancy from, 89
victim response to/recovery from, 169
Sexual assault, elder victims of, 191–198
    abuse by unrelated care providers,
        192
    advocacy for, 196
    APS for, 192, 195
    CJ system and, 195
    cognitive dysfunction/impairment/
        dementia and, 193
    development of trust by health care
        worker, 194
    etiology of, 192–193
    general principles of, 193
    genitalia inspection in, 195
    history of, 193–194
    incestuous abuse, 148, 152, 192
    intervention, 195–196
    marital/partner abuse, 192
    physical assessment, 194–195
    prevalence of, 192
    prevention, 196–198
    rape-related trauma symptoms of,
        193–194
    RRA, in elder care settings, 192
    STI presence and, 194–195
    stranger/acquaintance assault, 192
Sexual assault, female victims of,
        165–182
    assessment of, 171–177
    diagnostic testing, 176–177
    documentation of injury in, 178
    etiology of, 170–171
    fear of retaliation and, 170
    follow up care for, 179
    history, 172–174
    injury, common locations of, 175
    intervention, 177–179
    mandatory reporting, lack of, 177

physical assessment of, 174–176
physical injuries from, 171
pregnancy test, 176
prevalence of, 169–170
prevention, 179–180
psychological trauma from, 171
TEARS genital injuries, 175–176
Sexual assault, male victims of, 183–190
    advocacy for, 186
    assessment of, 185–188
    denial of/lack of support for, 184
    diagnostic testing, 188
    documentation of injury in, 188
    etiology of, 185
    general principles of, 185–186
    history and, 186–187
    intervention, 188–189
    myths about, 184
    physical assessment, 187–188
    prevalence of, 183–185
    prevention, 189
    in prison population, 183–184
    safety concerns and, 184
    self-blame in, 185
    services, lack of for, 184
    sexual consequences of, 187
    stigma/shame/embarrassment of,
        186–187
    underreporting of, 184–185
Sexual Assault in the First Degree, 168
Sexual assault nurse examiners (SANE),
        180
Sexual assault response team (SART),
        50, 180
Sexually deviant pathway, to sexual
        offending, 316–319
Sexually transmitted disease. *See* Sexually
        transmitted infections
Sexually transmitted infections (STIs), 4,
        176, 269, 271
    of elder victim of sexual assault,
        194–195
    of incarcerated female offenders, 345
Sexual masochism, 316
    hypoxyphilia/asphyxiophilia, 399–400
Sexual Misconduct, 168
Sexual offense pathway, 315–320

Sexual sadism, 316, 318–319

Sexual violence. *See also* Adult perpetrators, of sexual violence; Older adult
perpetrators of sexual violence;
Sexual abuse/assault
adult perpetrators of, 315–335
involuntary deviant sexual intercourse,
167
older adult perpetrators of,
337–339
rape, 23, 167, 170, 178, 179–180,
193–194, 321–323
sodomy, 167, 168
statutory rape, 167
WHO definition of, 167

Shaekelford, T., 144

Short Screening Scale for PTSD, 93

Silohu, H., 88

Simon, T., 99

Sixth Amendment, 44, 45, 48

Social effects, of violence, 94

Sodomy, 167, 168

Somatic symptoms, of adult survivors of
child sexual abuse, 4

Sommers, M., 175

SORAG. *See* Sex Offender Risk Appraisal
Guide

Specimen analysis
by crime laboratory, 35
evidence, labeling of, 37

Speltz, K., 324

Spitzberg, B., 220

Stable 2007 risk assessment, 328

Stalking, 99, 217–225
assessment of, 220–222
etiology of, 219–220
evidence collection/documentation
of, 223–224
gender difference in, 218–219
intervention, 222–224
in IPV, 118, 221–222
juvenile, 219
legal definition of, 217
Mullen typology of, 219–220
orders of protection for, 223
prevalence of, 218–219
types of, 217, *220*

Stalking Resource Center, Stalking Incident and Behavior Log of, 223

Static-99 risk assessment, 326–327

Static 2002 risk assessment, 326, 327

STIs. *See* Sexually transmitted infections

Stockholm syndrome
conditions for, 93
as psychological effect of violence,
93–94
treatment for, 93–94

Stop Violence Against Women, 88

Strangulation, 29, 124

Stress. *See* Professional stress

Stress management, 78–80
for caregiver, 114, 148–149, 150, 310,
319
EAP for, 80
individual, 78–79
institutional, 80

Stress-related disorders, 77

Structured clinical assessment, 257

Stuart, 256

Subpoena, of expert witness, 49

Substance abuse
biopsychosocial influences on, 237
childhood physical/sexual abuse and,
85
of female offenders, 343
IPV, of older adults and, 132
of offender, in community, 279
red flag signs/symptoms for, 239
risk and, 257
TCs for, 243
treatment programs, for female
offenders, 347–348

Substance Abuse and Mental Health
Services Administration, 395–396

Substance abuse offending, 235–244
alcohol-usage offenses, 236
assessment of, 238–241
drug-defined offenses, 235
drug-related offenses, 235
drug-using lifestyle offenses, 235–236
etiology of, 237
general principles, of assessment,
238–239
history/physical assessment for, 239

intervention, 241–242
IPV and, 136–137, 237
prevalence of, 236–237
prevention, 242–243
screening for, in Criminal justice setting, 241
screening for, in health care settings, 240–241
Substance dependence, 236
Suicidal ideation, 391, 407
Suicide, 3, 391–398
assessment of, 394–396
diagnostic testing, 396
etiology of, 393
history/physical assessment of, 394–396
intervention, 396
male rates of, 6
prevalence of, 392
prevention, 397–398
warning signs, 395–396
Suspect, 43

T
TBI. *See* Traumatic brain injury syndrome
TEARS, on genital injuries, 175–176
Teaster, P.B., 192
Testamentary competency, 59–60
Testimony, in trial, 56
Therapeutic communities (TCs), for substance abuse, 243
Therapy phases, for IPV perpetrators, 292–293
Thoennes, N., 169, 170, 183
Tjaden, P., 169, 170, 183
Trace evidence, 36–37, 40
Trafficking in Persons and Worker Exploitation Task Force, 205
Trafficking Victims Protection Act (2000), 199
Transgenerational violence, elder abuse by family member and, 148, 149
Transvestic fetishism, 316
Trauma, of victims, 3
ASD from, 89–90
documentation/quotations of, 210

Trauma Screening Questionnaire (TSQ), 92–93
Traumatic brain injury syndrome (TBI), 250
screenings/evaluations/treatment for, 268
supervision/treatment issues of, 267
Trial, 46–47
testimony in, 56
voir dire and, 50, 56
TSQ. *See* Trauma Screening Questionnaire
Tuberculosis (TB), 4, 269

U
United States v. Frye, 54
University of Iowa Department of Family Medicine Elder Mistreatment/Elder Abuse, screening tools of, 155–156
U.S. Preventive Services Task Force (USPSTF), 396
USPSTF. *See* U.S. Preventive Services Task Force

V
VAWA. *See* Violence Against Women
Verbal abuse, in IPV, 117
Vicarious traumatization, 75–76, 332
Victim. *See also* Personal injury victim; Sexual assault, elder victims of; Sexual assault, female victims of; Sexual assault, male victims of; Victim service programs
advocacy center, 126
advocate for, 97
with Alzheimer's, responding to, 107–108
behaviors/feelings of, 3–4
compensation, 99–100
with developmental disabilities, responding to, 109–114
grooming of, by child sexual abuser, 323
of human trafficking, 199–207
interventions for adult/older adult, 95–98
mental illness and, 4, 108–109, 247

needs, 95–97
path, in CJ system, 47–48, 227
of personal injury, 207–215
physical effects, of violence on, 87–89
psychological effects, of violence on,
89–96
reaction, from stalking, 222
rights, 95–98, 230–231
secrecy of assault by, 4
social effects, of violence on, 94
trauma of, 3, 89–90, 210
Victimization effects, on adult/older
adult, 4, 6, 85–101
description of, 85–87
interventions and, 95–98
order of protection and, 98–99
physical effects, of violence, 87–89
psychological effects, of violence,
89–96
social effects, of violence, 94
victim compensation and, 99–100
victim rights and, 95–98
Victims Assistance Training Program, of
OVC, 228
Victim service programs, 100, 227–232
CBOs, 228–229
criminal justice-based services,
229–231
FBOs, 229
reservation-based services, 231–232
Violence. *See also* Adult perpetrators, of
sexual violence; Intimate Partner
Violence, of adults; Intimate Partner Violence, of LGBT; Intimate
Partner Violence, of older adults;
Older adult perpetrators of sexual
violence; Sexual violence
against adult males, 86
aggravating factors for, 358
American Indian rate of, 232
crime rates, 4
cycle/continuum of, 3–8, 5
effect of, on older adults, 86
financial cost of, 99
in health care settings, 65–71
health problem of, 3, 4–7
human, animal cruelty v., 354–356

impact of, 3–4
as learned behavior, 5, 7
of offender, in community, 279
physical effects, on victim, 87–89
psychological effects, on victim, 89–96
social effects, on victim, 94
substance abuse and, 236
Violence Against Women Act (VAWA),
immigration status and, 17
Violence Risk Appraisal Guide (VRAG),
258, 326
Violence risk assessment, 253–258
clinical/actuarial/structured clinical
approaches to, 257, 326–328
etiology of, 254–257
Voir dire, 50, 56
Voyeurism, 316, 317
VRAG. *See* Violence Risk Appraisal
Guide

W
Walker, R., 126
Ward, T., 319
Weapon, prisoner creation of, 266
WEB. *See* Women's Experience with
Battering
Weisz, V., 144
Wernicke-Korsakoff syndrome, 250
Westfal, R.E., 189
West Virginia Foundation for Rape Infor-
mation and Services, 189
Whitaker, D., 333
White, M., 140, 144
WHO. *See* World Health Organization
Wisner, C., 94
Women
health of offender, in community,
280–281
prisoners, 342
victims, 6, 87–88, 104
Women's Experience with Battering
(WEB) scale, 131
Woods, S., 88
Worden, J.W., 407
Workplace violence
BLS on homicides and, 66
with criminal intent, 65

customer/client intent, 65
employer responsibility in, 66
personal relationship, 66
prevalence of, 66–67
prevention, 69–70
risk factors for, 67–68
stalking and, 224
worker-on-worker, 66

World Health Organization (WHO), 6
disability definition by, 103
on FGM, 14
on IPV social/economic costs, 94

Z
Zink, T., 94
Zoophilia, 358, 360